3Ts in Gastrointestinal Microbiome Era: Technology, Translational Research and Transplant

3Ts in Gastrointestinal Microbiome Era: Technology, Translational Research and Transplant

Editors

Rinaldo Pellicano
Sharmila Fagoonee

MDPI • Basel • Beijing • Wuhan • Barcelona • Belgrade • Manchester • Tokyo • Cluj • Tianjin

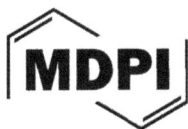

Editors
Rinaldo Pellicano
Unit of Gastroenterology
Molinette-SGAS Hospital
Turin, Italy

Sharmila Fagoonee
Institute for Biostructure and Bioimaging
National Research Council
Molecular Biotechnology Center
Turin, Italy

Editorial Office
MDPI
St. Alban-Anlage 66
4052 Basel, Switzerland

This is a reprint of articles from the Special Issue published online in the open access journal *Journal of Clinical Medicine* (ISSN 2077-0383) (available at: https://www.mdpi.com/journal/jcm/special_issues/Gastrointestinal_Microbiome).

For citation purposes, cite each article independently as indicated on the article page online and as indicated below:

LastName, A.A.; LastName, B.B.; LastName, C.C. Article Title. *Journal Name* **Year**, *Volume Number*, Page Range.

ISBN 978-3-0365-2796-3 (Hbk)
ISBN 978-3-0365-2797-0 (PDF)

© 2021 by the authors. Articles in this book are Open Access and distributed under the Creative Commons Attribution (CC BY) license, which allows users to download, copy and build upon published articles, as long as the author and publisher are properly credited, which ensures maximum dissemination and a wider impact of our publications.

The book as a whole is distributed by MDPI under the terms and conditions of the Creative Commons license CC BY-NC-ND.

Contents

About the Editors vii

Abraham Ajayi, Tolulope Jolaiya and Stella Smith
Evolving Technologies in Gastrointestinal Microbiome Era and Their Potential
Clinical Applications
Reprinted from: *J. Clin. Med.* **2020**, *9*, 2565, doi:10.3390/jcm9082565 1

Taku Morita, Keiichi Mitsuyama, Hiroshi Yamasaki, Atsushi Mori, Tetsuhiro Yoshimura, Toshihiro Araki, Masaru Morita, Kozo Tsuruta, Sayo Yamasaki, Kotaro Kuwaki, Shinichiro Yoshioka, Hidetoshi Takedatsu and Takuji Torimura
Gene Expression of Transient Receptor Potential Channels in Peripheral Blood Mononuclear
Cells of Inflammatory Bowel Disease Patients
Reprinted from: *J. Clin. Med.* **2020**, *9*, 2643, doi:10.3390/jcm9082643 15

Amir Mari, Fadi Abu Baker, Mahmud Mahamid, Wisam Sbeit and Tawfik Khoury
The Evolving Role of Gut Microbiota in the Management of Irritable Bowel Syndrome:
An Overview of the Current Knowledge
Reprinted from: *J. Clin. Med.* **2020**, *9*, 685, doi:10.3390/jcm9030685 27

Gian Paolo Caviglia, Alessandra Tucci, Rinaldo Pellicano, Sharmila Fagoonee, Chiara Rosso, Maria Lorena Abate, Antonella Olivero, Angelo Armandi, Ester Vanni, Giorgio Maria Saracco, Elisabetta Bugianesi, Marco Astegiano and Davide Giuseppe Ribaldone
Clinical Response and Changes of Cytokines and Zonulin Levels in Patients with Diarrhoea-Predominant Irritable Bowel Syndrome Treated with *Bifidobacterium Longum* ES1 for 8 or 12 Weeks:
A Preliminary Report
Reprinted from: *J. Clin. Med.* **2020**, *9*, 2353, doi:10.3390/jcm9082353 41

Camille Brehin, Damien Dubois, Odile Dicky, Sophie Breinig, Eric Oswald and Matteo Serino
Evolution of Gut Microbiome and Metabolome in Suspected Necrotizing Enterocolitis: A
Case-Control Study
Reprinted from: *J. Clin. Med.* **2020**, *9*, 2278, doi:10.3390/jcm9072278 53

Davide Giuseppe Ribaldone, Gian Paolo Caviglia, Amina Abdulle, Rinaldo Pellicano, Maria Chiara Ditto, Mario Morino, Enrico Fusaro, Giorgio Maria Saracco, Elisabetta Bugianesi and Marco Astegiano
Adalimumab Therapy Improves Intestinal Dysbiosis in Crohn's Disease
Reprinted from: *J. Clin. Med.* **2019**, *8*, 1646, doi:10.3390/jcm8101646 67

Jaroslaw Bilinski, Mikolaj Dziurzynski, Pawel Grzesiowski, Edyta Podsiadly, Anna Stelmaszczyk-Emmel, Tomasz Dzieciatkowski, Lukasz Dziewit and Grzegorz W. Basak
Multimodal Approach to Assessment of Fecal Microbiota Donors Based on Three
Complementary Methods
Reprinted from: *J. Clin. Med.* **2020**, *9*, 2036, doi:10.3390/jcm9072036 77

Stefano Bibbò, Carlo Romano Settanni, Serena Porcari, Enrico Bocchino, Gianluca Ianiro, Giovanni Cammarota and Antonio Gasbarrini
Fecal Microbiota Transplantation: Screening and Selection to Choose the Optimal Donor
Reprinted from: *J. Clin. Med.* **2020**, *9*, 1757, doi:10.3390/jcm9061757 93

Simona Panelli, Enrica Capelli, Giuseppe Francesco Damiano Lupo, Annalisa Schiepatti, Elena Betti, Elisabetta Sauta, Simone Marini, Riccardo Bellazzi, Alessandro Vanoli, Annamaria Pasi, Rosalia Cacciatore, Sara Bacchi, Barbara Balestra, Ornella Pastoris, Luca Frulloni, Gino Roberto Corazza, Federico Biagi and Rachele Ciccocioppo
Comparative Study of Salivary, Duodenal, and Fecal Microbiota Composition Across Adult Celiac Disease
Reprinted from: *J. Clin. Med.* **2020**, *9*, 1109, doi:10.3390/jcm9041109 . . . . **107**

Malene R. Spiegelhauer, Juozas Kupcinskas, Thor B. Johannesen, Mindaugas Urba, Jurgita Skieceviciene, Laimas Jonaitis, Tove H. Frandsen, Limas Kupcinskas, Kurt Fuursted and Leif P. Andersen
Transient and Persistent Gastric Microbiome: Adherence of Bacteria in Gastric Cancer and Dyspeptic Patient Biopsies after Washing
Reprinted from: *J. Clin. Med.* **2020**, *9*, 1882, doi:10.3390/jcm9061882 . . . . **127**

Marcantonio Gesualdo, Felice Rizzi, Silvia Bonetto, Stefano Rizza, Federico Cravero, Giorgio Maria Saracco and Claudio Giovanni De Angelis
Pancreatic Diseases and Microbiota: A Literature Review and Future Perspectives
Reprinted from: *J. Clin. Med.* **2020**, *9*, 3535, doi:10.3390/jcm9113535 . . . . **151**

Marilena Durazzo, Arianna Ferro and Gabriella Gruden
Gastrointestinal Microbiota and Type 1 Diabetes Mellitus: The State of Art
Reprinted from: *J. Clin. Med.* **2019**, *8*, 1843, doi:10.3390/jcm8111843 . . . . **171**

Emidio Scarpellini, Sharmila Fagoonee, Emanuele Rinninella, Carlo Rasetti, Isabella Aquila, Tiziana Larussa, Pietrantonio Ricci, Francesco Luzza and Ludovico Abenavoli
Gut Microbiota and Liver Interaction through Immune System Cross-Talk: A Comprehensive Review at the Time of the SARS-CoV-2 Pandemic
Reprinted from: *J. Clin. Med.* **2020**, *9*, 2488, doi:10.3390/jcm9082488 . . . . **185**

Yixi He, Binyin Li, Dingya Sun and Shengdi Chen
Gut Microbiota: Implications in Alzheimer's Disease
Reprinted from: *J. Clin. Med.* **2020**, *9*, 2042, doi:10.3390/jcm9072042 . . . . **209**

About the Editors

Rinaldo Pellicano (MD) is a Gastroenterologist at Molinette Hospital and San Giovanni Antica Sede (SGAS) Outpatient Clinic (Azienda Ospedaliero-Universitaria Città della Salute e della Scienza) in Turin, Italy. He obtained his specialist degree in Gastroenterology and Digestive Endoscopy at the University of Turin. His main research activities are related to 1) the characterization and role of microbioma in gastrointestinal and extra-gastrointestinal diseases 2) the role of Helicobacter pylori infection in the pathogenesis of gastroduodenal and extra-gastroduodenal manifestations; 3) the cure of Helicobacter pylori infection with conventional and innovative treatments; 4) possible association between occult HCV infection and cryptogenic chronic hepatitis; 5) cure of patients with chronic hepatitis of viral and non-viral etiology; 6) cure of patients with inflammatory bowel diseases. Dr. Pellicano has been appointed as lecturer for several courses at the University of Turin, including Management of Inflammatory Bowel Diseases (Master of Coloproctology). He performs numerous editorial duties, such as 1) Chief Editor of Minor Gastroenterology; 2) Subspeciality Editor of Minerva Medica and PanMinerva Medica; 3) Editorial Board Member of several journals, including Medicina; World Journal of Gastroenterology; International Journal of Celiac Disease; Medicines; Biomedical Research and Therapy; 4) reviewer of several scientific journals. His scientific publications can be found on PubMed (https://pubmed.ncbi.nlm.nih.gov/?term=Pellicano+Rinaldo&size=200) and his books and chapters on his webpage (http://rinaldopellicano.blogspot.com/).

Sharmila Fagoonee (PhD) is a Researcher at the Institute of Biostructure and Bioimaging of the Italian National Research Council and Molecular Biotechnology Center in Turin, Italy. After her BSc (hons) in Biology in Mauritius and MSc in Cellular Biology in Bordeaux, France, she got her PhD in Cell and Molecular Biology at the University of Turin. She has been appointed as a lecturer for courses on Regenerative Medicine at the University of Turin regarding the master's course in Stem Cells and Regenerative Medicine and Cell Factory Management, Advanced Training Course in Regenerative Medicine, Italian Regenerative Medicine Infrastructure—IRMI, and Cell Biology courses for the MSc in Molecular Biotechnology. Using a multidisciplinary approach including advanced molecular techniques such as RNA-seq and large-scale proteomics, as well as in vitro and in vivo studies, her two main current research areas regard 1) regenerative medicine: adult stem cells-based therapy for human metabolic diseases; identify circulating extracellular vesicles-based biomarkers for the early diagnosis of liver fibrosis, and for predicting the progression of liver fibrosis to hepatocellular carcinoma; evaluation of nephropathy arising from cholestasis. 2) Post-transcriptional regulation of gene expression, in particular investigating the molecular mechanisms underlying the role of the RNA binding proteins and splicing factors, ESRP1 and 2, in human diseases. As part of her editorial activities, she has been recently appointed as Chief Editor of Minerva Biotechnology and Biomolecular Research and is an Editorial Board Member of Journal of Clinical Medicine; World Journal of Gastroenterology and Biomedical Research and Therapy, as well as a reviewer of several journals.

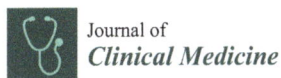

Review

Evolving Technologies in Gastrointestinal Microbiome Era and Their Potential Clinical Applications

Abraham Ajayi [1] Tolulope Jolaiya [2] and Stella Smith [1,3,*

1. Department of Molecular Biology and Biotechnology, Nigerian Institute of Medical Research, Yaba, Lagos 101212, Nigeria; ajayiabraham2013@gmail.com
2. Department of Microbiology, University of Lagos, Akoka 101212, Nigeria; oshuntee@yahoo.com
3. Department of Biological Sciences, Mountain Top University, Ogun 110106, Nigeria
* Correspondence: stellasmith@nimr.gov.ng; Tel.: +234-803-705-8989

Received: 18 June 2020; Accepted: 4 August 2020; Published: 7 August 2020

Abstract: The human gastrointestinal microbiota (GIM) is a complex and diverse ecosystem that consists of community of fungi, viruses, protists and majorly bacteria. The association of several human illnesses, such as inflammatory bowel disease, allergy, metabolic syndrome and cancers, have been linked directly or indirectly to compromise in the integrity of the GIM, for which some medical interventions have been proposed or attempted. This review highlights and gives update on various technologies, including microfluidics, high-through-put sequencing, metabolomics, metatranscriptomics and culture in GIM research and their applications in gastrointestinal microbiota therapy, with a view to raise interest in the evaluation, validation and eventual use of these technologies in diagnosis and the incorporation of therapies in routine clinical practice.

Keywords: gastrointestinal; microbiota; technology; therapy; high-throughput

1. Introduction

The human gastrointestinal tract is one of the most complex and diverse ecosystem known, with a plethora of fungi, viruses, bacteria and protists. This community of commensals usually dominated by bacteria is often referred to as microbiota, and their collective genome is termed the microbiome. The gut microbiota play critical role in the health of the host, which include but is not limited to the maturation of the immune system, the prevention of pathogenic infection, the alteration of intestinal morphology and angiogenesis, the fermentation of undigested polysaccharides and the synthesis and conversion of bioactive compounds [1–4].

Perturbations or dysbiosis of the gut microbiota as a result of diet, drug intake or environmental changes can result in severe health challenges with fatal outcomes. Diseases such as irritable bowel syndrome (IBS); obesity; inflammatory bowel disease (IBD), which includes ulcerative colitis (UC) and Crohn's disease; cancer; and inflammatory disorders (diseases associated with abnormal function of the immune system and chronic inflammation) are associated with the perturbation of the gut microbiota [5,6]. An array of other diseases, such as neurodegenerative disorders (Alzheimer's disease and the autism spectrum disorder), chronic kidney disease, diabetes and atherosclerotic cardiovascular disease, as summarized in Table 1, have been linked to the dysbiosis of the gut [7–9]. The focus of this review is centered on gastrointestinal diseases associated with the alteration of the gut microbiota, and recent technologies used in the study of gastrointestinal microbiota, with the view to identifying their potential applications in clinical practice.

Table 1. Summary of Diseases/Metabolic Syndrome, Microbial Indicators of Healthy and Dysfunctional Gut.

Subject	Metabolic Syndrome/Disease	Correlated Clinical Indicator	Indicator Microbe (Healthy Metabolic State)	Indicator Microbe (Dysfunctional Metabolic State)	Reference
Adult (Male & Female)	Prediabetes or type 2 diabetes mellitus	Impaired lipid & glucose metabolism	*Clostridia* and *Rikenellaceae* members	*Holdemania* & *Blautia* genera	[10]
Adult	Obesity	NI	Balance population of *Bacteroidetes* & *Firmicutes*	Few *Bacteroidetes* & more *Firmicutes*	[11]
Adult	Alzheimer's Disease	Low Mini-Mental State Examination score, APOE ε4 carriers, high Clinical Dementia Rating and Activity of Daily Living scores	Normal gut microbiota population comprising *Firmicutes*, *Proteobacteria*, *Bacteroidetes* and *Actinobacteria*	Significant decrease in the population of *Negativicutes* and *Bacteroidia*	[12,13]
Children	Autism	NI	Moderate level of *Clostridium histolyticum*, normal population of *Firmicutes*, *Bacteroidetes*	Lower levels of *Prevotella*, *Coprococcus*, *Veillonellaceae*, *Firmicutes* and *Bifidobacterium* and higher levels of *Clostridium histolyticum*, *Desulfovibrio*, *Lactobacillus*, *Sarcina Clostridium*, *Bacteroidetes* and *Caloramator*	[14]
Adult	Early chronic kidney disease	abnormal kidney structure, urinary albumin excretion rate ≥30 mg/24 h, glomerular filtration rate, 30–90 mL/minute/1.73 m²	Abundance of *Roseburia* and other genera	Abundance of *Ruminococcus* and other genera	[9]
Adult	Atherosclerotic cardiovascular disease	stable angina, unstable angina, or acute myocardial infarction, ≥50% stenosis in single or multiple vessel	Higher population of *Bacteroides* and *Prevotella*	Relative reduction in *Bacteroides* and *Prevotella* and enrichment in *Streptococcus* spp. and *Escherichia*, *Klebsiella* spp., *Enterobacter aerogenes*	[15]

NI: Not Indicated.

2. Methods

The literature on gut microbiota, diseases associated with perturbation of the gut microbiota and technologies used in gut microbiome research were searched through Google Scholar and PubMed/MEDLINE. The final search date was 29 February, 2020. Search strings such as "gut microbiome", "gastrointestinal microbiota", "microbiota dysbiosis and metabolic syndrome" and "technologies in microbiota research" were used. The search comprised original and review articles written in English. Retrieved articles were reviewed and sorted to eliminate duplicates and unwanted articles.

3. Results and Discussion

From the early start scientists used traditional culture and isolation techniques to study the flora of the body but today, improved methods including high-throughput culturing methods, high-throughput sequencing, microfluidics, human fecal transplant (Figure 1) approaches are being used in the study and treatment of the human microbiome ecosystem, so as to examine their role in inducing disease and to map out remedy against infective bacteria [16–19].

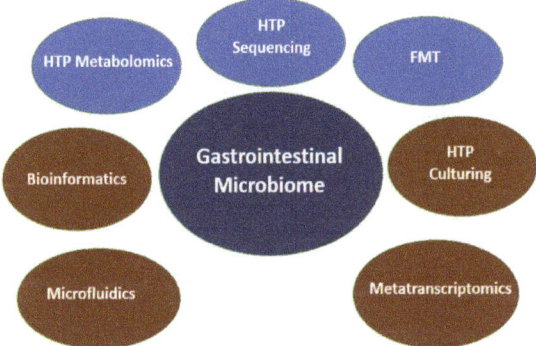

Figure 1. Various technologies used in the study of gastrointestinal microbiome. HTTP: high-throughput, FMT: fecal microbiota transplantation.

3.1. The Human Gut and Its Microbiota

Prior to its birth, it is presumed that the unborn is free of microbial flora, and that at birth, the infant first comes in contact with the resident microbial flora of the mothers' vagina if birth was through the natural birth canal, or the microbial flora of the mothers' skin if birth was through cesarean section [20–22]. Although some studies [23–25] have suggested the early inoculation of the fetus with bacteria and bacteria DNA through the placenta. The study by de Goffau et al. [26] reported that the human placenta has no microbiome. Detected bacteria were acquired during labor and delivery. After birth, according to the findings of Koenig et al. [27], there were apparent chaotic shifts of microbiome from that endowed with genes facilitating lactate utilization and plant polysaccharide metabolism mediated by milk-based diet to increase in *Bacteroidetes* initiated by introduction of solid food that prepares the infant gut for adult diet. However, in the findings of Differding et al. [28], the early introduction of infants to complementary food was associated with altered gut microbiota composition and butyric acid concentration, which have been previously identified as precursors to oxidative stress, immune disorder and obesity in childhood.

The microbiome of the adult gut accommodates various communities of phylotypes belonging to the phyla *Actinobacteria, Proteobacteria, Bacteroidetes, Fusobacteria, Firmicutes* and *Verrucomicrobia* [2]. Most of these phyla are present in the stomach, small intestine and colon. However, the colon is more populated with several genera belonging to the afore mentioned phyla, including the genus *Akkemansia* that belongs to the phylum *Verrucomicrobia*, which has been found to be limited in patients with obesity, inflammatory bowel disease and other metabolic syndromes, while it is in abundance in the biopsies of healthy individuals [2,29]. As has been reported in several studies, dietary types and pattern shapes and determines the diversity of the gut microbiome. In the submission of Amabebe et al. [30], high fat and carbohydrate diet builds a gut microbiota that is predominated by *Methanobrevibacter*, *Firmicutes* (*Clostridium*) and *Prevotella* and deficient in bacteria such as *Bacteroides*, *Lactobacillus*, *Akkermansia* and *Bifidobacterium*. Barone et al. [31], in their study brought to the fore the impact of modern Paleolithic diet (MPD) that consist of vegetables, seeds, lean meat, fruits, eggs, nuts and fish on the gut microbiome. They observed that the gut microbiome of urban Italians adhering to MPD showed an ample degree of biodiversity with high relative abundance of fat-loving and bile tolerant microorganisms. As have been mentioned earlier, perturbations or dysbiosis in combination with altered permeability are crucial mechanisms that mediate disease manifestation [32]. Fecal microbiota transplantation (FMT) has gained relevance in recent times in the treatment and correction of gut infections or disorders that might have resulted from the depletion of resident microbiota and infection by pathogenic bacteria. Huge successes have been recorded in FMT therapy, with about 92% efficacy reported in the treatment of recurrent *Clostridium difficile* infection [33]. In a recent study by Zou et al. [34], it was shown that patients with Crohn's disease and ulcerative colitis that had FMT were in remission after three days of transplant with notable bacterial colonization of the gut. FMT therapy has been extended to the treatment of lifestyle and other diseases, such as diabetes, metabolic syndrome, Parkinson's disease, obesity and cancer. FMT entails transfer of gut microbiota in feces of a healthy donor to recipient patient to correct/treat a disorder or gastrointestinal disease [35–37]. Although the level of success of this procedure, is yet to be wide spread due to some constraints identified by Cammarota et al. [38], including difficulties with donor recruitment, lack of dedicated centers and issues pertaining to safety monitoring and regulation, hence, the proposal for the provision of stool banks to bridge the gap of FMT in clinical practice.

The afore mentioned technique offers a natural option to routine medical treatments of chronic ailments by providing direct and effective remedy preventing dysbiosis in the host, thereby improving health conditions [39,40].

3.2. Technologies in Gastrointestinal Microbiome Study

Since the structure, composition and diversity of the human gut microbiota has been correlated with the health status of humans, it could be presumed that the future of combating certain ailments is through exploring individualized gastrointestinal microbiome as the gastrointestinal microbiome era heralds. In the past, scientists have used culture independent techniques such as electrophoresis based methods, including denaturing gradient gel electrophoresis (DGGE), temperature gradient gel electrophoresis (TGGE) and PCR based methods, such as terminal restriction fragment length polymorphism (T-RFLP) and random amplified polymorphic DNA (RAPD), to study the community structure, diversity and genetic relatedness of bacteria in communities. Fluorescence in situ hybridization (FISH) is a cytogenetic technique that has been used in the study of individual microbes within gut microbiota, such as *Listeria monocytogenes*, *Salmonella* species, *Helicobacter pylori* and *Yersinia enterocoliticai*, which are gut pathogens [41–44]. Russmann et al. [45] used FISH in the diagnosis of *Helicobacter pylori* cultured isolates, and the same technique was used to proffer antibiotic treatment options. These methods had a lot of drawbacks, including the need for specific probes, low resolution, specificity and sensitivity. However, advances in sequencing and culture technologies have paved the way to analyzing big data arising from exploration of the rich microbiome ecosystem of the gut, which is evident in several studies, as shown in Table 2. Such technologies are high-throughput sequencing, microfluidics, high-throughput metabolomics, assays engineered organoids derived from human stem cells and high-throughput culturing [46]. They have far reaching advantages over the older or traditional technology already mentioned, but with some limitations as well (summary in Table 3). The pros and cons of these technologies are described below.

Table 2. Studies on Microbiome, Outcomes and Methods Employed.

Subject	Methods Employed	Outcome	Reference
Association between breast milk oligosaccharides and fecal microbiota in healthy breast fed infants	16S rRNA genes sequencing of V4 region using the Illumina Hiseq 2000 platform, porous graphitized carbon–ultra high-performance liquid chromatography (PGC–UPLC-MS) and bioinformatics (QIIME)	Microbiota composition strongly influenced by infant age, associated mode of delivery and breast milk	[47]
Dynamics and stabilization of the human gut microbiome during the first year of life	Metagenomics (DNA extraction from stool samples and preparation of DNA library using Illumina Hiseq2000) and bioinformatics (SOAPdenovo2, GeneMark v2.7, NCBI database)	Nutrition has a far reaching influence on infant microbiota composition and function with halting of breast-feeding other than introduction of solid food	[48]
Determining the diversity of human gut microbiota	Culture with enrichment, 16S rRNA gene sequencing of V3 region using the Illumina Miseq platform and bioinformatics (QIIME)	Use of enriched culture method enhanced the culturability of bacteria identified by 16S sequencing of the microbiota of the human gut	[49]
Impact of diet during pregnancy on maternal microbiota clusters and its influence on neonatal microbiota and infant growth during the first 18 months of life	16S rRNA gene sequencing of V3-V4 region using Miseq Illumina platform. Bioinformatics (QIIME, LEfSe, Calypso online platform)	Diet is an important perinatal factor in the initial phase of life and have significant impact on neonatal microbiome	[50]
Heritable components of the human fecal microbiome are associated with visceral fat	Measuring of body composition by dual-energy X-ray absorptiometry, 16S rRNA gene sequencing of V4 region on Illumina Miseq platform and bioinformatics (QIIME 1.7.0, PICRUSt v1.0.0, STAMP)	There was significant association of adiposity-OTU abundance with host genetic variations indicating possible role of host genes in influencing the link between obesity and fecal microbiome	[51]
Succession of microbial consortia in the developing infant gut microbiome	454-pyrosequencing of 16S rRNA gene, GC-MS analysis of SCFA, quantitative PCR and bioinformatics (QIIME, MG-RAST, NCBI database)	Revealed shifts in microbiome associated with life events	[26]
Identification of uncultured bacteria that are metabolic responders in a microbiota	Massively parallel single-cell genome sequencing technique (SAG-gel Platform), 16S rRNA gene sequencing of V3-V4 using Illumina Miseq 2 × 300bp platform and bioinformatics (QIIME2 v.2019.1). Determination of the concentration of SCFA was done by GC-mass spectrophotometry	Functions of uncultured bacteria in the microbiota were elucidated	[52]
Study of human gut colonization linked to in utero by microbial communities in the amniotic fluid and placenta	Culture, Gradient Gel Electrophoresis (DGGE), 16S rRNA gene pyrosequencing of V1-V3 region, quantitative PCR and bioinformatics (PICRUSt, QIIME, LEfSe)	The microbiota composition of infant gut at the age of 3-4 days begins to look like that detected in colostrum hence, the presumption that colonization is initiated prenatally by a distinct microbiota in the amniotic fluid and placenta	[53]

Table 3. Summary of the Potential Clinical Application of Various Technologies and Their Advantages and Disadvantages.

Technology/Methodology	Advantage	Disadvantage	Potential Clinical Application
Metagenomics (High-through sequencing)	• Provides information on culturable and 'non-culturable' or yet to be cultured microorganisms. • Captures both viable and unviable species of microorganisms. • Essential details of diversity and community structure of the gut microbiota is provided	• Further studies on microorganisms present in the microbiota is not possible since direct extraction of DNA is employed restricting physical access to the microorganisms.	• Could be used by clinicians for the proper diagnosis of gastrointestinal diseases with overlapping clinical presentation. Or for identifying microbiological markers that predict the presence of certain diseases.
High-throughput Metabolomics	• Provides information on the various metabolites of gut resident microorganisms and how it correlates to disease conditions. • Specific metabolites identified could serve as biomarkers • Can be used for measuring and evaluating the effect of dietary intake on the gut microbiota	• Loss of metabolites of some members of the microbiota due to sample handling. • Drawback in its use for personalized medicine/nutrition because of the existence of variability in human microbiota and their metabolites.	• Monitoring metabolites of gut microbiota using high-throughput metabolomics can help in the early diagnosis and management of metabolic syndromes that has been linked with the gut microbiota. • Can guide physicians on recommending dietary intake to patients.
High-throughput Metatranscriptomics	• Captures active members of the microbiota • Gives insight into the functions of various members of the gut microbiota • Can provide information on how members of the microbiota respond to changes within their environment	• Since RNA is not as stable as DNA, handling of sample can results in biases in finial results analyzed. • There is still a shortfall in metadata in repositories to which the enormous data generated from metatranscriptomics of the gut can match since this technology is still evolving	• Can identify how the function of a microbe in the gut influence the severity or progression of a disease • Can be used to monitor the interaction of the gut microbiota and host's mucosal immune system
Microfluidics	• Provide miniaturized platform for in vitro simulation, cultivation and manipulation of gut microbiota. • Make possible selective targeting and culture of important members of the gut microbiota. • Permit the combination of culture, DNA extraction, amplification and sequencing on a single platform.	• Human gut on chip might not give optimal performance as in natural human gut.	• This technology can be deployed clinically to monitor perturbation of gut microbiota in good time and enable precision in intervention by manipulating and stimulating the growth of beneficial or essential gut health promoting bacteria. • Microfluidics in microbiome studies can guide in the prescription of antibiotics.
High-throughput Culturing	• Culture gives access to the in-depth study of individual microorganisms that are cultured from the gut microbiota providing information on structure, morphology, physiology, growth conditions, inter & intra species interactions. • Culture captures only viable bacteria population. • Enable enumeration of bacteria species present	• Laborious and time consuming. • Limited number of members of the microbiota are accounted for since majority of them are 'non-culturable' or yet to be cultured. • Technique may be expensive due to the array of materials and specialized laboratory needed.	• Could provide avenue for precise treatment of gut diseases resulting from dysbiosis of specific species of bacteria and enable formulation of probiotics

3.3. 16S rRNA Gene Amplicon Sequencing

The in-depth study of the gut microbiome has been made possible through metagenomic approaches employing high-throughput sequencing technologies. Metagenomics entails the sequencing of total community DNA, which provides information on the richness, community structure and function of microbial species to be evaluated [54]. Sequencing of the hypervariable region of the 16S rRNA gene in combination with bioinformatics has been widely used to decipher the microbial composition of a community in an ecosystem like the gut. Using 16S rDNA illumina sequencing, Pires et al. [4] were able to characterize the gut microbiome of individuals living in the Amazon, which revealed huge variation in composition, compared to people living in industrialized settings. Similarly, Barone et al. [31] used information from 16S rRNA gene sequencing to explain gut microbiome response to a modern Paleolithic diet in a Western lifestyle context. Previous studies have also accessed and studied pediatric gut microbiome using 454 pyrosequencing of *16S rRNA* genes [27,55]. The use of 16S rRNA sequencing in evaluating the microbial composition of a microbiota has its various imperfections which whole genome shotgun sequencing (WGSS) has taken care of. WGSS has been used in several gastrointestinal microbiome studies. Vogtmann et al. [56] reported the reproducibility using WGSS in the study of the association of colorectal cancer and the human gut microbiome. Several bioinformatics platforms and tools, including Quantitative Insight Into Microbial Ecology (QIIME), Phylogenetic Investigation of Communities by Reconstruction of Unobserved States (PICRUSt), STatistical Analyses of Metagenomic Profiles (STAMP) [51], Linear Discriminant Analysis with Effect Size (LEfSe) [12] CLAssifier based on Reduced k-mers (CLARK), Mothur, Kraken [57] to mention a few that exist for analyzing the enormous genetic data that is generated from gastrointestinal microbiome studies. These tools help in predicting/assigning microbial taxonomy and give insight into the diversity, richness and composition of microbial species in a microbiota [58]. The enormous data obtained from metagenomic study of gut microbiota can be employed by clinicians for proper diagnosis or prediction of gastrointestinal diseases and guide antibiotic therapy in clinical settings. Vila et al. [6], demonstrated through analyzing metagenomic data of the gut microbiota of patients that IBD could be differentiated from IBS with microbial taxonomic makers, since both conditions have overlapping clinical manifestation that requires colonoscopy (an invasive procedure) for an accurate diagnosis by a clinician. Furthermore, in the same study, they were able to capture, from the same data, the resistome of the patients. A major limitation of this approach is the bias in the composition of databases to which comparisons are made.

3.4. Microfluidics

A major challenge in gastrointestinal microbiome research is the existence of the microbiota as a community in which most members are yet to be cultivated thus making it difficult to identify what species is doing what within the ecosystem. Microfluidics technology is providing a platform where single microbial cells within the gastrointestinal microbiota can be tracked, studied and manipulated. Liu and Walther-Antonio [58] identified two powerful microfluidics that have the potential applications in cell sorting, cell culture, cell screening, genome application, metabolic screening/analyses and gene expression. A recent study by Chijiwa et al. [52] used single cell sequencing based on an SAG-gel platform that employed microfluidic droplet generator to unravel the metabolic function of uncultivated bacterial species in intestinal microbiome, in which the fermentation of dietary fiber resulting in the production of short-chain fatty acid from ingested fibers was evaluated. This technique enabled the thorough study of specific bacterial species and deciphering their specific function that contributes to the health of the gastrointestinal tract. Another interesting innovation in the area of microfluidics in microbiome research is the development of organs on chip. This has allowed the design of experiments that captures minute complexities of microenvironment with extraordinary resolution, giving details of the microbial diversity, structure and functions of the microbiota of specific organs of the human system [59]. The development of a primary human small intestine on a chip using biopsy derived organoids by Kasendra et al. [60] (as shown in Figure 2), in which they suggested that its potential use in the study of infection, metabolism, drug pharmacokinetics and nutrition can be a viable and efficient tool in studying human gastrointestinal microbiota. Another principal application of microfluidics is in the study of antibiotic susceptibility of bacterial cells in real time. Cama et al. [61] in their study demonstrated the rapid quantification of antibiotic accumulation in Gram negative bacteria.

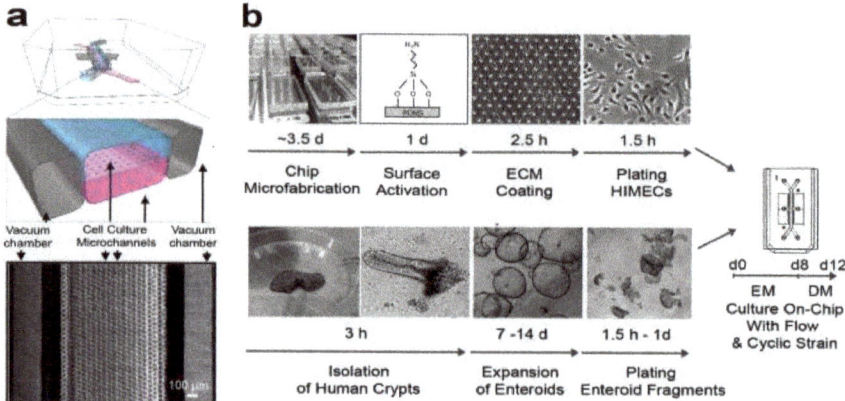

Figure 2. Primary human intestine chip manufacturing outline. (**a**) A cross-sectional view from the top of the chip and a phase contrast micrograph of the chip viewed from the bottom showing the upper (epithelial; blue) and lower (microvascular; pink) cell culture microchannels separated by a porous, Extracellular Matrix (ECM)-coated, Polydimethylsiloxane (PDMS) membrane sandwiched in-between. (**b**) An outline in developing microfluidic co-cultures of primary human intestinal epithelium and intestinal microvascular endothelium in the intestine chip. Source: Kasendra et al. [60] (*Scientific Reports*, Springer Nature) Licensed under CC BY 4.0.

By employing a combination of time-lapse auto-fluorescence microscopy and single-cell microfluidics, this technology could help reduce the overprescription of antibiotics, which is known to drive resistance. Beyond the aforementioned potential application of microfluidics, it also has clinical application in understanding the pathogenesis of gastrointestinal diseases, diagnosis, drug delivery and personalized or individualized medicine.

3.5. High-Throughput Metabolomics

High-throughput metabolomics (HTM) is becoming a popular method for studying various metabolites resulting from activities of bacterial populations in microbiota. Metabolomics is the process of assessing the metabolite profile in any given sample or ecosystem [62]. This has been made possible by using methods such as high throughput mass spectrometry. Koening et al. [27] used gas chromatography-mass spectrometry (GC-MS) to measure the concentration of short chain fatty acids (acetate, butyrate and propionate) in fecal samples, which was then correlated with bacterial diversity of the gut microbiota of infants. Similarly, Pires et al. [4] used mass spectrometry with direct infusion (DI-MS) on a Fourier transform ion cyclotron resonance instrument, to evaluate the chemical ecology of the gut environment of urban and rural dwellers of the Amazon. The use of HTM in gastrointestinal microbiome study has been used to demystify the role of short chain fatty acid (propionic acid) in ameliorating multiple sclerosis disease in humans. Duscha et al. [63] investigated variations in microbiota and their associated short chain fatty acid metabolites and the effect of dietary propionic acid on immune-regulatory elements using high-performance liquid chromatography-tandem mass spectrometry (LC-MS/MS). It was revealed that propionic acid was greatly reduced in the serum and feces of multiple sclerosis patients compared with healthy controls. Conversely, the accumulation of specific short chain fatty acids has been associated with obesity, because they become additional source of energy, thereby altering the balance of energy regulation [64]. Other metabolites, including polyunsaturated fatty acids linked with regulating several processes within the brain, bile acids, such as lithocholic acid, ursodeoxycholic acid and tauroursodeoxycholic acid and amino acid neurotransmitters such as glycine, aspartic acid, glutamic acid and gamma-aminobutyric acid (GABA), are metabolic products of the activities of gut microbiota, which have been profiled by mass spectrometry based metabolomics [65]. Wilson and Forse [66] also developed an electronic-nose technology for early disease detection in microbial dysbiosis. These electronic-nose technologies have multi-sensor arrays and are able to analyze chemicals. Their invention could detect new groups of volatile organic compounds that are biomarkers metabolites also known as dysbiosis-associated disease markers, thereby providing a link between human ailments and resident microbes. The technology is noninvasive as it uses breath as sampling method. Gut metabolome is undoubtedly a peculiar candidate for the clinical diagnosis and management of gastrointestinal diseases. However, it comes with attendant limitations. Smirnov et al. [67] identified some limitations of metabolomics in gut microbiota research, including problems with sample handling, resulting in the loss of some metabolites due to freezing and thawing; drawbacks in personalized medicine/nutrition, due to the existence of variability in human microbiota and their metabolites; choice of adequate animal model and equipment. Improvement in sample handling and processing will prevent the loss of vital metabolites that otherwise would have not been accounted for. Furthermore, creating a database of metabolites associated with various members of the gut microbiota will enhance the use of gut metabolome in assigning biomarkers for the purpose of diagnosis, treatment and management of gastrointestinal diseases by physicians.

3.6. Metatranscriptomics

Metatranscriptomics is another technique that has been employed in gut microbiota studies leveraging the technological advances in RNA sequencing (RNA-seq) [68]. Metatranscriptomics entails retrieving, sequencing and analyzing total messenger RNA (mRNA) or microRNA (from a microbial ecosystem), to ascertain what genes are expressed within that community [69]. In practice, the retrieved or extracted RNA is converted into a complimentary DNA (cDNA) using a reverse transcriptase and oligo (dT) primers or random hexamers, after which libraries are constructed and sequenced. However, semi direct RNA sequencing, bypassing the conversion of RNA to cDNA, has also been developed. Metatranscriptomics is apt in human gut microbiota exploration, as it shows the real-time functional activities of microbiomes and is better positioned in associating gut microorganisms with host performance [70]. Furthermore, it provides a window through which active pathways are identified, and shows how expressed functions have a role in disease severity and progression [71]. This technology also gives insight into the interaction of the gut microbiota and mucosal immune system, which can help physicians track malfunctions in the host's physiology [68].

3.7. High-Throughput Culturing

Several bacterial culture techniques have been developed overtime making it possible to culture a reasonable number of gut bacteria that had not been cultivated in the past. One such culture technique is culturomics. Culturomics, according to Lagier et al. [72], is a culturing technique that employs multiple culture conditions and matrix-assisted laser desorption/ionization time of flight (MALDI-TOF) and 16S rRNA gene amplification/sequencing for identification, as shown in Figure 3. Traore et al. [73] isolated 1162 bacteria strains by culturomics in a study that compared the gastrointestinal microbiota of Africans to the West. Goodman et al. [74] reported the use of gut microbiota medium (GMM) with high-throughput anaerobic culturing techniques in combination with metagenomics in characterizing extensive personal human gut microbiota culture collection and manipulation in gnotobiotic mice. Similarly, Lau et al. [49] revealed that using culture-enriched molecular profiling consisting of 66 culture conditions in conjunction with 16S rRNA gene sequencing was able to yield a robust data on the diversity of the microbiota that were present in sampled human feces. High-throughput culture methods have obvious advantages of enhancing the culturability of otherwise 'non-culturable' bacterial population, hence, giving room for the in-depth study of identified species. This technique is quite elaborate requiring specialized laboratories and it is space and time consuming. Harnessing the enormous potentials of high-throughput culturing techniques will provide clinicians with the platform for precise treatment of gut associated diseases resulting from perturbation, since implicated microbiota members can be cultured. Additionally, in the formulation and administration of probiotics, this technique can be useful. Furthermore, the morphology, physiology and biochemistry of individual microorganism can be studied and their response/interaction with drugs easily evaluated, thereby enabling the proper treatment of gut diseases.

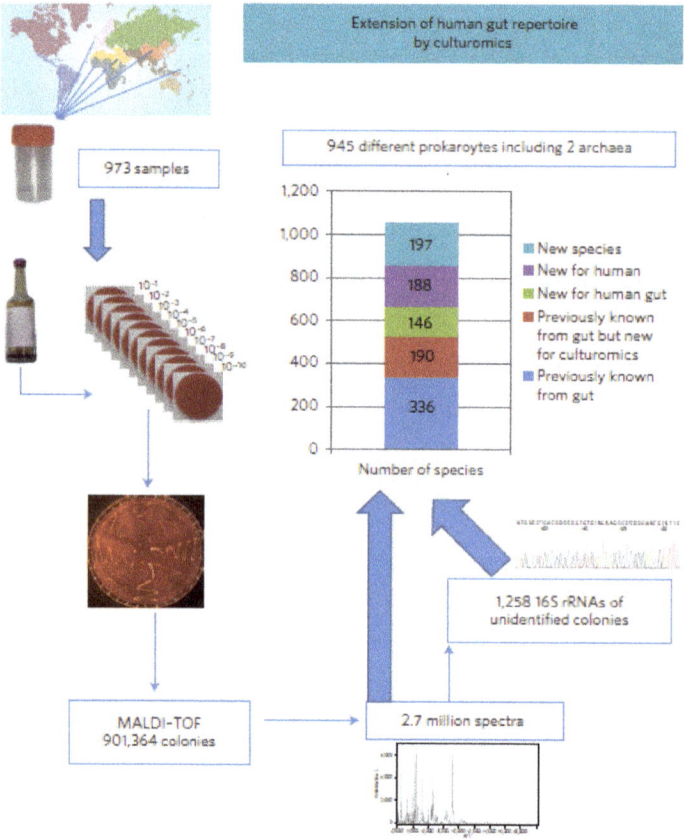

Figure 3. A stepwise outline of culturomics, enabling the culture of previously uncultured bacterial species in the human gut. Source: Lagier et al. [72] (*Nature Microbiology*, Macmillan Publishers Limited) Licensed under CC BY 4.0.

4. Future Perspectives and Conclusions

Although research in gut microbiota is still evolving, already available data and methods of exploring this complex ecosystem has helped to sharpen our knowledge and understanding of the microbiome and how it affects human health. Several studies and technologies that have focused on interactions between the gut microbiome and diet have revealed how the introduction of new micro-organisms and their change over time have opened up opportunities for their future intervention, as well as diagnostic tools based on the microbiome. These methods have been used to identify the yet-to-be cultured microbes of the gut microbiota, using the activity of various microbial metabolites for the purpose of pathogen identification. In addition, gut microbiome studies have been used in fecal microbial transplant for the treatment and correction of gut infections/disorders.

These techniques have therefore been proven to provide efficient information on the gut microbiome and how it evolves over time, thereby generating rich data sets that have been useful for treatment of yet to be identified pathogens, while enabling faster and more accurate diagnosis even from non-invasive sampling. Finally, the gut microbiome research has upped the ante on genomic technologies, because genomes of the gut microbiomes are sequenced to give us a better understanding of the gut microbiome.

Author Contributions: Conceptualization, S.S.; Methodology, A.A.; Data curation, S.S., A.A., and T.J.; writing original draft preparation, S.S., A.A., and T.J.; writing-review and editing, A.A. and S.S. All authors have read and agreed to the published version of the manuscript.

Funding: This research received no external funding.

Conflicts of Interest: The authors declare no conflict of interest.

References

1. Matsuki, T.; Tanaka, R. Function of the human gut microbiota. In *The Human Microbiota and Microbiome*; CABI Publishing: Cardiff, UK, 2014; pp. 90–106.
2. Blaut, M. Composition and function of the gut microbiome. In *The Gut Microbiome in Health and Disease*; Springer Science and Business Media LLC: Berlin, Germany, 2018; pp. 5–30.
3. Valdes, A.; Walter, J.; Segal, E.; Spector, T. Role of the gut microbiota in nutrition and health. *BMJ* **2018**, *361*, k2179. [CrossRef] [PubMed]
4. Pires, E.S.; Hardoim, C.C.P.; Miranda, K.R.; Secco, D.A.; Lobo, L.A.; de Carvalho, D.P.; Han, J.; Borchers, C.H.; Ferreira, R.B.R.; Salles, J.F.; et al. The gut microbiome and metabolome of two riparian communities in the amazon. *Front. Microbiol.* **2019**, *10*. [CrossRef] [PubMed]
5. Karkman, A.; Lehtimäki, J.; Ruokolainen, L. The ecology of human microbiota: Dynamics and diversity in health and disease. *Ann. N. Y. Acad. Sci.* **2017**, *1399*, 78–92. [CrossRef]
6. Vila, A.V.; Imhann, F.; Collij, V.; Jankipersadsing, S.A.; Gurry, T.; Mujagic, Z.; Kurilshikov, A.; Bonder, M.J.; Jiang, X.; Tigchelaar, E.F.; et al. Gut microbiota composition and functional changes in inflammatory bowel disease and irritable bowel syndrome. *Sci. Transl. Med.* **2018**, *10*, eaap8914. [CrossRef] [PubMed]
7. Wang, X.; Sun, G.; Feng, T.; Zhang, J.; Huang, X.; Wang, T.; Xie, Z.; Chu, X.; Yang, J.; Wang, H.; et al. Sodium oligomannate therapeutically remodels gut microbiota and suppresses gut bacterial amino acids-shaped neuroinflammation to inhibit Alzheimer's disease progression. *Cell Res.* **2019**, *29*, 787–803. [CrossRef] [PubMed]
8. Kang, D.-W.; Adams, J.B.; Gregory, A.C.; Borody, T.; Chittick, L.; Fasano, A.; Khoruts, A.; Geis, E.; Maldonado, J.; McDonough-Means, S.; et al. Microbiota Transfer Therapy alters gut ecosystem and improves gastrointestinal and autism symptoms: An open-label study. *Microbiome* **2017**, *5*, 10. [CrossRef] [PubMed]
9. Hu, Q.; Wu, K.; Pan, W.; Zeng, Y.; Hu, K.; Chen, D.; Huang, X.; Zhang, Q. Intestinal flora alterations in patients with early chronic kidney disease: A case-control study among the Han population in southwestern China. *J. Int. Med. Res.* **2020**, *48*, 300060520926033. [CrossRef]
10. Lippert, K.; Kedenko, L.; Antonielli, L.; Gemeier, C.; Leitner, M.; Kautzky-Willer, A.; Paulweber, B.; Hackl, E.; Kedenko, I. Gut microbiota dysbiosis associated with glucose metabolism disorders and the metabolic syndrome in older adults. *Benef. Microbes* **2017**, *8*, 545–556. [CrossRef]
11. Ley, R.E.; Turnbaugh, P.J.; Klein, S.; Gordon, J.I. Microbial ecology: Human gut microbes associated with obesity. *Nature* **2006**, *444*, 1022–1023. [CrossRef]
12. Zhuang, Z.-Q.; Shen, L.-L.; Li, W.-W.; Fu, X.; Zeng, F.; Gui, L.; Lv, Y.; Cai, M.; Zhu, C.; Tan, Y.-L.; et al. Gut Microbiome is Altered in Patients with Alzheimer's Disease. *J. Alzheimer's Dis.* **2018**, *63*, 1337–1346. [CrossRef]
13. He, Y.; Li, B.; Sun, D.; Chen, S. Gut microbiota: Implications in Alzheimer's disease. *J. Clin. Med.* **2020**, *9*, 2042. [CrossRef] [PubMed]
14. Li, Q.; Han, Y.; Dy, A.B.C.; Hagerman, R.J. The Gut Microbiota and Autism Spectrum Disorders. *Front. Cell. Neurosci.* **2017**, *11*, 120. [CrossRef] [PubMed]

15. Jie, Z.; Xia, H.; Zhong, S.-L.; Feng, Q.; Li, S.; Liang, S.; Zhong, H.; Liu, Z.; Gao, Y.; Zhao, H.; et al. The gut microbiome in atherosclerotic cardiovascular disease. *Nat. Commun.* **2017**, *8*, 845. [CrossRef] [PubMed]
16. Feeney, A.; Sleator, R.D. The human gut microbiome: The ghost in the machine. *Future Microbiol.* **2012**, *7*, 1235–1237. [CrossRef] [PubMed]
17. Khosravi, A.; Mazmanian, S.K. Disruption of the gut microbiome as a risk factor for microbial infections. *Curr. Opin. Microbiol.* **2013**, *16*, 221–227. [CrossRef]
18. Sommer, M.O. Advancing gut microbiome research using cultivation. *Curr. Opin. Microbiol.* **2015**, *27*, 127–132. [CrossRef]
19. Dabke, K.; Hendrick, G.; Devkota, S. The gut microbiome and metabolic syndrome. *J. Clin. Investig.* **2019**, *129*, 4050–4057. [CrossRef]
20. Barko, P.C.; McMichael, M.A.; Swanson, K.S.; Williams, D.A. The gastrointestinal microbiome. *J. Vet. Intern. Med.* **2018**, *32*, 9–25. [CrossRef]
21. Dominguez-Bello, M.G.; Costello, E.K.; Contreras, M.; Magris, M.; Hidalgo, G.; Fierer, N.; Knight, R. Delivery mode shapes the acquisition and structure of the initial microbiota across multiple body habitats in newborns. *Proc. Natl. Acad. Sci. USA* **2010**, *107*, 11971–11975. [CrossRef]
22. Shao, Y.; Forster, S.C.; Tsaliki, E.; Vervier, K.; Strang, A.; Simpson, N.; Kumar, N.; Stares, M.D.; Rodger, A.; Brocklehurst, P.; et al. Stunted Microbiota and Opportunustic pathogens colonization in caesarean-section birth. *Nature* **2019**, *574*, 117–121. [CrossRef]
23. Satokari, R.; Gronroo, T.; Laitinen, K.; Salminen, S.; Isolauri, E. Bifidobacterium and Lactobacillus DNA in the human placenta. *Lett. Appl. Microbiol.* **2009**, *48*, 8–12. [CrossRef] [PubMed]
24. Aagaard, K.; Ma, J.; Antony, K.M.; Ganu, R.; Petrosino, J.; Versalovic, J. The placenta harbors a unique microbiome. *Sci. Transl. Med.* **2014**, *6*, 237ra65. [CrossRef] [PubMed]
25. Yu, K.; Rodriguez, M.D.; Paul, Z.; Gordon, E.; Rice, K.; Triplett, W.E.; Keller-Wood, M.; Wood, C.E. Proof of principle: Physiological transfer of small numbers of bacteria from mother to fetus in late-gestation pregnant sheep. *PLoS ONE* **2019**, *14*, e0217211. [CrossRef] [PubMed]
26. De Goffau, M.C.; Lager, S.; Sovio, U.; Gaccioli, F.; Cook, E.; Peacock, S.J.; Parkhill, J.; Charnock-Jones, D.S.; Smith, G.C.S. Human placenta has no microbiome but can contain pathogens. *Nature* **2019**, *572*, 329–334. [CrossRef]
27. Koenig, J.E.; Spor, A.; Scalfone, N.; Fricker, A.D.; Stombaugh, J.; Knight, R.; Angenent, L.T.; Ley, R.E. Succession of microbial consortia in the developing infant gut microbiome. *Proc. Natl. Acad. Sci. USA* **2011**, *108*, 4578–4585. [CrossRef]
28. Differding, M.K.; Benjamin-Neelon, S.E.; Hoyo, C.; Østbye, T.; Mueller, N.T. Timing of complementary feeding is associated with gut microbiota diversity and composition and short chain fatty acid concentrations over the first year of life. *BMC Microbiol.* **2020**, *20*, 56. [CrossRef]
29. Cozzolino, A.; Vergalito, F.; Tremonte, P.; Iorizzo, M.; Lombardi, S.J.; Sorrentino, E.; Luongo, D.; Coppola, R.; Marco, R.D.; Succi, M. Preliminary evaluation of the safety and probiotic potential of *Akkermansiamuciniphila* OSM 22959 in comparison with *Lactobacillus rhamnosus* GG. *Microorganisms* **2020**, *8*, 189. [CrossRef]
30. Amabebe, E.; Robert, F.O.; Agbalalah, T.; Orubu, E.S.F. Microbial dysbiosis-induced obesity: Role of gut microbiota in homeostasis of energy metabolism. *Br. J. Nutr.* **2020**, *3*, 1–23. [CrossRef]
31. Barone, M.; Turroni, S.; Rampelli, S.; Soverini, M.; D'Amico, F.; Biagi, E.; Brigidi, P.; Troiani, E.; Candela, M. Gut microbiome response to a modern Paleolithic diet in a western lifestyle context. *PLoS ONE* **2019**, *14*, e0220619. [CrossRef]
32. Caviglia, G.P.; Rosso, C.; Ribaldone, D.G.; Dughera, F.; Fagoonee, S.; Astegiano, M.; Pellicano, R. Physiopathology of intestinal barrier and the role of Zonulin. *Minerva Biotecnol.* **2019**, *31*, 83–92. [CrossRef]
33. Kim, K.O.; Gluck, M. Fecal Microbiota Transplantation: An Update on Clinical Practice. *Clin. Endosc.* **2019**, *52*, 137–143. [CrossRef] [PubMed]
34. Zou, M.; Jie, Z.; Cui, B.; Wang, H.; Feng, Q.; Zou, Y.; Zhang, X.; Yang, H.; Wang, J.; Zhang, F.; et al. Faecalmicrobiota transplantation results in bacterial strain displacement in patients with inflammatory bowel diseases. *FEBS Open Bio* **2019**, *10*, 41–55. [CrossRef] [PubMed]
35. Bibbò, S.; Settanni, C.R.; Porcari, S.; Bocchino, E.; Ianiro, G.; Cammarota, G.; Gasbarrin, A. Fecal Microbiota Transplantation: Screening and Selection to Choose the Optimal Donor. *J. Clin. Med.* **2020**, *9*, 1757. [CrossRef]
36. Sbahi, H.; Di Palma, J.A. Faecalmicrobiota transplantation: Applications and limitations in treating gastrointestinal disorders. *BMJ Open Gastroenterol.* **2016**, *3*, e000087. [CrossRef] [PubMed]

37. Antushevich, H. Faecalmicrobita transplantation in disease therapy. *Clin. Chim. Acta* **2019**, *503*, 90–98. [CrossRef]
38. Cammarota, G.; Ianiro, G.; Kelly, C.R.; Mullish, B.H.; Allegretti, J.R.; Kassam, Z.; Putignani, L.; Fischer, M.; Keller, J.J.; Castello, S.P.; et al. International consensus conference on stool banking for faecalmicrobiota transplantation in clinical practice. *Gut* **2019**, *68*, 2111–2121. [CrossRef]
39. Belizário, J.E.; Faintuch, J.; Garay-Malpartida, M. Gut Microbiome Dysbiosis and Immunometabolism: New Frontiers for Treatment of Metabolic Diseases. *Mediat. Inflamm.* **2018**, *2037838*, 1–12. [CrossRef]
40. Wong, A.C.; Levy, M. New approaches to microbiome-based therapies. *mSystems* **2019**, *4*, e00122-19. [CrossRef]
41. Guimaraes, N.; Azevedo, N.F.; Figueiredo, C.; Keevil, C.W.; Vieira, M. Development and application of a novel peptide nucleic acid probe for the specific detection of Helicobacter pylori in gastric biopsy specimen. *Clin. Microbiol.* **2007**, *45*, 3089–3094. [CrossRef]
42. Baysal, A.H. Comparison of conventional culture method and fluorescent in situ hybridization technique from detection of Listeria Spp. In ground beef, turkey and chicken breast fillets in Izmir, Turkey. *J. Food Prot.* **2014**, *77*, 2021–2030. [CrossRef]
43. Becattini, S.; Littmann, E.R.; Carter, R.A.; Kim, S.G.; Morjaria, S.M.; Ling, L.; Gyaltshen, Y.; Fontana, E.; Taur, Y.; Leiner, I.M.; et al. Commensal Microbesprovide First Line Defence Against Listeria monocytogenes Infection. *J. Exp. Med.* **2017**, *214*, 1973–1989. [CrossRef] [PubMed]
44. Prudent, E.; Raoult, D. Fluorescent in situ hybridization, a complementary molecular tool for the clinical diagnosis of infectious diseases by intracellular and fastidious bacteria. *FEMS Microbiol. Rev.* **2019**, *43*, 88–107. [CrossRef]
45. Russmann, H.; Adler, K.; Haas, R.; Gebert, B.; Koletzko, S.; Heesemann, J. Rapid and accurate Determination of genotypic clarithromycin resistance in cultured Helicobacter pylori by fluorescent in situ hybridization. *J. Clin. Microbial.* **2001**, *39*, 4142–4144. [CrossRef] [PubMed]
46. Arnold, J.W.; Roach, J.; Azcarate-Peril, M.A. Emerging technologies for gut microbiome research. *Trends Microbiol.* **2016**, *24*, 887–901. [CrossRef]
47. Borewicz, K.; Gu, F.; Saccenti, E.; Hechler, C.; Beijers, R.; de Weerth, C.; van Leeuwen, S.S.; Schols, H.A.; Smidt, H. The association between breast milk oligosaccharides and faecal microbiota in healthy breastfed infants at two, six, and twelve weeks of age. *Sci. Rep.* **2020**, *10*, 4270. [CrossRef] [PubMed]
48. Backhed, F.; Roswall, J.; Peng, Y.; Feng, Q.; Jia, H.; Kovatcheva, P.-D.; Li, Y.; Xia, Y.; Xie, H.; Zhong, H.; et al. Dynamics and Stabilization of the Human Gut Microbiome during the First Year of Life. *Cell Host Microbe* **2015**, *17*, 690–703. [CrossRef]
49. Lau, J.T.; Whelan, F.J.; Herath, I.; Lee, C.H.; Collins, S.M.; Bercik, P.; Surette, M.G. Capturing the diversity of the human gut microbiota through culture-enriched molecular profiling. *Genome Med.* **2016**, *8*, 72. [CrossRef]
50. García-Mantrana, I.; Selma-Royo, M.; González, S.; Parra-Llorcac, A.; Martínez-Costad, C.; Collado, M.C. Distinct maternal microbiota clusters are associated with diet during pregnancy: Impact on neonatal microbiota and infant growth during the first 18 months of life. *Gut Microbes* **2020**, *11*, 962–978. [CrossRef]
51. Beaumont, M.; Goodrich, J.K.; Jackson, M.A.; Yet, I.; Davenport, E.R.; Vieira, S.-S.; Debelius, J.; Pallister, T.; Mangino, M.; Raes, J.; et al. Heritable components of the human fecal microbiome are associated with visceral fat. *Genome Biol.* **2016**, *17*, 189. [CrossRef]
52. Chijiwa, R.; Hoskawa, M.; Kogawa, M.; Nishikawa, Y.; Ide, K.; Sakanashi, C.; Takahashi, K.; Takeyama, H. Single-cell genomics of uncultured bacteria reveals dietary fiber responders in the mouse gut microbiota. *Microbiome* **2020**, *8*, 5. [CrossRef]
53. Collado, M.C.; Rautava, S.; Aakko, J.; Isolauri, E.; Salminen, S. Human gut colonization may be initiated in utero by distinct microbial communities in the placenta and amniotic fluid. *Sci. Rep.* **2016**, *6*, 23129. [CrossRef] [PubMed]
54. Albenberg, L.; Kelsen, J. Advances in gut microbiome research and relevance to pediatric diseases. *J. Pediatr.* **2016**, *178*, 16–20. [CrossRef] [PubMed]
55. Saulnier, D.M.; Riehle, K.; Mistretta, T.A.; Diaz, M.-A.; Mandal, D.; Raza, S.; Weidler, E.M.; Qin, X.; Coarfa, C.; Milosavljevic, A.; et al. Gastrointestinal microbiome signatures of pediatric patients with irritable bowel syndrome. *Gastroenterology* **2011**, *141*, 1782–1791. [CrossRef] [PubMed]

56. Vogtmann, E.; Hua, X.; Zeller, G.; Sunagawa, S.; Voigt, A.Y.; Hercog, R.; Weidler, E.M.; Qin, X.; Coarfa, C.; Milosavljevic, A.; et al. Colorectal cancer and the human gut microbiome: Reproducibility with whole genome shotgun sequencing. *PLoS ONE* **2016**, *11*, e0155362. [CrossRef] [PubMed]
57. Siegwald, L.; Caboche, S.; Even, G.; Viscoglisoi, E.; Audebert, C.; Chabe, M. The impact of bioinformatics pipelines on microbiota studies: Does the analytical "Microscope" affect the biological interpretation? *Microorganisms* **2019**, *7*, 393. [CrossRef] [PubMed]
58. Liu, Y.; Walther-Antonio, M. Microfluidics: A new tool for microbial single cell analyses in human microbiome studies. *Biomicrofluidics* **2017**, *11*, 061501. [CrossRef]
59. Udayasuryan, B.; Slade, D.J.; Verbridge, S.S. *Microfluidics in Microbiome and Cancer Research*; Wiley: Hoboken, NJ, USA, 2019; pp. 281–317.
60. Kasendra, M.; Tovaglieri, A.; Sontheimer, A.-P.; Jalili-Firoozinezhad, S.; Bein, A.; Chalkiadaki, A.; Scholl, W.; Zhang, C.; Rickner, H.; Bein, A.; et al. Development of a primary human Small Intestine-on-a-Chip using biopsy-derived organoids. *Sci. Rep.* **2018**, *8*, 2871. [CrossRef]
61. Cama, J.; Voliotis, M.; Metz, J.; Smith, A.; Iannucci, J.; Keyser, U.F.; Atanasova, K.T.; Pagliara, S. Single-cell microfluidics facilitates the rapid quantification of antibiotic accumulation in Gramnegative bacteria. *Lab Chip* **2020**, *20*, 2765–2775. [CrossRef]
62. Sarangi, A.N.; Goel, A.; Aggarwal, R. Methods for studying gut microbita: A primer for physicians. *J. Clin. Exp. Hepatol.* **2019**, *9*, 62–73. [CrossRef]
63. Duscha, A.; Gisevius, B.; Hirschberg, S.; Yissachar, N.; Stangl, G.J.; Eilers, E.; Bader, V.; Haase, S.; Kaisler, J.; David, C.; et al. Propionic acid shapes the multiple sclerosis disease course by an immunomodulatory mechanism. *Cell* **2020**, *180*, 1–14.
64. Murugesan, S.; Nirmalkar, K.; Hoyo-Vadillo, C.; García-Espitia, M.; Ramírez-Sánchez, D.; García-Mena, J. Gut microbiome production of short-chain fatty acids and obesity in children. *Eur. J. Clin. Microbiol. Infect. Dis.* **2017**, *37*, 621–625. [CrossRef] [PubMed]
65. Luan, H.; Wang, X.; Cai, Z. Mass spectrometry-based metabolomics: Targeting the crosstalk between gut microbiota and brain in neurodegenerative disorders. *Mass Spectrom. Rev.* **2017**, *38*, 1–12. [CrossRef] [PubMed]
66. Wilson, A.D.; Forse, L.B. Development of Electronic-Nose technologies for early disease detection based on microbial dysbiosis. *Proceedings* **2019**, *4*, 32. [CrossRef]
67. Maier, T.V.; Walker, A.; Heinzmann, S.S.; Forcisi, S.; Martinez, I.; Walter, J.; Kopplin, P.S. Challenges of metabolomics in human gut microbiota research. *Int. J. Med. Microbiol.* **2016**, *306*, 266–279.
68. Bashiardes, S.; Zilberman-Schapira, G.; Elinav, E. Use of Metatranscriptomics in Microbiome Research. *Bioinform. Biol. Insights* **2016**, *10*, 19–25. [CrossRef] [PubMed]
69. Gosalbes, M.J.; Durban, A.; Pignatelli, M.; Abellan, J.J.; Jimenez-Hernandez, N.; Perez-Cobas, A.E.; Latorre, A.; Moya, A. Metatranscriptomic Approach to Analyze the Functional Human Gut Microbiota. *PLoS ONE* **2011**, *6*, e17447. [CrossRef]
70. Li, F.; Hitch, T.C.A.; Chen, Y.; Creevey, C.J.; Guan, L.L. Comparative metagenomic and metatranscriptomic analyses reveal the breed effect on the rumen microbiome and its associations with feed efficiency in beef cattle. *Microbiome* **2019**, *7*, 6. [CrossRef]
71. Shakya, M.; Lo, C.C.; Chain, P.S.G. Advances and Challenges in Metatranscriptomic Analysis. *Front. Genet.* **2019**, *10*, 904. [CrossRef]
72. Lagier, J.-C.; Khelaifia, S.; Alou, M.T.; Ndongo, S.; Dione, N.; Hugon, P.; Caputo, A.; Cadoret, F.; Traore, S.I.; Secck, E.H.; et al. Culture of previously uncultured members of the human gut microbiota by culturomics. *Nat. Microbiol.* **2016**, *1*, 16203. [CrossRef]
73. Traore, S.I.; Bilen, M.; Cadoret, F.; Khelaifa, S.; Million, M.; Raoult, D.; Lagier, J.C. Study of huma gastrointestinal microbiota by culturomics in Africa. *Med. Sante Trop.* **2019**, *29*, 366–370.
74. Goodman, A.L.; Kallstrom, G.; Faith, J.J.; Reyes, A.; Moore, A.; Dantas, G.; Gordon, J.I. Extensive personal human gut microbiota culture collection characterized and manipulated in gnobiotic mice. *Proc. Natl. Acad. Sci. USA* **2011**, *108*, 6252–6257. [CrossRef] [PubMed]

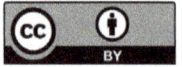 © 2020 by the authors. Licensee MDPI, Basel, Switzerland. This article is an open access article distributed under the terms and conditions of the Creative Commons Attribution (CC BY) license (http://creativecommons.org/licenses/by/4.0/).

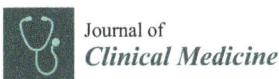

Article

Gene Expression of Transient Receptor Potential Channels in Peripheral Blood Mononuclear Cells of Inflammatory Bowel Disease Patients

Taku Morita [1], Keiichi Mitsuyama [1,2,*], Hiroshi Yamasaki [1,2], Atsushi Mori [1,2], Tetsuhiro Yoshimura [1,2], Toshihiro Araki [1,2], Masaru Morita [1,2], Kozo Tsuruta [1,2], Sayo Yamasaki [1], Kotaro Kuwaki [1,2], Shinichiro Yoshioka [1,2], Hidetoshi Takedatsu [1,2] and Takuji Torimura [1]

[1] Department of Medicine, Division of Gastroenterology, School of Medicine, Kurume University, 67 Asahi-Machi, Kurume 830-0011, Japan; morita_taku@med.kurume-u.ac.jp (T.M.); yamasaki_hiroshi@kurume-u.ac.jp (H.Y.); mori_atsushi@med.kurume-u.ac.jp (A.M.); yoshimura_tetsuhiro@med.kurume-u.ac.jp (T.Y.); araki_toshihiro@med.kurume-u.ac.jp (T.A.); morita_masaru@med.kurume-u.ac.jp (M.M.); tsuruta_kouzou@med.kurume-u.ac.jp (K.T.); yasumoto_sayo@med.kurume-u.ac.jp (S.Y.); kuwaki_koutarou@kurume-u.ac.jp (K.K.); yoshioka_shinichirou@kurume-u.ac.jp (S.Y.); takedatsu_hidetoshi@med.kurume-u.ac.jp (H.T.); tori@med.kurume-u.ac.jp (T.T.)

[2] Inflammatory Bowel Disease Center, Kurume University Hospital, 67 Asahi-Machi, Kurume 830-0011, Japan

* Correspondence: ibd@med.kurume-u.ac.jp; Tel.: +81-942-31-7561

Received: 11 July 2020; Accepted: 12 August 2020; Published: 14 August 2020

Abstract: We examined the expression profile of transient receptor potential (TRP) channels in peripheral blood mononuclear cells (PBMCs) from patients with inflammatory bowel disease (IBD). PBMCs were obtained from 41 ulcerative colitis (UC) patients, 34 Crohn's disease (CD) patients, and 30 normal subjects. mRNA levels of TRP channels were measured using the quantitative real-time polymerase chain reaction, and correlation tests with disease ranking, as well as laboratory parameters, were performed. Compared with controls, TRPV2 and TRPC1 mRNA expression was lower, while that of TRPM2, was higher in PBMCs of UC and CD patients. Moreover, TRPV3 mRNA expression was lower, while that of TRPV4 was higher in CD patients. TRPC6 mRNA expression was higher in patients with CD than in patients with UC. There was also a tendency for the expression of TRPV2 mRNA to be negatively correlated with disease activity in patients with UC and CD, while that of TRPM4 mRNA was negatively correlated with disease activity only in patients with UC. PBMCs from patients with IBD exhibited varying mRNA expression levels of TRP channel members, which may play an important role in the progression of IBD.

Keywords: crohn's disease; mononuclear cells; transient receptor potential channel; ulcerative colitis

1. Introduction

Inflammatory bowel disease (IBD), consisting primarily of ulcerative colitis (UC) and Crohn's disease (CD), represents a group of chronic inflammatory disorders involving the gastrointestinal tract. Its pathogenesis is complex; however, current research suggests that an intricate network of multiple interacting mechanisms in genetically susceptible individuals may orchestrate the dysregulation of immune and inflammatory responses [1,2].

The transient receptor potential (TRP) channel family, a diverse family of proteins that are reportedly expressed throughout the human body, have emerged as a novel and interrelated system to detect and respond to various environmental stimuli including mechanical, thermal, or chemical stimuli. With this function, they are likely to be sensors for monitoring specific responses to different exogenous and endogenous chemical and physical stimuli [3–6]. Members of the TRP superfamily are classified according to their amino acid sequences and structural similarities into canonical (TRPC), vanilloid (TRPV), melastatin (TRPM), ankyrin (TRPA), polycystin (TRPP), and mucolipin (TRPML) subfamilies [3–5]. It was recently revealed that the role of TRP channels reaches beyond the control of neuropeptide release from sensory nerves as they are also expressed in immune and resident tissue cells, such as epithelial cells, where they modulate many functions including cytokine production and migration. Therefore, a vital interplay between these cells appears to maintain homeostasis in the intestine, while the disruption of this interplay may be involved in the development and maintenance of IBD [7–10].

In the gut wall of IBD patients, immune cells migrating from systemic circulation release various inflammatory and immunoregulatory molecules, such as cytokines and free radicals, that modulate intestinal inflammation and tissue damage [11]. Therefore, peripheral blood mononuclear cells (PBMCs) are of particular interest due to their involvement in inflammatory and immune cell function. PBMCs may be in contact with multiple stimuli within the blood that have the potential to release TRP channels, resulting in modulation of intestinal inflammation. Therefore, an evaluation of TRP channel expression in PBMCs from IBD patients may provide insights regarding the disease pathogenesis; while changes in their expression level may mirror intestinal inflammation. Recently, the expression of these TRP channel members in PBMCs have been reported in healthy subjects and patients with various diseases [12–15]. However, to date no data regarding their expression in PBMCs from patients with IBD has been reported.

TRPV1–TRPV4; TRPM2, TRPM4, and TRPM5; and TRPC1 as well as TRPC3–TRPC7, are the most relevant TRP channels in immune cells under normal and specific disease conditions [12–15]. Therefore, this study focused on the expression profiles of these TRP channel members in PBMCs obtained from patients with IBD. Furthermore, the relationships between TRP channel levels and the disease activity index, as well as other laboratory parameters were investigated.

2. Materials and Methods

2.1. Ethical Considerations

This study was approved by the Ethical Committee of Kurume University (14253, 25 March 2015). Written informed consent was obtained from each subject before enrollment in the study.

2.2. Patients

This study was conducted at Kurume University Hospital between September 2011 and May 2016. A total of 105 subjects, including 41 patients with UC, 34 with CD, and 30 healthy subjects were enrolled. Prior to commencing the study, 19 subjects were excluded due to an insufficient sample volume. The patient diagnosis was based on characteristic clinical, endoscopic, radiological, and histological features. The patient characteristics and the medical therapy they received are summarized in Table 1.

2.3. Clinical Evaluations

For the evaluation of disease activity, clinical activity in patients with UC was graded using the partial Mayo score (PMS), with the inactive disease defined as a score ≤2, with no individual sub-score >1 point [16]. Patients with CD were graded according to the CD activity index (CDAI) comprised of eight factors, each added after adjustment with a weighted factor, with the inactive disease defined as a score <150 points [17].

Table 1. Patient characteristics.

	Healthy Volunteers	Ulcerative Colitis	Crohn's Disease	p-Value
	(n = 30)	(n = 41)	(n = 34)	
Sex, male/female	13/17	19/22	12/12	0.61
Age, years	39	41	35	0.17
(median, IQR)	(32–44)	(29–58)	(27–47)	
Area involved		total colitis/ left-side colitis/ proctitis 26/8/7	ileitis/ ileocolitis/ colitis 4/23/7	
Disease duration, months		81	106	0.19
(median, IQR)		(60.5–171.5)	(60.9–274.2)	
Treatments				
No medication		2 (4.9)	0 (0.0)	0.19
5-aminosalicylic acid (%)		36 (87.8)	25 (73.5)	0.11
Prednisolone (%)		7 (17.1)	3 (8.8)	0.3
Immunomodulator (%)		7 (17.1)	9 (26.5)	0.32
Leukocytapheresis (%)		2 (4.9)	0 (0.0)	0.19
Nutrition therapy (%)		0 (0.0)	21 (61.8)	<0.01
Anti-tumor necrosis factor (%)		3 (7.3)	24 (70.6)	<0.01
Surgery (%)		0 (0.0)	15 (44.1)	<0.01

IQR: Interquartile range.

2.4. Determination of Laboratory Parameters

Blood samples were collected from all patients and were used to measure the following laboratory parameters: Total leukocyte count, serum levels of hemoglobin, albumin, and C-reactive protein (CRP).

2.5. Separation of PBMCs and RNA Extraction

Blood samples (10 mL) were obtained by cubital venous puncture and collected in standard sterile polystyrene vacuum tubes with heparin. First, freshly drawn blood was diluted at a ratio of 1:2.5 with a phosphate buffered saline. PBMCs were isolated from the diluted blood by a Ficoll-Paque (GE Healthcare, Uppsala, Sweden) density gradient centrifugation according to the manufacturer's instructions. PBMCs were pelleted, snap-frozen on dry ice, and stored at −80 °C until use [18]. RNA was extracted from PBMC samples following the protocol described for the TRIzol reagent (Invitrogen, Carlsbad, CA, USA). The quantity and purity of the RNA were determined for all samples on a Nanodrop ND-1000 spectrophotometer (Thermo Scientific, Waltham, MA, USA). The average yield was 23,000 ng. The purity, as measured by the A260/280 ratio, was between 1.91 and 1.95 [18].

2.6. Measurement of TRP Channel mRNA Expression Using Real-Time Quantitative Polymerase Chain Reaction (Real-Time qPCR)

Total RNA was converted into cDNA using the ReverTra Ace qPCR RT kit (Toyobo, Osaka, Japan). The generated cDNAs (25 ng) were stored at −20 °C. cDNA was added to the TaqMan Gene Expression Master Mix (Applied Biosystems, Foster City, CA, USA). qPCR reactions (20 µL) composed of 2 µL cDNA template, TaqMan Universal PCR Master Mix (2×, Thermo Fisher Scientific, Foster City, CA, USA), TaqMan assay (20×, Thermo Fisher Scientific), and H_2O. RT-PCR was performed using the StepOne Real-Time PCR System (Applied Biosystems). Reactions, run in triplicate, were incubated at 50 °C for 2 min and 95 °C for 10 min, followed by 40 cycles of 95 °C for 15 s and 60 °C for 1 min. The TaqMan probe and primer sets for the target genes used in this study are shown in Table 2.

Table 2. Details of TaqMan probes and primers used in this study.

Gene	Accession Number	Assay
GAPDH	NM_001256799.2	Hs02786624_g1
	NM_001289745.1	
	NM_001289746.1	
	NM_002046.5	
TRPV1	NM_018727.5	Hs00218912_m1
	NM_080704.3	
	NM_080705.3	
	NM_080706.3	
TRPV2	NM_016113.4	Hs00901648_m1
TRPV3	NM_001258205.1	Hs00376854_m1
	NM_145068.3	
TRPV4	NM_001177428.1	Hs01099348_m1
	NM_001177431.1	
	NM_001177433.1	
	NM_021625.4	
	NM_147204.2	
TRPM2	NM_001320350.1	Hs01066091_m1
	NM_001320351.1	
	NM_001320352.1	
	NM_003307.3	
TRPM4	NM_001195227.1	Hs00214167_m1
	NM_001321281.1	
	NM_001321282.1	
	NM_001321283.1	
	NM_001321285.1	
	NM_017636.3	
TRPM5	NM_014555.3	Hs00175822_m1
TRPC1	NM_001251845.1	Hs00608195_m1
	NM_003304.4	
TRPC3	NM_001130698.1	Hs00162985_m1
	NM_003305.2	
TRPC4	NM_001135955.1	Hs01077392_m1
	NM_001135956.1	
	NM_001135957.1	
	NM_001135958.1	
	NM_003306.1	
TRPC5	NM_012471.2	Hs00202960_m1
TRPC6	NM_004621.5	Hs00988479_m1
TRPC7	NM_001167576.1	Hs00220638_m1
	NM_001167577.2	
	NM_020389.2	

GAPDH: Glyceraldehyde 3-phosphate dehydrogenase; TRP: Transient receptor potential.

GAPDH was used as the reference gene. Ct values for GAPDH mRNA of an individual PBMC per sample were calculated. The mean was calculated from experiments performed in duplicate. For data analysis, the StepOne software v2.1 was used. Data representing the relative expression of detected mRNA normalized to GAPDH mRNA was used as a calibrator for comparative analysis. RT-qPCR was performed in accordance with the Minimum Information for Publication of Quantitative Real-Time PCR Experiments (MIQE) guidelines [19,20]. The relative expression data was calculated according to the $2^{-\Delta\Delta Ct}$ method.

2.7. Statistical Analyses

Results were analyzed using the JMP v12 statistical package (SAS Institute, Cary, NC, USA). The normality of distribution was assessed using the Shapiro–Wilk test. As mRNA levels of each TRP channel were all not normally distributed, statistical analyses were performed using Mann–Whitney U and Kruskal–Wallis H tests and correlation analysis was performed using Spearman's rank correlation test. The Bonferroni-corrected Mann–Whitney U test was used to evaluate inter-group comparisons of the mean differences according to their distribution. Data are shown as the mean ± standard deviation (SD) or as correlation coefficients.

3. Results

3.1. TRP Channel Levels in IBD

The expression of TRP channels in PBMCs from the IBD and control groups are summarized in Figure 1. The observed fold changes in all TRP channel members were very small. However, when compared with mRNA expression levels in PBMCs from healthy controls (TRPV2, 1.54 ± 0.44; TRPV3, 0.15 ± 0.08; TRPV4, 0.95 ± 0.39; TRPM2, 1.54 ± 0.63; TRPC1, 1.73 ± 0.64), those of TRPV2 and TRPC1 were lower in both UC (1.11 ± 0.39 (0.72-fold), $p < 0.0001$ and 1.15 ± 0.65 (0.66-fold), $p = 0.0002$, respectively) and CD (1.18 ± 0.34 (0.77-fold), $p = 0.0014$ and 1.24 ± 0.65 (0.72-fold), $p = 0.0021$, respectively) groups, those of TRPM2 were higher in both UC (2.20 ± 0.76 (1.43-fold), $p < 0.0001$) and CD (2.28 ± 0.86 (1.47-fold), $p < 0.0001$) groups, those of TRPV3 were lower only in the CD group (0.09 ± 0.06 (0.58-fold), $p = 0.001$), and those of TRPV4 were higher only in the CD (1.40 ± 0.72 (1.48-fold), $p = 0.0067$) group.

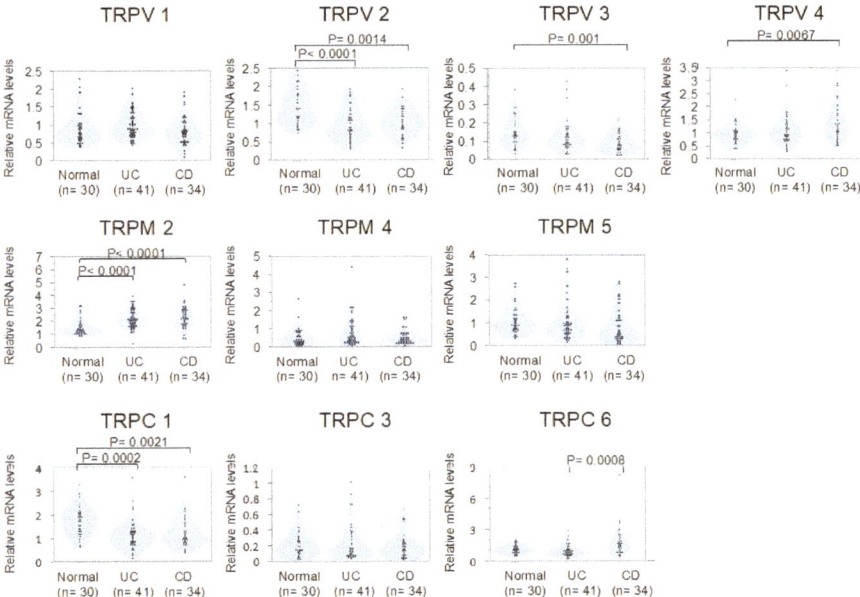

Figure 1. Expression of transient receptor potential (TRP) channels in healthy subjects, patients with ulcerative colitis (UC) and Crohn's disease (CD). Bars represent mean ± SD. N: Number of subjects. Inter-group significance, Bonferroni-corrected Mann–Whitney U test, $p < 0.01$.

Further, TRPC6 mRNA expression was higher in the CD group (1.68 ± 1.41 (1.79-fold), $p = 0.0008$) than in the UC group (0.94 ± 0.55).

In addition, the mRNA expression levels of each TRP channel in PBMCs from healthy controls were variable. We found that TRPV3 had the lowest (0.15-fold relative to GAPDH) and TRPC1 had the highest (1.73-fold relative to GAPDH) expression.

3.2. Relationship between TRP Channel Levels and Disease Activity

Figure 2 shows the relationship between the expression of each TRP channel member and the clinical disease progression, assessed using PMS for UC patients, and CDAI for CD patients. There was a tendency observed for the mRNA expression of TRPV2 to negatively correlate with disease activity in both UC and CD groups, while that of TRPM4 was negatively correlated with disease activity in only the UC group. However, the significance of these correlations is questionable since the R^2 values were <0.1.

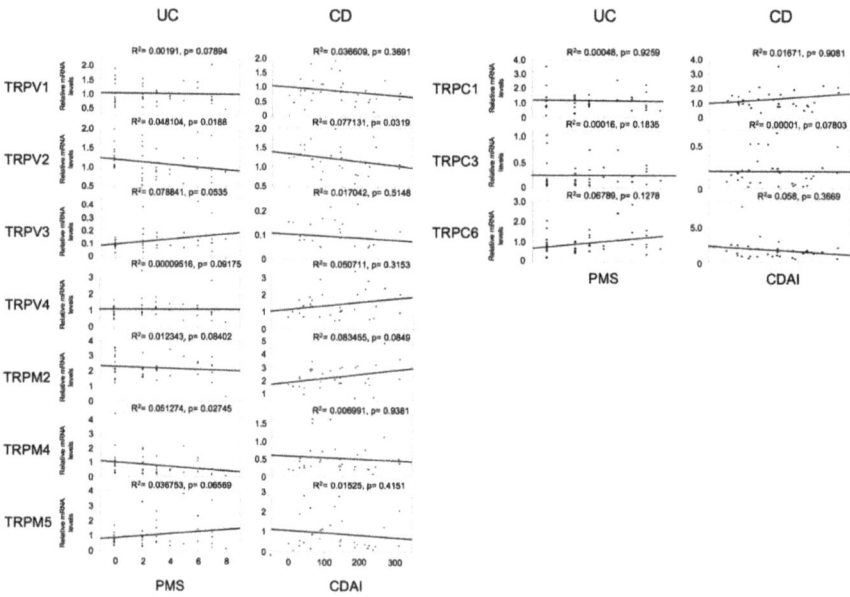

Figure 2. Correlation between TRP channel expression and clinical disease progression in patients with ulcerative colitis (UC) and Crohn's disease (CD). Clinical disease progression was assessed using the partial Mayo score (PMS) for patients with UC and the CD activity index (CDAI) for patients with CD. N: Number of patients.

3.3. Correlation between Expression of TRP Channels and Clinical Parameters

Table 3 summarizes the correlation coefficients and significance values for comparisons between the expression of each TRP channel member and the indicated laboratory parameters. In the UC group, mRNA expression of TRPV2 and TRPV3 negatively correlated with the leukocyte count, while that of TRPV4 and TRPM5 positively correlated with the serum albumin and hemoglobin levels, respectively. In the CD group, the expression of TRPV4 positively correlated with the CRP level.

3.4. Relationship between TRP Channel Expression and Medical Treatment

We also assessed the relationship between each TRP channel member and medical treatment received by the patient. Since the number of patients in each group was fairly small, no significant association was found between individual TRP channel members and specific medical treatments (Supplementary Figure S1).

Table 3. Correlation coefficients and significance of differences between each transient receptor potential (TRP) channel expression and laboratory parameters in patients with ulcerative colitis (UC) or Crohn's disease (CD).

	UC				CD			
	CRP	Alb	WBC	Hb	CRP	Alb	WBC	Hb
TRPV1	0.011	0.009	−0.206	0.116	−0.174	0.224	−0.275	0.0461
TRPV2	−0.111	−0.01	−0.500 **	−0.151	−0.275	0.039	−0.205	−0.199
TRPV3	0.089	0.079	−0.399 *	0.129	−0.216	0.346	−0.146	0.1235
TRPV4	0.105	0.432 *	−0.027	0.341	0.355 *	−0.229	0.167	0.1165
TRPM2	−0.282	−0.095	0.285	−0.213	0.315	−0.064	0.032	0.0448
TRPM4	−0.011	−0.03	0.161	−0.196	−0.125	0.004	−0.193	0.0211
TRPM5	−0.07	0.24	−0.013	0.378 *	−0.268	0.283	−0.344	−0.128
TRPC1	−0.125	0.031	0.033	−0.062	0.327	−0.295	0.262	−0.132
TRPC3	−0.177	−0.044	0.296	0.11	−0.182	−0.009	0.197	−0.196
TRPC6	0.038	−0.106	0.052	−0.121	−0.057	0.347	0.056	0.515 **

Alb: Albumin; CRP: C-reactive protein; Hb: Hemoglobin; WBC: White blood cell. * $p < 0.05$, ** $p < 0.005$.

4. Discussion

Recently, it was revealed that TRP channels are expressed throughout the human body, including in immune cells, sensory nerves, and resident tissue cells [4–7]. Saunders et al. examined the expression of TRPV1 and TRPV2 in PBMCs from healthy subjects and speculated that as they have a role in the detection of noxious stimuli in the blood or under pathological conditions, their upregulation acts as an indicator of inflammation [13,21]. However, to the best of our knowledge, the current study is the first to explore the relationships among the gene expression profiles of TRP channel members in PBMCs from patients with IBD.

TRPV1, a polymodal receptor involved in inflammation and nociception, plays an important role in visceral hypersensitivity [22]. Reportedly, TRPV1-immunoreactivity in colonic tissue is increased, and is correlated with the severity of abdominal pain in patients with IBD [22,23]. More recently, TRPV1 was shown to be expressed in CD4+ T cells, where it regulates cell activation and proinflammatory properties in IBD [24]. Meanwhile, a TRPV1 antagonist suppressed colitis and colorectal distension in animal models [25]. In a study, two-fold upregulation of the TRPV1 gene was found in PBMCs of patients hyposensitive to capsaicin, pain, and thermal stimuli [14]. However, in the present study, we did not observe any significant differences in TRPV1 expression in PBMCs from patients with IBD compared to healthy controls. Hence, further studies are needed to determine the role of the TRPV1 pathway in PBMCs from IBD patients using protein or functional data.

TRPV2 triggers a wide range of physiological actions including changes in the innate and adaptive immune system. It is expressed in granulocytes and monocytes/macrophages and contributes to phagocytosis, migration, and inflammatory cytokine production [26]. In PBMCs, the increased expression of TRPV2 was closely correlated with childhood asthma [15]. In TRPV2-knockout mice, colitis was less severe due to the reduced infiltration of macrophages [27], suggesting that the TRPV2 pathway plays a key role in the development of colitis. Our study showed that TRPV2 expression in PBMCs decreased in patients with UC and CD and was inversely correlated with disease activity. Based on these findings, a reduction in TRPV2 expression in PBMCs may hypothetically dampen the proinflammatory response and could possibly reduce the severity of intestinal inflammation. However, further investigations are required to confirm this hypothesis.

TRPV3 is broadly expressed in intestinal epithelial cells, possibly for nutrient sensing and digestion [28,29]; however, its precise function is not well understood. With the exception of one study reporting its association with a higher risk of colorectal cancer, none others have investigated the role of TRPV3 in gut disease [30]. Interestingly, a recent study demonstrated a decrease in the proliferation rate of oral epithelial cells in TRPV3-knockout mice [31], suggesting that TRPV3 may contribute to oral wound repair. Our data revealed that TRPV3 expression was only decreased in PBMCs of patients with CD, however, its function in PBMCs requires further investigation.

TRPV4 is expressed and is functional in intestinal epithelial cells, glial cells, and CD45+ leukocytes; its activation in the gut causes increased intracellular calcium concentrations and chemokine release [28]. Studies have indicated a strong role for TRPV4 in IBD with elevated expression of TRPV4 observed in the intestinal tissue of patients with UC and CD [32]. In animal models of colitis, TRPV4 activation causes inflammation [32], and its blockade alleviates inflammation [33]. In this study, we found that the expression of TRPV4 was also upregulated in PBMCs and was correlated with the CRP level in patients with CD. Although the correlations were quite weak, and conclusions cannot be drawn based on mRNA levels without protein and modulation data, our data suggests a potential role for leukocyte TRPV4 in the pathophysiology of CD.

Recent studies have also revealed the involvement of TRPM2 in various aspects of immunity [34]. In a colitis model, TRPM2 has been implicated in inflammatory pathways, specifically as a key participant in chemokine production [35]. Contrary to this proinflammatory action, TRPM2-knockout mice exhibited decreased survival after liver infection with *Listeria monocytogenes* [36]. Thus, TRPM2 may be detrimental or beneficial depending on the underlying disease. Although no information is available on TRPM2 expression in the intestinal tissue, its upregulation in PBMCs of patients with UC and CD is of particular interest as a participant in disease pathogenesis and as a promising marker for disease activity.

TRPM4 plays a predominant role as a negative feedback mechanism during calcium oscillations, which may be important for differential gene expression in T cells [37]. A recent study showed that TRPM4 plays an important role in the immune surveillance processes. It is essential for the proper functioning of monocytes/macrophages and the efficiency of the subsequent response to infection [38], as well as the migration of dendritic cells [39]. At present, no information is available on the role of TRPM4 in gut disease. Our study showed no alteration in TRPM4 expression in PBMCs from either UC or CD patients, however, further investigation is needed.

Knowledge of the role of TRPM5, predominantly expressed by tuft cells that are an intestinal epithelial subset [40], in gut disease is limited [41]. A recent report showed that the disruption of chemosensory signaling through the loss of TRPM5 abrogates the expansion of tuft cells [42]. Interestingly, the ablation of doublecortin-like kinase 1 (DCLK), a marker of tuft cells, in the colonic epithelium exacerbates colitis in mice [43,44]. This finding suggests that TRPM5 plays an important role in regulating the intestinal inflammatory response and epithelial integrity. Another study showed that the number of DCLK1-positive cells decreased in intestinal tissue from patients with celiac disease [45]. Meanwhile, our study found no alteration in TRPM5 expression in PBMCs from either UC or CD patients, warranting further investigation.

The TRPC subfamily comprises six members (TRPC1, TRPC3–7) in humans, many of which are ubiquitously expressed in tissues and modulate a multitude of cellular responses [46]. Of these, TRPC1, TRPC3, and TRPC6 were detectable in this study. As TRPC1 controls the release of interleukin-1 from macrophages [47] and that of tumor necrosis factor-α from mast cells [48], its decreased expression in PBMCs from patients with UC and CD seen in our study may enhance disease development. Moreover, the expression of TRPC6 was upregulated in PBMCs from patients with CD but not those with UC in this study. These results, together with those of a previous study reporting increased TRPC6 mRNA levels in stenotic areas of patients with CD [49], suggest that TRPC6 may be associated with excessive CD fibrosis.

To date, the mechanisms of TRP channel expression in PBMCs from patients with IBD remain elusive. TRP channels in PBMCs may respond to multiple stimuli present in the peripheral circulation of these patients. The different expression levels of these TRP channels may suggest a possible role as an indicator of inflammation at secondary sites, as well as involvement in IBD pathophysiology. Additionally, the difference in expression of TRPV channels in UC and CD patients may result from differences in the disease pathogenesis. Recent studies have also shown that lipopolysaccharide (LPS) activates several members of the TRP channel family, such as TRPV4 and TRPA1, as well as the Toll-like receptor 4 (TLR4), suggesting the role of TRP channels as sensors of bacterial endotoxins, and therefore, as crucial players in innate immunity. Moreover, since TRP channel and TLR expression overlap in many cell types, including immune cells and epithelial cells, it would be of interest to explore the crosstalk between intracellular signaling pathways initiated by TLR activation and TRP channel activation in patients with IBD [50]. Understanding the involvement of TRP channel members in IBD will be crucial to evaluate the potential for manipulating TRP activity as a therapeutic intervention [51,52].

As the majority of our patients were receiving medications, we assessed whether medical treatment may affect the expression of TRP channel family in PBMCs. A subgroup analysis among patients with untreated and treated IBD showed that the use of medications had no significant effect on mRNA levels of any TRP. Future studies sequentially assessing mRNA levels of TRPs in the same patient are required to confirm this lack of association.

This study had certain limitations. First, it was conducted at a single center and involved a limited number of patients, which could cause a β-error, particularly for the analysis of the medical treatment. Second, as this study analyzed the gene expression of all PBMCs, the PBMC subsets that actually express TRP channels remain to be determined. Third, this study characterized the TRP expression at the mRNA level only. To support any conclusion on the role of TRP channels in PBMCs in IBD, the evaluation of TRP channel protein levels (enzyme-linked immunosorbent assay or immunocytochemistry), as well as modulation experiments (specific activation/inhibition, knockdown/knockout in vitro, and/or in animal models) are required. Fourth, the changes in expression levels and correlation strengths observed were very small, hence, careful attention should be paid in interpreting the data. Fifth, correlations between each TRP channel and laboratory parameters did not clearly implicate functional relationships, particularly in TRPV3, TRPV4, and TRPM5 in UC, therefore, follow up studies are needed. Finally, this study analyzed leukocytes obtained from the peripheral circulation, and not from the diseased intestine. A comparison of gene expression at these two sites could help advance our understanding of the pathophysiology of IBD.

The present results indicate, for the first time, that PBMCs from patients with IBD express different mRNA levels of TRP channel members, which may play an important role in the progression of IBD. Furthermore, their expression levels in PBMCs are a promising marker for IBD. Further studies are needed to determine the clinical and pathogenic role of TRP channels in IBD.

Supplementary Materials: The following are available online at http://www.mdpi.com/2077-0383/9/8/2643/s1, Figure S1: Comparison of TRP channel expression according to the current use of medications in patients with (a) ulcerative colitis (UC) and (b) Crohn's disease (CD) (b). Some of the patients received more than one category of treatment. Bars represent the median. 5ASA: 5-aminosalicylic acid; PSL: Prednisolone; IM: Immunomodulator; TNF: Tumor necrosis factor.

Author Contributions: K.M. designed the research; T.M., K.M., H.Y., A.M., T.Y., T.A., M.M., K.T., S.Y. (Sayo Yamasaki), K.K., S.Y. (Shinichiro Yoshioka), and H.T. performed the study and analyzed the data; K.M. and T.T. supervised the project; T.M. and K.M. co-wrote the manuscript. All authors have read and agreed to the published version of the manuscript.

Funding: This research was supported partly by a Grant-in-Aid from the Ministry of Science and Education and by Health and Labour Sciences Research Grants for research on intractable diseases from the Ministry of Health, Labour, and Welfare of Japan.

Conflicts of Interest: The authors declare no conflict of interest.

References

1. Khor, B.; Gardet, A.; Xavier, R.J. Genetics and pathogenesis of inflammatory bowel disease. *Nature* **2011**, *474*, 307–317. [CrossRef]
2. Maloy, K.J.; Powrie, F. Intestinal homeostasis and its breakdown in inflammatory bowel disease. *Nature* **2011**, *474*, 298–306. [CrossRef] [PubMed]
3. Moran, M.M.; McAlexander, M.A.; Biro, T.; Szallasi, A. Transient receptor potential channels as therapeutic targets. *Nat. Rev. Drug Discov.* **2011**, *10*, 601–620. [CrossRef] [PubMed]

4. Billeter, A.T.; Hellmann, J.L.; Bhatnagar, A.; Polk, H.C., Jr. Transient receptor potential ion channels: Powerful regulators of cell function. *Ann. Surg.* **2014**, *259*, 229–235. [CrossRef] [PubMed]
5. Parenti, A.; De Logu, F.; Geppetti, P.; Benemei, S. What is the evidence for the role of TRP channels in inflammatory and immune cells? *Br. J. Pharmacol.* **2016**, *173*, 953–969. [CrossRef]
6. Sousa-Valente, J.; Andreou, A.P.; Urban, L.; Nagy, I. Transient receptor potential ion channels in primary sensory neurons as targets for novel analgesics. *Br. J. Pharmacol.* **2014**, *171*, 2508–2527. [CrossRef]
7. Kaneko, Y.; Szallasi, A. Transient receptor potential (TRP) channels: A clinical perspective. *Br. J. Pharmacol.* **2014**, *171*, 2474–2507. [CrossRef]
8. Nilius, B.; Owsianik, G.; Voets, T.; Peters, J.A. Transient receptor potential cation channels in disease. *Physiol. Rev.* **2007**, *87*, 165–217. [CrossRef]
9. Allais, L.; De Smet, R.; Verschuere, S.; Talavera, K.; Cuvelier, C.A.; Maes, T. Transient Receptor Potential Channels in Intestinal Inflammation: What Is the Impact of Cigarette Smoking? *Pathobiology* **2017**, *84*, 1–15. [CrossRef]
10. Zielinska, M.; Jarmuz, A.; Wasilewski, A.; Salaga, M.; Fichna, J. Role of transient receptor potential channels in intestinal inflammation and visceral pain: Novel targets in inflammatory bowel diseases. *Inflamm. Bowel Dis.* **2015**, *21*, 419–427. [CrossRef]
11. Rugtveit, J.; Brandtzaeg, P.; Halstensen, T.S.; Fausa, O.; Scott, H. Increased macrophage subset in inflammatory bowel disease: Apparent recruitment from peripheral blood monocytes. *Gut* **1994**, *35*, 669–674. [CrossRef] [PubMed]
12. Schwarz, E.C.; Wolfs, M.J.; Tonner, S.; Wenning, A.S.; Quintana, A.; Griesemer, D.; Hoth, M. TRP channels in lymphocytes. In *Transient Receptor Potential (TRP) Channels*; Springer: Berlin/Heidelberg, Germany, 2007; pp. 445–456. [CrossRef]
13. Saunders, C.I.; Kunde, D.A.; Crawford, A.; Geraghty, D.P. Expression of transient receptor potential vanilloid 1 (TRPV1) and 2 (TRPV2) in human peripheral blood. *Mol. Immunol.* **2007**, *44*, 1429–1435. [CrossRef] [PubMed]
14. Spinsanti, G.; Zannolli, R.; Panti, C.; Ceccarelli, I.; Marsili, L.; Bachiocco, V.; Frati, F.; Aloisi, A.M. Quantitative Real-Time PCR detection of TRPV1-4 gene expression in human leukocytes from healthy and hyposensitive subjects. *Mol. Pain* **2008**, *4*, 1744–8069. [CrossRef] [PubMed]
15. Cai, X.; Yang, Y.C.; Wang, J.F.; Wang, Q.; Gao, J.; Fu, W.L.; Zhu, Z.Y.; Wang, Y.Y.; Zou, M.J.; Wang, J.X.; et al. Transient receptor potential vanilloid 2 (TRPV2), a potential novel biomarker in childhood asthma. *J. Asthma* **2013**, *50*, 209–214. [CrossRef]
16. Schroeder, K.W.; Tremaine, W.J.; Ilstrup, D.M. Coated oral 5-aminosalicylic acid therapy for mildly to moderately active ulcerative colitis. A randomized study. *N. Engl. J. Med.* **1987**, *317*, 1625–1629. [CrossRef]
17. Best, W.R.; Becktel, J.M.; Singleton, J.W. Rederived values of the eight coefficients of the Crohn's Disease Activity Index (CDAI). *Gastroenterology* **1979**, *77*, 843–846. [CrossRef]
18. Boyd, M.; Thodberg, M.; Vitezic, M.; Bornholdt, J.; Vitting-Seerup, K.; Chen, Y.; Coskun, M.; Li, Y.; Lo, B.Z.S.; Klausen, P.; et al. Characterization of the enhancer and promoter landscape of inflammatory bowel disease from human colon biopsies. *Nat. Commun.* **2018**, *9*, 1–19. [CrossRef]
19. Santos, F.; Marini, N.; Santos, R.S.D.; Hoffman, B.S.F.; Alves-Ferreira, M.; de Oliveira, A.C. Selection and testing of reference genes for accurate RT-qPCR in rice seedlings under iron toxicity. *PLoS ONE* **2018**, *13*, e0193418. [CrossRef]
20. Bustin, S.A.; Benes, V.; Garson, J.A.; Hellemans, J.; Huggett, J.; Kubista, M.; Mueller, R.; Nolan, T.; Pfaffl, M.W.; Shipley, G.L.; et al. The MIQE guidelines: Minimum information for publication of quantitative real-time PCR experiments. *Clin. Chem.* **2009**, *55*, 611–622. [CrossRef]
21. Vandewauw, I.; Owsianik, G.; Voets, T. Systematic and quantitative mRNA expression analysis of TRP channel genes at the single trigeminal and dorsal root ganglion level in mouse. *BMC Neurosci.* **2013**, *14*, 21. [CrossRef]
22. Yiangou, Y.; Facer, P.; Dyer, N.H.; Chan, C.L.; Knowles, C.; Williams, N.S.; Anand, P. Vanilloid receptor 1 immunoreactivity in inflamed human bowel. *Lancet* **2001**, *357*, 1338–1339. [CrossRef]
23. Akbar, A.; Yiangou, Y.; Facer, P.; Brydon, W.G.; Walters, J.R.; Anand, P.; Ghosh, S. Expression of the TRPV1 receptor differs in quiescent inflammatory bowel disease with or without abdominal pain. *Gut* **2010**, *59*, 767–774. [CrossRef] [PubMed]

24. Bertin, S.; Aoki-Nonaka, Y.; Lee, J.; de Jong, P.R.; Kim, P.; Han, T.; Yu, T.; To, K.; Takahashi, N.; Boland, B.S.; et al. The TRPA1 ion channel is expressed in CD4+ T cells and restrains T-cell-mediated colitis through inhibition of TRPV1. *Gut* **2017**, *66*, 1584–1596. [CrossRef] [PubMed]
25. Miranda, A.; Nordstrom, E.; Mannem, A.; Smith, C.; Banerjee, B.; Sengupta, J.N. The role of transient receptor potential vanilloid 1 in mechanical and chemical visceral hyperalgesia following experimental colitis. *Neuroscience* **2007**, *148*, 1021–1032. [CrossRef]
26. Santoni, G.; Farfariello, V.; Liberati, S.; Morelli, M.B.; Nabissi, M.; Santoni, M.; Amantini, C. The role of transient receptor potential vanilloid type-2 ion channels in innate and adaptive immune responses. *Front. Immunol.* **2013**, *4*, 34. [CrossRef]
27. Issa, C.M.; Hambly, B.D.; Wang, Y.; Maleki, S.; Wang, W.; Fei, J.; Bao, S. TRPV2 in the development of experimental colitis. *Scand. J. Immunol.* **2014**, *80*, 307–312. [CrossRef]
28. De Petrocellis, L.; Orlando, P.; Moriello, A.S.; Aviello, G.; Stott, C.; Izzo, A.A.; Di Marzo, V. Cannabinoid actions at TRPV channels: Effects on TRPV3 and TRPV4 and their potential relevance to gastrointestinal inflammation. *Acta Physiol. (Oxf.)* **2012**, *204*, 255–266. [CrossRef]
29. Ueda, T.; Yamada, T.; Ugawa, S.; Ishida, Y.; Shimada, S. TRPV3, a thermosensitive channel is expressed in mouse distal colon epithelium. *Biochem. Biophys. Res. Commun.* **2009**, *383*, 130–134. [CrossRef]
30. Hoeft, B.; Linseisen, J.; Beckmann, L.; Muller-Decker, K.; Canzian, F.; Husing, A.; Kaaks, R.; Vogel, U.; Jakobsen, M.U.; Overvad, K.; et al. Polymorphisms in fatty-acid-metabolism-related genes are associated with colorectal cancer risk. *Carcinogenesis* **2010**, *31*, 466–472. [CrossRef]
31. Aijima, R.; Wang, B.; Takao, T.; Mihara, H.; Kashio, M.; Ohsaki, Y.; Zhang, J.Q.; Mizuno, A.; Suzuki, M.; Yamashita, Y.; et al. The thermosensitive TRPV3 channel contributes to rapid wound healing in oral epithelia. *FASEB J.* **2015**, *29*, 182–192. [CrossRef]
32. D'Aldebert, E.; Cenac, N.; Rousset, P.; Martin, L.; Rolland, C.; Chapman, K.; Selves, J.; Alric, L.; Vinel, J.P.; Vergnolle, N. Transient receptor potential vanilloid 4 activated inflammatory signals by intestinal epithelial cells and colitis in mice. *Gastroenterology* **2011**, *140*, 275–285. [CrossRef] [PubMed]
33. Fichna, J.; Mokrowiecka, A.; Cygankiewicz, A.I.; Zakrzewski, P.K.; Malecka-Panas, E.; Janecka, A.; Krajewska, W.M.; Storr, M.A. Transient receptor potential vanilloid 4 blockade protects against experimental colitis in mice: A new strategy for inflammatory bowel diseases treatment? *Neurogastroenterol. Motil.* **2012**, *24*, e557–e560. [CrossRef] [PubMed]
34. Foroutan, F.; Jokerst, J.V.; Gambhir, S.S.; Vermesh, O.; Kim, H.W.; Knowles, J.C. Sol-gel synthesis and electrospraying of biodegradable $(P_2O_5)_{55}$-$(CaO)_{30}$-$(Na_2O)_{15}$ glass nanospheres as a transient contrast agent for ultrasound stem cell imaging. *ACS Nano* **2015**, *9*, 1868–1877. [CrossRef] [PubMed]
35. Yamamoto, S.; Shimizu, S.; Kiyonaka, S.; Takahashi, N.; Wajima, T.; Hara, Y.; Negoro, T.; Hiroi, T.; Kiuchi, Y.; Okada, T.; et al. TRPM2-mediated Ca^{2+} influx induces chemokine production in monocytes that aggravates inflammatory neutrophil infiltration. *Nat. Med.* **2008**, *14*, 738–747. [CrossRef]
36. Knowles, H.; Heizer, J.W.; Li, Y.; Chapman, K.; Ogden, C.A.; Andreasen, K.; Shapland, E.; Kucera, G.; Mogan, J.; Humann, J.; et al. Transient Receptor Potential Melastatin 2 (TRPM2) ion channel is required for innate immunity against Listeria monocytogenes. *Proc. Natl. Acad. Sci. USA* **2011**, *108*, 11578–11583. [CrossRef]
37. Launay, P.; Cheng, H.; Srivatsan, S.; Penner, R.; Fleig, A.; Kinet, J.P. TRPM4 regulates calcium oscillations after T cell activation. *Science* **2004**, *306*, 1374–1377. [CrossRef]
38. Serafini, N.; Dahdah, A.; Barbet, G.; Demion, M.; Attout, T.; Gautier, G.; Arcos-Fajardo, M.; Souchet, H.; Jouvin, M.H.; Vrtovsnik, F.; et al. The TRPM4 channel controls monocyte and macrophage, but not neutrophil, function for survival in sepsis. *J. Immunol.* **2012**, *189*, 3689–3699. [CrossRef]
39. Barbet, G.; Demion, M.; Moura, I.C.; Serafini, N.; Leger, T.; Vrtovsnik, F.; Monteiro, R.C.; Guinamard, R.; Kinet, J.P.; Launay, P. The calcium-activated nonselective cation channel TRPM4 is essential for the migration but not the maturation of dendritic cells. *Nat. Immunol.* **2008**, *9*, 1148–1156. [CrossRef]
40. Harris, N. The enigmatic tuft cell in immunity. *Science* **2016**, *351*, 1264–1265. [CrossRef]
41. Bezencon, C.; le Coutre, J.; Damak, S. Taste-signaling proteins are coexpressed in solitary intestinal epithelial cells. *Chem. Senses* **2007**, *32*, 41–49. [CrossRef]
42. Gerbe, F.; Sidot, E.; Smyth, D.J.; Ohmoto, M.; Matsumoto, I.; Dardalhon, V.; Cesses, P.; Garnier, L.; Pouzolles, M.; Brulin, B.; et al. Intestinal epithelial tuft cells initiate type 2 mucosal immunity to helminth parasites. *Nature* **2016**, *529*, 226–230. [CrossRef] [PubMed]

43. Qu, D.; Weygant, N.; May, R.; Chandrakesan, P.; Madhoun, M.; Ali, N.; Sureban, S.M.; An, G.; Schlosser, M.J.; Houchen, C.W. Ablation of Doublecortin-Like Kinase 1 in the Colonic Epithelium Exacerbates Dextran Sulfate Sodium-Induced Colitis. *PLoS ONE* **2015**, *10*, e0134212. [CrossRef] [PubMed]
44. Steele, S.P.; Melchor, S.J.; Petri, W.A., Jr. Tuft Cells: New Players in Colitis. *Trends Mol. Med.* **2016**, *22*, 921–924. [CrossRef] [PubMed]
45. Leppanen, J.; Helminen, O.; Huhta, H.; Kauppila, J.H.; Miinalainen, I.; Ronkainen, V.P.; Saarnio, J.; Lehenkari, P.P.; Karttunen, T.J. Doublecortin-like kinase 1-positive enterocyte-A new cell type in human intestine. *APMIS* **2016**, *124*, 958–965. [CrossRef] [PubMed]
46. Nilius, B.; Owsianik, G. The transient receptor potential family of ion channels. *Genome Biol.* **2011**, *12*, 218. [CrossRef] [PubMed]
47. Py, B.F.; Jin, M.; Desai, B.N.; Penumaka, A.; Zhu, H.; Kober, M.; Dietrich, A.; Lipinski, M.M.; Henry, T.; Clapham, D.E.; et al. Caspase-11 controls interleukin-1beta release through degradation of TRPC1. *Cell Rep.* **2014**, *6*, 1122–1128. [CrossRef]
48. Medic, N.; Desai, A.; Olivera, A.; Abramowitz, J.; Birnbaumer, L.; Beaven, M.A.; Gilfillan, A.M.; Metcalfe, D.D. Knockout of the Trpc1 gene reveals that TRPC1 can promote recovery from anaphylaxis by negatively regulating mast cell TNF-alpha production. *Cell Calcium* **2013**, *53*, 315–326. [CrossRef]
49. Kurahara, L.H.; Sumiyoshi, M.; Aoyagi, K.; Hiraishi, K.; Nakajima, K.; Nakagawa, M.; Hu, Y.; Inoue, R. Intestinal myofibroblast TRPC6 channel may contribute to stenotic fibrosis in Crohn's disease. *Inflamm. Bowel Dis.* **2015**, *21*, 496–506. [CrossRef]
50. Boonen, B.; Alpizar, Y.A.; Meseguer, V.M.; Talavera, K. TRP Channels as Sensors of Bacterial Endotoxins. *Toxins (Basel)* **2018**, *10*, 326. [CrossRef]
51. Holzer, P. Transient receptor potential (TRP) channels as drug targets for diseases of the digestive system. *Pharmacol. Ther.* **2011**, *131*, 142–170. [CrossRef]
52. Boesmans, W.; Owsianik, G.; Tack, J.; Voets, T.; Vanden Berghe, P. TRP channels in neurogastroenterology: Opportunities for therapeutic intervention. *Br. J. Pharmacol.* **2011**, *162*, 18–37. [CrossRef] [PubMed]

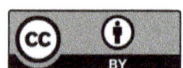

© 2020 by the authors. Licensee MDPI, Basel, Switzerland. This article is an open access article distributed under the terms and conditions of the Creative Commons Attribution (CC BY) license (http://creativecommons.org/licenses/by/4.0/).

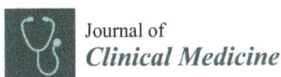

Review

The Evolving Role of Gut Microbiota in the Management of Irritable Bowel Syndrome: An Overview of the Current Knowledge

Amir Mari [1,*], Fadi Abu Baker [2], Mahmud Mahamid [1,3], Wisam Sbeit [4] and Tawfik Khoury [1,4]

1. Gastroenterology and Endoscopy Units, The Nazareth Hospital, EMMS, Nazareth, Faculty of Medicine in the Galilee, Bar-Ilan University, Safed 1311502, Israel; mahmudmahamid@yahoo.com (M.M.); tawfikkhoury1@hotmail.com (T.K.)
2. Gastroenterology Department, Hillel Yaffe Medical Center, Hadera 38100, Israel; fa_fd@hotmail.com
3. Gastroenterology Department, Sharee Zedek Medical Center, Jerusalem 9103102, Israel
4. Gastroenterology Department, Galilee Medical Center, Nahariya, Israel, Faculty of Medicine in the Galilee, Bar-Ilan University, Safed 1311502, Israel; wisams@gmc.gov.il
* Correspondence: amir.mari@hotmail.com; Tel.: +972-50987-0611

Received: 7 February 2020; Accepted: 2 March 2020; Published: 4 March 2020

Abstract: The intestinal microbiota is one of the most rapidly evolving areas in biology and medicine. Extensive research in the last decade has escalated our understanding of the role of the microbiota in the pathogenesis of several intestinal and extra-intestinal disorders. Marked by high prevalence, substantial morbidity, and enormous costs, irritable bowel syndrome (IBS) is an important chronic gastrointestinal disorder that is widely encountered by gastroenterologists. Despite advances in our understanding of its pathophysiology, curative interventions have yet to be discovered, and therapeutic approaches remain symptom-driven. Recently, accumulating evidence has enlightened the possible impact of an imbalanced gut microbiome in the pathogenesis of IBS. In fact, several studies have documented altered microbiota in patients, while others have shown that IBS severity was associated with a distinct microbiota signature. These findings may pave the way for the use of microbiota manipulation strategies as an attractive option for IBS management, and may have an essential role in efforts to reduce the societal and economic effects of this ever-growing disorder. In this review, we have outlined the results of the latest research on the association between microbiota and IBS and their implications for the clinical management of affected patients.

Keywords: gut; microbiome; IBS

1. Introduction

Irritable bowel syndrome (IBS) is a common functional gastrointestinal disorder characterized by chronic recurrent abdominal pain, changes in bowel habits, and other symptoms such as bloating and flatulence. Based on the Rome IV criteria, four subtypes of IBS exist depending on the predominant stool pattern, including IBS with constipation (IBS-C), IBS with diarrhea (IBS-D), IBS with mixed bowel habits (IBS-M), and unclassified IBS [1,2]. IBS has a global prevalence of approximately 11% and is associated with several comorbidities, such as anxiety, depression, fibromyalgia, migraines, chronic pelvic pain, and others [3,4]. IBS is a major socioeconomic burden because affected patients utilize more healthcare resources with reduced work productivity when compared to the healthy population [5]. IBS is a complex heterogeneous condition with a multifactorial pathogenesis. Proposed mechanisms involved in the pathogenesis of IBS include visceral hypersensitivity, gut–brain axis alterations, disorders in the epithelial barrier integrity leading to abnormal mucosal intestinal permeability, changed intestinal motility, immune system activation, food intolerance, low-grade inflammation, altered enteroendocrine pathways signaling, genetic basis (e.g., mutation in the SC5NA gene encoding a sodium channel ion; a number of single-nucleotide polymorphism studies have also identified polymorphisms in genes associated with IBS pathogenesis including genes coding for serotonin signaling, immune regulation, and epithelial barrier function), and the evolving concept of dysbiosis in the gut microbiota (Figure 1) [6–15].

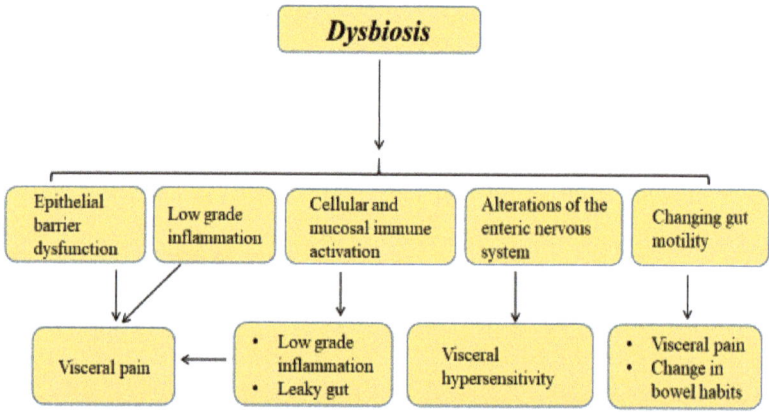

Figure 1. Role of the microbiome in irritable bowel syndrome (IBS).

Gastrointestinal (GI) microbiota are the most relevant microbial community in the body and belong to the so-called microbiota which includes all microorganisms living in the human body. The intestinal microbiota includes bacteria, archaea, fungi, eukaryotes, and viruses. Most of the bacteria in the GI tract are represented in four main bacterial phyla: Firmicutes, Bacteroidetes, Proteobacteria, and Actinobacteria [16,17]. Trillions of microorganisms reside in the GI tract, with the highest density in the colon. However, most of them remain uncharacterized. Since this number is approximately equal to 10 times the total number of body cells, the interest in microbiota study for intestinal and extra-intestinal diseases is not surprising [18–22]. Advances in molecular biology techniques have significantly contributed to microbiome research. The most common technique to analyze the composition of the gut bacteria is marker gene sequencing, generally using the 16S rRNA gene [23–25]. Advantages of this method are related to its simplicity and low cost.

The aim of this review is to overview the most up-to-date literature about the evolving role of gut microbiome manipulation in IBS management, with a focus on probiotics, prebiotics, antibiotics, and fecal transplantation.

2. Methods

A search for studies published before January 2020 was performed in the PubMed and Embase databases. All authors participated in the search process. We looked for the terms "irritable bowel syndrome", "microbiota", "treatment", "prebiotic", "probiotic", "synbiotic", "FODMAP", "meta-analysis", "randomized", "clinical", "bifidobacteria", "lactobacillus", "firmicutes", "bacteroidetes", "methane", "methanogen", "diet", "fecal transplantation", "bacteriophage", and "fungi", mainly focusing on the literature that describes effects on microbiota, clinical studies, and therapeutic effects in IBS. The search was restricted to articles in the English language.

3. The Microbiome in IBS

A rash of research activity in this field from the last decade has led to the evidence that a disruption in the biodiversity, richness, and composition of the gut microbiota—a process named dysbiosis—plays a key function in the pathogenesis of IBS [26]. Dysbiosis can take place through several mechanisms: the overgrowth or vanishing of specific bacteria species, alterations in the relative richness of bacteria, and lastly, by mutation or gene transfer [27].

In IBS patients, GI dysbiosis has been associated with a visceral increased perception of pain and enhanced mucosal permeability that is provoked by the defective mucosal epithelial barrier, interfering with gut immune homeostasis and subsequently promoting gut inflammation and enhancing cellular and mucosal immune activation [28,29]. Moreover, it has also been associated with changing gut motility, low-grade chronic inflammation, alterations of the enteric nervous system, and vagal afferents neurons as well as brain functions [30–32]. In opposition, gut microbiota can be affected by the brain activity on intestinal motility, secretion, and immune function, generating the microbiota–gut–brain axis [12,33].

Microbiological and infectious bases of IBS pathogenesis have been previously established by several groups. Halvorson et al. reported a seven-fold increased risk of post-infectious IBS after acute infectious gastroenteritis [34]. Moreover, therapeutic interventions that manipulate the gut microbiota such as antibiotics, prebiotics, probiotics, and fecal microbial transplantation have been linked to improvements in IBS symptoms [35–37]. Several studies aiming to characterize and map the microbiome signature of IBS have shown divergent results. Nonetheless, data suggest that there is a relative richness of proinflammatory bacterial species containing Enterobacteriaceae, with a parallel decline in *Lactobacillus* and *Bifidobacterium* [38,39]. A decreased percentage of *Lactobacillus* and *Bifidobacterium* species has also been described in the IBS microbiota, leading to disturbances in short-chain fatty acid production and in immunologic and bactericidal activity, with a negative effect on microbiota function and stability [40–46]. Interestingly, the Firmicutes/Bacteroidetes ratio is a possible indicator of bacterial population shifts, and both high and low ratios of Firmicutes/Bacteroidetes have been reported in IBS patients [47–50]. These contrasts may be explained by differences in technical methods and subtypes of IBS, as well as the severity of IBS [38]. Several groups examined gut microbiota in different subtypes of IBS and compared the microbiota texture between different IBS subtypes as well as different IBS symptoms [48,51,52]. A study by Ringel-Kulka et al. using fecal samples from 60 patients with IBS and 20 healthy controls revealed major variances in the microbiota between the different subtypes of IBS based on clinical symptoms of abdominal bloating and bowel habits (IBS-D, IBS-C, or IBS-M type) [53]. A study examining both fecal and colonic mucosal microbiota in patients with chronic constipation found that their mucosal microbiota differed from those of the controls, with a higher abundance of Bacteroidetes species in the patients than in the controls. However, although the profile of the colonic mucosal microbiota discriminated between these two cohorts with a high level of accuracy, this finding was independent of colonic transit time. In contrast, the profile of the fecal microbiota was associated with colonic transit, but not with the clinical diagnosis of constipation [54]. Putting all of this together, numerous evidence is emerging regarding the link between microbiota and IBS pathogenesis, making microbiota manipulation strategies an attractive option for IBS management.

4. Therapeutic Interventions for Microbiome Manipulation in IBS

4.1. Probiotics

Historically, the theory of probiotics was described by Elie Metchnikoff in 1908, who observed that fermented foods—principally those fermented by lactic acid bacteria—had favorable effects on human wellbeing and longevity. According to the most updated definition based on the Food and Agriculture Organization as well as the World Health Organization, probiotics are defined as "live microorganisms that, when administered in adequate amounts, confer a health benefit on the host" [55]. Probiotics related to IBS pathogenesis are mainly those containing *Lactobacillus* and *Bifidobacterium* species [56]. Tentatively, probiotics may promote a favorable modulation of altered gut microbiota by several mechanisms: reducing the number of competing pathogens by both the production of antimicrobial substances and interfering in intestinal mucosal adhesion [57,58], modulating the metabolism of biliary salts [59], reducing low-grade inflammation [60], and regulating immune activation as well as gut motility [61]. Several meta-analyses of randomized controlled trials (RCTs) that assessed the effects of single probiotic strains, compared to a placebo in relieving IBS related symptoms [35,59,62], have concluded that probiotics are more efficient when compared to placebos in relieving global IBS symptoms including bloating abdominal pain. In safety terms, all studies have reported comparable rates of adverse events to the placebo arms. In an Iranian IBS cohort, Jafari and colleagues observed the effects of combinations of strains of *Bifidobacterium*, *Lactobacillus*, and *Streptococcus* genera [63]. The main finding was that 85% of patients in the probiotic group reported satisfactory relief of general symptoms compared with 47% in the control group ($p < 0.01$). In general terms, probiotics seem to have favorable effects on improving IBS symptoms, with an excellent safety profile. Nonetheless, more randomized controlled trials are warranted to better define some concerns such as treatment duration and optimal strain, and to better study personalized treatment.

4.2. Prebiotics

Since 2007, prebiotics have been defined as a "nonviable food component that confers a health benefit on the host associated with modulation of the microbiota" [64]. Prebiotics are basically classified as disaccharides or oligosaccharides and are resistant to enzymatic and chemical breakdown until they reach the colon, where they are fermented by colonic bacteria, stimulating the generation of microbial metabolic products such as short-chain fatty acids (acetate, butyrate, and propionate) [65]. Short-chain fatty acids give several benefits to the colonocytes, such as an energy source, regulation of electrolytes and water absorption, enhanced blood flow, and oxygenation [66]. Moreover, probiotics may promote host health and modulation of GI motility, reduction in visceral hypersensitivity, downregulation of low-grade mucosal immune activation, improvement of epithelial permeability, enhancement of gut–brain communication, and restoration of intestinal dysbiosis. Thus, these data provide a mechanistic rationale for a role of prebiotics in managing IBS symptoms. Indeed, several clinical studies have examined prebiotics' performance in ameliorating symptoms of functional bowel disorders. A handful of RCTs evaluating the efficacy and safety of prebiotics in IBS [67,68] have been performed. In 1999, a small, double-blind crossover trial of oligofructose published by Hunter and colleagues [69] showed no therapeutic value in IBS patients. One year later, a randomized double-blind trial on almost 100 patients with IBS receiving either fructo-oligosaccharide or placebo for 12 weeks reported no statistically significant improvement in symptoms [70]. The first study to report a beneficial effect was a cross-over, single-blinded trial including 60 Rome II-defined IBS patients. Patients were randomized for four weeks to receive a low or high dose of trans-galacto-oligosaccharide or placebo. Both the low and high-dose arms experienced a significant improvement in stool consistency ($p < 0.05$), flatulence ($p < 0.05$), and bloating ($p < 0.05$) as well as a reduction in mean subjective global assessment (The subjective global assessment of relief was recorded at weekly intervals during the course of the study scored from 1–5. 1 = completely relieved, 2 = considerably relieved, 3 = somewhat relieved, 4 = unchanged, and 5 = worse) [71].

Interestingly, the prebiotic but not the placebo significantly enhanced fecal bifidobacteria [71]. A 12-week administration of partially hydrolyzed guar gum in a randomized, double-blind, placebo-controlled study led to a significant improvement in bloating and gasses scores with no effect on other reported IBS symptoms or quality of life scores, leading the authors to support its administration for IBS patients with an expected clinical effect on bloating and gasses [72]. In safety terms, all studies reported comparable rates of adverse events to the placebo arms. In conclusion, prebiotic use in IBS patients have yielded mixed to positive results, but further studies to address the combination, duration, and different aspects of effects on IBS are still warranted.

4.3. Non-Absorbable Antibiotics

Non-absorbable antibiotics, mainly rifaximin, have been shown to be safe and effective for the treatment of IBS with the diarrhea predominant type. Rifaximin, a rifamycin derivative, is a broad-spectrum, non-absorbable antibiotic which targets aerobic and anaerobic bacteria residing in the GI tract. Less than 1% of rifaximin is absorbed in the systemic circulation, making it very safe with extremely low toxicity and adverse events rates [73]. The proposed mechanisms of action of the non-absorbable antibiotics are the reduction of the amount of inhabitant GI bacteria, changes in bacterial structure, reduction of low-grade inflammation, and amelioration in gut permeability [74]. Rifaximin is the best-studied non-absorbable antibiotic for symptoms relief in IBS. The TARGET 1 and TARGET 2 trials, both designed as double-blinded, placebo-controlled, multi-center studies, have shown good efficacy of rifaximin for IBS symptoms relief [75]. In TARGET 1 and TARGET 2, a total number of 1258 patients with mild to moderate symptoms of IBS were randomized either to receive rifaximin 550 mg three times a day for 14 days or a placebo. Relief of IBS symptoms, after one month from the end of treatment, was reported more significantly among patients in the rifaximin group compared with those in the placebo group (40.7% vs. 31.7%, $p < 0.001$), with a comparable adverse events occurrence in both groups [75]. TARGET 3, a randomized, placebo-controlled study including 2579 patients with IBS, revealed that the durability of symptoms relief among patients with IBS-D responding to a 14-day course of rifaximin was reduced by 50% after 70 days from the end of treatment [76]. With a second treatment course, the most significant benefit was the relief of stool urgency and abdominal bloating [76].

4.4. Fecal Microbiota Transplantation

Fecal microbiota transplant (FMT), also known as a stool transplant, is the process of transplantation of fecal bacteria from a healthy individual into a recipient. FMT involves the restoration of the colonic microflora by introducing healthy bacterial flora through the infusion of stool (e.g., via colonoscopy, enema, rogastric tube or by mouth in the form of a capsule containing freeze-dried material) obtained from a healthy donor. To date, FMT has been approved for the treatment of resistant *Clostridium difficile* infections [77,78], and in this context, it has been shown to be an effective therapy [79]. However, its therapeutic effect among IBS patients is still emerging. As reported above, in the last few years, several studies have underlined the role of dysbiosis among patients with IBS, with lower *Lactobacillus* spp. in IBS-D and increased loads of *Veillonella* spp., and genera *Coprococcus*, *Collinsella*, and *Coprobacillus* [42,80]. Other data revealed a decrease in the biodiversity of microbiota in the fecal composition of IBS-D patients [51]. Therefore, targeting the gut microbiota composition might be a promising therapy in IBS. However, among IBS patients, FMT has shown conflicting results. A previous randomized controlled study showed beneficial effects of FMT on IBS symptoms. In this study, 55 patients with IBS-D or IBS-M received 50–80 g of feces mixed with 200 mL of isotonic saline and 50 mL of 85% glycerol, administered to the cecum by colonoscopy, and were compared to 28 patients who received a placebo. Patients treated with FMT showed a significant clinical response at three months compared to those in the placebo group (65% vs. 43%, $p = 0.049$) [39]. These findings were further confirmed by other recent studies showing a positive effect on IBS symptoms after transplant, as 70–85% and 45–60% of patients reported symptomatic relief in the first three months and six months after FMT, respectively [81,82]. On the contrary, a recent study including 52 IBS adult patients who were randomized to either active FMT or placebo capsules administered for 12 months did not show beneficial effects favoring FMT at three months. In fact, a significant improvement in IBS symptom scores was observed at three months favoring the placebo ($p = 0.012$), and after three months, the results obtained by an IBS quality of life questionnaire were in favor of the placebo ($p = 0.003$) [83]. Moreover, a recent meta-analysis including eight single-arm trials (SATs) and 5 RCTs did not report beneficial effects of FMT among patients with IBS (relative risk = 0.93, 95%, confidence interval (CI confidence interval) 0.50–1.75, $p = 0.83$ for RCT), while in the SAT 59.5% of patients (95% CI 49.1–69.3) showed a significant improvement [84]. Given the controversies regarding the published data, FMT-based treatments for IBS are still not widely accepted among gastroenterologists, as they are concerned about effectiveness and safety profile [85]. Therefore, the role of FMT must be further addressed by randomized, double-blind, placebo-controlled studies. Recent international consensus of stool banking for FMT have involved experts from Europe, North America, and Australia who proposed consensus guideline statements regarding several issues in stool banking, including the selection of donors and screening objectives, collection and processing of stool samples, monitoring of outcomes, ethical issues, and the evolving role of FMT in *Clostridioides difficile* infection and other diseases encountered in daily clinical practice [86]. Figure 2 demonstrates the established and evolving therapeutic options for IBS.

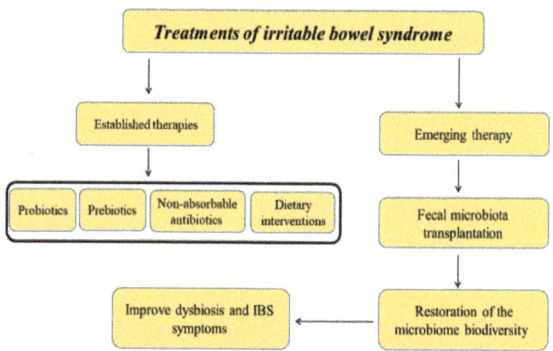

Figure 2. Treatments of irritable bowel syndrome (IBS) by targeting the gut microbiome.

4.5. Dietary Intervention

Dietary modifications constitute one of the first choices of treatment for IBS patients [87]. Indeed, a careful history may reveal patterns of symptoms linked to specific food consumption. Although debatable, a high-fiber diet has traditionally been encouraged particularly in IBS-C patients, given the absence of serious side effects and its potential benefit [88,89]. In recent years, there has been a growing clinical and scientific interest in the use of a diet low in FODMAPs (fermentable oligosaccharides, disaccharides, monosaccharides, and polyols) in IBS patients. Since its introduction, reports in the literature including several RCTs have reported the efficacy of a low-FODMAP diet in improving global IBS symptoms, visceral pain, bloating, and quality of life [90–96]. However, large and long-term RCTs are still lacking, and various concerns have been raised including diet complexity and cost, risk of nutritional deficiencies, and importantly, an unclear impact on gut microbiome [97–99].

A focus on the role of a gluten-free diet (GFD) in IBS has grown recently, with studies demonstrating the induction of symptoms following gluten consumption in IBS patients [100]. However, evidence to support gluten avoidance in IBS has been conflicting. Moreover, a recent report has suggested that fructans rather than gluten protein are responsible for the symptomatic improvement reported in a gluten-free diet [101]. Further studies are required to evaluate the effect of a GFD on nutritional status, gut microbiota, and long-term outcomes.

5. Conclusions

In conclusion, in the current review we have provided a focused summary of the latest literature on the potential role of gut dysbiosis in the pathogenesis of IBS and discussed the translation of microbiota-modifying strategies as a novel therapeutic option for this disorder (Figure 1). There is strong growing evidence supporting microbiome-based therapeutic approaches with dietary intervention, probiotics, prebiotics, non-absorbable antibiotics, and FMTs for the treatment of IBS (Table 1). Nonetheless, more knowledge is needed to better address the role of microbiome-based therapeutic interventions in the clinical management of IBS. Several future microbiome-based therapeutic options are being explored and investigated, including genetic engineering of bacteria, personalized microbiota manipulation, postbiotics, and bacteriophage therapy.

Table 1. Summary of the meta-analysis studies reporting efficacy of therapeutic interventions in irritable bowel syndrome (IBS) based on overall global IBS symptoms.

Reference	Number Studies	Number Patients	Primary Endpoint as Dichotomous Variable (RR ± 95% CI) Clinical Improvement	Primary Endpoint as Dichotomous Variable (RR ± 95% CI) Symptoms Persistence	p-Value
Meta-Analysis of RCT Studies of Probiotics vs. Placebo					
Didari T., 2015 [59]	15	1793	2.43 ± 1.13–5.21	-	0.02
Zhang Y., 2016 [35]	21	1639	1.82 ± 1.27–2.6	-	<0.001
Liang D., 2019 [102]	14	1695	1.27 ± 1.13–1.44	-	<0.001
McFarland L.V., 2008 [103]	23	1404	0.77 pooled ± 0.62–0.94	-	<0.001
Connell M., 2018 [104]	5	243	1.39 ± 0.99–1.98	-	0.06
Ford A.C., 2014 [63]	23	2575	-	0.79 ± 0.7–0.89	<0.0001
Tiequn B., 2015 [105]	6	273	17.62 pooled ± 5.12–60.65 for adults	-	<0.00001
		167	3.71 pooled ± 1.05–13.11 for children	-	0.04
Ritchie M.L., 2012 [106]	16	-	0.77 ± 0.65–0.92	-	-
Horvath A., 2011 [107]	3	167	1.7 ± 1.27–2.27	-	0.0004
Hoveyda N., 2009 [108]	7	425	1.6 ± 1.2–2.2	-	0.0007
Moayyedi P., 2010 [109]	10	918	-	0.71 ± 0.57–0.88	0.002
Nikfar S., 2008 [110]	8	1011	1.22 ± 1.07–1.4	-	0.004
McFarland L.V., 2008 [103]	20	1404	0.77 pooled ± 0.62–0.94	-	<0.001
Meta-Analysis of RCT Studies of Prebiotics vs. Placebo					
Wilson B., 2019 [67]	11	729	OR 0.62 ± 0.07–5.69	-	0.67
Ford A.C., 2018 [68]		Trials for prebiotics were sparse and no definite conclusions could be drawn			
Ford A.C., 2014 [63]					
Meta-Analysis of RCT Studies of Fecal Microbiota Transplantation vs. Placebo					
Myneedu K., 2019 [84]	5	262	0.93 ± 0.5–1.75	-	0.83
Xu D., 2019 [111]	4	254	0.93 ± 0.48–1.79	-	0.83
Ianiro G., 2019 [112]	5	267	-	0.98 ± 0.58–1.66	0.94
Meta-Analysis of RCT Studies of Non-Absorbable Antibiotics Rifaximin vs. Placebo					
Ford A.C., 2018 [68]	5	3610	-	0.84 ± 0.79–0.9	0.0002
Li J., 2016 [113]	4	1803	1.19 ± 1.08–1.32	-	0.0008
Menees S.B., 2012 [75]	5	1803	1.57 ± 1.22–2.01	-	<0.001

RCT: Randomized Controlled Trials; CI: Confidence Interval; pooled: Pooled RR.

Author Contributions: Conceptualization, A.M. and T.K.; methodology, A.M., F.A.B., M.M., W.S., T.K.; software, A.M., T.K.; validation, A.M., T.K. and M.M.; formal analysis, T.K., F.A.B.; investigation, A.M., T.K.; resources, A.M.; project administration, A.M. All authors have read and agreed to the published version of the manuscript.

Funding: This study did not receive any specific grant from funding agencies in the public, commercial, or not-for-profit sectors.

Conflicts of Interest: The authors declare no conflicts of interest regarding this manuscript.

References

1. Mearin, F.; Lacy, B.E.; Chang, L.; Chey, W.D.; Lembo, A.J.; Simren, M.; Spiller, R. Bowel Disorders. *Gastroenterology* **2016**. [CrossRef]
2. Simren, M.; Palsson, O.S.; Whitehead, W.E. Update on Rome IV Criteria for Colorectal Disorders: Implications for Clinical Practice. *Curr. Gastroenterol. Rep.* **2017**, *19*, 15. [CrossRef] [PubMed]
3. Canavan, C.; West, J.; Card, T. The epidemiology of irritable bowel syndrome. *Clin. Epidemiol.* **2014**, *6*, 71–80. [CrossRef] [PubMed]
4. Adriani, A.; Ribaldone, D.G.; Astegiano, M.; Durazzo, M.; Saracco, G.M.; Pellicano, R. Irritable bowel syndrome: The clinical approach. *Panminerva. Med.* **2018**, *60*, 213–222. [CrossRef]
5. Buono, J.L.; Mathur, K.; Averitt, A.J.; Andrae, D.A. Economic Burden of Irritable Bowel Syndrome with Diarrhea: Retrospective Analysis of a U.S. Commercially Insured Population. *J. Manag. Care Spec. Pharm.* **2017**, *23*, 453–460. [CrossRef]
6. Makker, J.; Chilimuri, S.; Bella, J.N. Genetic epidemiology of irritable bowel syndrome. *World J. Gastroenterol.* **2015**, *21*, 11353–11361. [CrossRef]
7. Powell, N.; Walker, M.M.; Talley, N.J. The mucosal immune system: Master regulator of bidirectional gut-brain communications. *Nat. Rev. Gastroenterol. Hepatol.* **2017**, *14*, 143–159. [CrossRef]
8. Pellissier, S.; Bonaz, B. The Place of Stress and Emotions in the Irritable Bowel Syndrome. *Vitam. Horm.* **2017**, *103*, 327–354. [CrossRef]
9. Deiteren, A.; de Wit, A.; van der Linden, L.; De Man, J.G.; Pelckmans, P.A.; De Winter, B.Y. Irritable bowel syndrome and visceral hypersensitivity: Risk factors and pathophysiological mechanisms. *Acta Gastroenterol. Belg.* **2016**, *79*, 29–38.
10. Mullin, G.E.; Shepherd, S.J.; Chander Roland, B.; Ireton-Jones, C.; Matarese, L.E. Irritable bowel syndrome: Contemporary nutrition management strategies. *JPEN J. Parenter. Enteral. Nutr.* **2014**, *38*, 781–799. [CrossRef]
11. Sundin, J.; Ohman, L.; Simren, M. Understanding the Gut Microbiota in Inflammatory and Functional Gastrointestinal Diseases. *Psychosom. Med.* **2017**, *79*, 857–867. [CrossRef] [PubMed]
12. Moloney, R.D.; Johnson, A.C.; O'Mahony, S.M.; Dinan, T.G.; Greenwood-Van Meerveld, B.; Cryan, J.F. Stress and the Microbiota-Gut-Brain Axis in Visceral Pain: Relevance to Irritable Bowel Syndrome. *CNS Neurosci. Ther.* **2016**, *22*, 102–117. [CrossRef]
13. Quigley, E.M.M. The Gut-Brain Axis and the Microbiome: Clues to Pathophysiology and Opportunities for Novel Management Strategies in Irritable Bowel Syndrome (IBS). *J. Clin. Med.* **2018**, *7*, 6. [CrossRef]
14. Fagoonee, S.; Pellicano, R. Does the Microbiota Play a Pivotal Role in the Pathogenesis of Irritable Bowel Syndrome? *J. Clin. Med.* **2019**, *8*, 1808. [CrossRef] [PubMed]
15. Gazouli, M.; Wouters, M.M.; Kapur-Pojskic, L.; Bengtson, M.B.; Friedman, E.; Nikcevic, G.; Demetriou, C.A.; Mulak, A.; Santos, J.; Niesler, B. Lessons learned–resolving the enigma of genetic factors in IBS. *Nat. Rev. Gastroenterol. Hepatol.* **2016**, *13*, 77–87. [CrossRef] [PubMed]
16. Gill, S.R.; Pop, M.; Deboy, R.T.; Eckburg, P.B.; Turnbaugh, P.J.; Samuel, B.S.; Gordon, J.I.; Relman, D.A.; Fraser-Liggett, C.M.; Nelson, K.E. Metagenomic analysis of the human distal gut microbiome. *Science* **2006**, *312*, 1355–1359. [CrossRef]
17. Backhed, F.; Fraser, C.M.; Ringel, Y.; Sanders, M.E.; Sartor, R.B.; Sherman, P.M.; Versalovic, J.; Young, V.; Finlay, B.B. Defining a healthy human gut microbiome: Current concepts, future directions, and clinical applications. *Cell Host. Microbe.* **2012**, *12*, 611–622. [CrossRef]
18. Ribaldone, D.G.; Caviglia, G.P.; Abdulle, A.; Pellicano, R.; Ditto, M.C.; Morino, M.; Fusaro, E.; Saracco, G.M.; Bugianesi, E.; Astegiano, M. Adalimumab Therapy Improves Intestinal Dysbiosis in Crohn's Disease. *J. Clin. Med.* **2019**, *8*, 1646. [CrossRef]

19. Masoodi, I.; Alshanqeeti, A.S.; Ahmad, S.; Alyamani, E.J.; Al-Lehibi, A.A.; Qutub, A.N.; Alsayari, K.N.; Alomair, A.O. Microbial dysbiosis in inflammatory bowel diseases: Results of a metagenomic study in Saudi Arabia. *Minerva. Gastroenterol. Dietol.* **2019**, *65*, 177–186. [CrossRef]
20. Bellocchi, C.; Fernandez-Ochoa, A.; Montanelli, G.; Vigone, B.; Santaniello, A.; Quirantes-Pine, R.; Borras-Linares, I.; Gerosa, M.; Artusi, C.; Gualtierotti, R.; et al. Identification of a Shared Microbiomic and Metabolomic Profile in Systemic Autoimmune Diseases. *J. Clin. Med.* **2019**, *8*, 1291. [CrossRef]
21. Korotkyi, O.H.; Vovk, A.A.; Dranitsina, A.S.; Falalyeyeva, T.M.; Dvorshchenko, K.O.; Fagoonee, S.; Ostapchenko, L.I. The influence of probiotic diet and chondroitin sulfate administration on Ptgs2, Tgfb1 and Col2a1 expression in rat knee cartilage during monoiodoacetate-induced osteoarthritis. *Minerva. Med.* **2019**, *110*, 419–424. [CrossRef]
22. Durazzo, M.; Ferro, A.; Gruden, G. Gastrointestinal Microbiota and Type 1 Diabetes Mellitus: The State of Art. *J. Clin. Med.* **2019**, *8*, 1843. [CrossRef] [PubMed]
23. Lloyd-Price, J.; Abu-Ali, G.; Huttenhower, C. The healthy human microbiome. *Genome Med.* **2016**, *8*, 51. [CrossRef]
24. Kim, Y.; Koh, I.; Rho, M. Deciphering the human microbiome using next-generation sequencing data and bioinformatics approaches. *Methods* **2015**, *79–80*, 52–59. [CrossRef]
25. Kuczynski, J.; Lauber, C.L.; Walters, W.A.; Parfrey, L.W.; Clemente, J.C.; Gevers, D.; Knight, R. Experimental and analytical tools for studying the human microbiome. *Nat. Rev. Genet.* **2011**, *13*, 47–58. [CrossRef] [PubMed]
26. Menees, S.; Chey, W. The gut microbiome and irritable bowel syndrome. *F1000Research* **2018**, *7*. [CrossRef] [PubMed]
27. Barbara, G.; Cremon, C.; Azpiroz, F. Probiotics in irritable bowel syndrome: Where are we? *Neurogastroenterol. Motil.* **2018**, *30*, e13513. [CrossRef] [PubMed]
28. Rea, K.; O'Mahony, S.M.; Dinan, T.G.; Cryan, J.F. The Role of the Gastrointestinal Microbiota in Visceral Pain. *Handb. Exp. Pharmacol.* **2017**, *239*, 269–287. [CrossRef] [PubMed]
29. Fukui, H. Increased Intestinal Permeability and Decreased Barrier Function: Does It Really Influence the Risk of Inflammation? *Inflamm. Intest. Dis.* **2016**, *1*, 135–145. [CrossRef]
30. Ohman, L.; Simren, M. Pathogenesis of IBS: Role of inflammation, immunity and neuroimmune interactions. *Nat. Rev. Gastroenterol. Hepatol.* **2010**, *7*, 163–173. [CrossRef]
31. Shi, N.; Li, N.; Duan, X.; Niu, H. Interaction between the gut microbiome and mucosal immune system. *Mil. Med. Res.* **2017**, *4*, 14. [CrossRef] [PubMed]
32. Donnachie, E.; Schneider, A.; Mehring, M.; Enck, P. Incidence of irritable bowel syndrome and chronic fatigue following GI infection: A population-level study using routinely collected claims data. *Gut* **2018**, *67*, 1078–1086. [CrossRef]
33. Kelly, J.R.; Kennedy, P.J.; Cryan, J.F.; Dinan, T.G.; Clarke, G.; Hyland, N.P. Breaking down the barriers: The gut microbiome, intestinal permeability and stress-related psychiatric disorders. *Front. Cell. Neurosci.* **2015**, *9*, 392. [CrossRef] [PubMed]
34. Halvorson, H.A.; Schlett, C.D.; Riddle, M.S. Postinfectious irritable bowel syndrome—A meta-analysis. *Am. J. Gastroenterol.* **2006**, *101*, 1894–1899. [CrossRef] [PubMed]
35. Zhang, Y.; Li, L.; Guo, C.; Mu, D.; Feng, B.; Zuo, X.; Li, Y. Effects of probiotic type, dose and treatment duration on irritable bowel syndrome diagnosed by Rome III criteria: A meta-analysis. *BMC Gastroenterol.* **2016**, *16*, 62. [CrossRef] [PubMed]
36. Valentin, N.; Camilleri, M.; Carlson, P.; Harrington, S.C.; Eckert, D.; O'Neill, J.; Burton, D.; Chen, J.; Shaw, A.L.; Acosta, A. Potential mechanisms of effects of serum-derived bovine immunoglobulin/protein isolate therapy in patients with diarrhea-predominant irritable bowel syndrome. *Physiol. Rep.* **2017**, *5*. [CrossRef]
37. El-Salhy, M.; Mazzawi, T. Fecal microbiota transplantation for managing irritable bowel syndrome. *Expert. Rev. Gastroenterol. Hepatol.* **2018**, *12*, 439–445. [CrossRef]
38. Rodino-Janeiro, B.K.; Vicario, M.; Alonso-Cotoner, C.; Pascua-Garcia, R.; Santos, J. A Review of Microbiota and Irritable Bowel Syndrome: Future in Therapies. *Adv. Ther.* **2018**, *35*, 289–310. [CrossRef]
39. Johnsen, P.H.; Hilpusch, F.; Cavanagh, J.P.; Leikanger, I.S.; Kolstad, C.; Valle, P.C.; Goll, R. Faecal microbiota transplantation versus placebo for moderate-to-severe irritable bowel syndrome: A double-blind, randomised, placebo-controlled, parallel-group, single-centre trial. *Lancet Gastroenterol. Hepatol.* **2018**, *3*, 17–24. [CrossRef]

40. Zhuang, X.; Xiong, L.; Li, L.; Li, M.; Chen, M. Alterations of gut microbiota in patients with irritable bowel syndrome: A systematic review and meta-analysis. *J. Gastroenterol. Hepatol.* **2017**, *32*, 28–38. [CrossRef]
41. Balsari, A.; Ceccarelli, A.; Dubini, F.; Fesce, E.; Poli, G. The fecal microbial population in the irritable bowel syndrome. *Microbiologica* **1982**, *5*, 185–194.
42. Malinen, E.; Rinttila, T.; Kajander, K.; Matto, J.; Kassinen, A.; Krogius, L.; Saarela, M.; Korpela, R.; Palva, A. Analysis of the fecal microbiota of irritable bowel syndrome patients and healthy controls with real-time PCR. *Am. J. Gastroenterol.* **2005**, *100*, 373–382. [CrossRef] [PubMed]
43. Carroll, I.M.; Chang, Y.H.; Park, J.; Sartor, R.B.; Ringel, Y. Luminal and mucosal-associated intestinal microbiota in patients with diarrhea-predominant irritable bowel syndrome. *Gut Pathog.* **2010**, *2*, 19. [CrossRef]
44. Kerckhoffs, A.P.; Samsom, M.; van der Rest, M.E.; de Vogel, J.; Knol, J.; Ben-Amor, K.; Akkermans, L.M. Lower Bifidobacteria counts in both duodenal mucosa-associated and fecal microbiota in irritable bowel syndrome patients. *World J. Gastroenterol.* **2009**, *15*, 2887–2892. [CrossRef]
45. Rajilic-Stojanovic, M.; Biagi, E.; Heilig, H.G.; Kajander, K.; Kekkonen, R.A.; Tims, S.; de Vos, W.M. Global and deep molecular analysis of microbiota signatures in fecal samples from patients with irritable bowel syndrome. *Gastroenterology* **2011**, *141*, 1792–1801. [CrossRef]
46. Duboc, H.; Rainteau, D.; Rajca, S.; Humbert, L.; Farabos, D.; Maubert, M.; Grondin, V.; Jouet, P.; Bouhassira, D.; Seksik, P.; et al. Increase in fecal primary bile acids and dysbiosis in patients with diarrhea-predominant irritable bowel syndrome. *Neurogastroenterol. Motil.* **2012**, *24*. [CrossRef]
47. Tap, J.; Derrien, M.; Tornblom, H.; Brazeilles, R.; Cools-Portier, S.; Dore, J.; Storsrud, S.; Le Neve, B.; Ohman, L.; Simren, M. Identification of an Intestinal Microbiota Signature Associated With Severity of Irritable Bowel Syndrome. *Gastroenterology* **2017**, *152*, 111–123. [CrossRef]
48. Jeffery, I.B.; O'Toole, P.W.; Ohman, L.; Claesson, M.J.; Deane, J.; Quigley, E.M.; Simren, M. An irritable bowel syndrome subtype defined by species-specific alterations in faecal microbiota. *Gut* **2012**, *61*, 997–1006. [CrossRef]
49. Jalanka-Tuovinen, J.; Salojarvi, J.; Salonen, A.; Immonen, O.; Garsed, K.; Kelly, F.M.; Zaitoun, A.; Palva, A.; Spiller, R.C.; de Vos, W.M. Faecal microbiota composition and host-microbe cross-talk following gastroenteritis and in postinfectious irritable bowel syndrome. *Gut* **2014**, *63*, 1737–1745. [CrossRef] [PubMed]
50. Lozupone, C.A.; Stombaugh, J.; Gonzalez, A.; Ackermann, G.; Wendel, D.; Vazquez-Baeza, Y.; Jansson, J.K.; Gordon, J.I.; Knight, R. Meta-analyses of studies of the human microbiota. *Genome Res.* **2013**, *23*, 1704–1714. [CrossRef] [PubMed]
51. Carroll, I.M.; Ringel-Kulka, T.; Keku, T.O.; Chang, Y.H.; Packey, C.D.; Sartor, R.B.; Ringel, Y. Molecular analysis of the luminal- and mucosal-associated intestinal microbiota in diarrhea-predominant irritable bowel syndrome. *Am. J. Physiol. Gastrointest. Liver Physiol.* **2011**, *301*, G799–G807. [CrossRef] [PubMed]
52. Carroll, I.M.; Ringel-Kulka, T.; Siddle, J.P.; Ringel, Y. Alterations in composition and diversity of the intestinal microbiota in patients with diarrhea-predominant irritable bowel syndrome. *Neurogastroenterol. Motil.* **2012**, *24*, 521–530. [CrossRef] [PubMed]
53. Ringel-Kulka, T.; Benson, A.K.; Carroll, I.M.; Kim, J.; Legge, R.M.; Ringel, Y. Molecular characterization of the intestinal microbiota in patients with and without abdominal bloating. *Am. J. Physiol. Gastrointest. Liver Physiol.* **2016**, *310*, G417–G426. [CrossRef] [PubMed]
54. Parthasarathy, G.; Chen, J.; Chen, X.; Chia, N.; O'Connor, H.M.; Wolf, P.G.; Gaskins, H.R.; Bharucha, A.E. Relationship Between Microbiota of the Colonic Mucosa vs. Feces and Symptoms, Colonic Transit, and Methane Production in Female Patients With Chronic Constipation. *Gastroenterology* **2016**, *150*, 367–379. [CrossRef] [PubMed]
55. Hill, C.; Guarner, F.; Reid, G.; Gibson, G.R.; Merenstein, D.J.; Pot, B.; Morelli, L.; Canani, R.B.; Flint, H.J.; Salminen, S.; et al. Expert consensus document. The International Scientific Association for Probiotics and Prebiotics consensus statement on the scope and appropriate use of the term probiotic. *Nat. Rev. Gastroenterol. Hepatol.* **2014**, *11*, 506–514. [CrossRef]
56. Wrighton, K.H. Mucosal immunology: Probiotic induction of tolerogenic T cells in the gut. *Nat. Rev. Immunol.* **2017**, *17*, 592. [CrossRef]
57. Simren, M.; Barbara, G.; Flint, H.J.; Spiegel, B.M.; Spiller, R.C.; Vanner, S.; Verdu, E.F.; Whorwell, P.J.; Zoetendal, E.G.; Rome Foundation, C. Intestinal microbiota in functional bowel disorders: A Rome foundation report. *Gut* **2013**, *62*, 159–176. [CrossRef]

58. Mayer, E.A.; Savidge, T.; Shulman, R.J. Brain-gut microbiome interactions and functional bowel disorders. *Gastroenterology* **2014**, *146*, 1500–1512. [CrossRef]
59. Didari, T.; Mozaffari, S.; Nikfar, S.; Abdollahi, M. Effectiveness of probiotics in irritable bowel syndrome: Updated systematic review with meta-analysis. *World J. Gastroenterol.* **2015**, *21*, 3072–3084. [CrossRef]
60. Joyce, S.A.; MacSharry, J.; Casey, P.G.; Kinsella, M.; Murphy, E.F.; Shanahan, F.; Hill, C.; Gahan, C.G. Regulation of host weight gain and lipid metabolism by bacterial bile acid modification in the gut. *Proc. Natl. Acad. Sci. USA* **2014**, *111*, 7421–7426. [CrossRef]
61. Bermudez-Brito, M.; Plaza-Diaz, J.; Munoz-Quezada, S.; Gomez-Llorente, C.; Gil, A. Probiotic mechanisms of action. *Ann. Nutr. Metab.* **2012**, *61*, 160–174. [CrossRef] [PubMed]
62. Jafari, E.; Vahedi, H.; Merat, S.; Momtahen, S.; Riahi, A. Therapeutic effects, tolerability and safety of a multi-strain probiotic in Iranian adults with irritable bowel syndrome and bloating. *Arch. Iran. Med.* **2014**, *17*, 466–470. [PubMed]
63. Ford, A.C.; Quigley, E.M.; Lacy, B.E.; Lembo, A.J.; Saito, Y.A.; Schiller, L.R.; Soffer, E.E.; Spiegel, B.M.; Moayyedi, P. Efficacy of prebiotics, probiotics, and synbiotics in irritable bowel syndrome and chronic idiopathic constipation: Systematic review and meta-analysis. *Am. J. Gastroenterol.* **2014**, *109*, 1547–1561, quiz 1546, 1562. [CrossRef] [PubMed]
64. Pineiro, M.; Asp, N.G.; Reid, G.; Macfarlane, S.; Morelli, L.; Brunser, O.; Tuohy, K. FAO Technical meeting on prebiotics. *J. Clin. Gastroenterol.* **2008**, *42*, S156–S159. [CrossRef] [PubMed]
65. Alvarez-Curto, E.; Milligan, G. Metabolism meets immunity: The role of free fatty acid receptors in the immune system. *Biochem. Pharmacol.* **2016**, *114*, 3–13. [CrossRef] [PubMed]
66. Roberfroid, M.; Gibson, G.R.; Hoyles, L.; McCartney, A.L.; Rastall, R.; Rowland, I.; Wolvers, D.; Watzl, B.; Szajewska, H.; Stahl, B.; et al. Prebiotic effects: Metabolic and health benefits. *Br. J. Nutr.* **2010**, *104*, S1–S63. [CrossRef]
67. Wilson, B.; Rossi, M.; Dimidi, E.; Whelan, K. Prebiotics in irritable bowel syndrome and other functional bowel disorders in adults: A systematic review and meta-analysis of randomized controlled trials. *Am. J. Clin. Nutr.* **2019**, *109*, 1098–1111. [CrossRef] [PubMed]
68. Ford, A.C.; Harris, L.A.; Lacy, B.E.; Quigley, E.M.M.; Moayyedi, P. Systematic review with meta-analysis: The efficacy of prebiotics, probiotics, synbiotics and antibiotics in irritable bowel syndrome. *Aliment. Pharmacol. Ther.* **2018**, *48*, 1044–1060. [CrossRef] [PubMed]
69. Hunter, J.O.; Tuffnell, Q.; Lee, A.J. Controlled trial of oligofructose in the management of irritable bowel syndrome. *J. Nutr.* **1999**, *129*, 1451S–1453S. [CrossRef]
70. Olesen, M.; Gudmand-Hoyer, E. Efficacy, safety, and tolerability of fructooligosaccharides in the treatment of irritable bowel syndrome. *Am. J. Clin. Nutr.* **2000**, *72*, 1570–1575. [CrossRef]
71. Silk, D.B.; Davis, A.; Vulevic, J.; Tzortzis, G.; Gibson, G.R. Clinical trial: The effects of a trans-galactooligosaccharide prebiotic on faecal microbiota and symptoms in irritable bowel syndrome. *Aliment. Pharmacol. Ther.* **2009**, *29*, 508–518. [CrossRef] [PubMed]
72. Niv, E.; Halak, A.; Tiommny, E.; Yanai, H.; Strul, H.; Naftali, T.; Vaisman, N. Randomized clinical study: Partially hydrolyzed guar gum (PHGG) versus placebo in the treatment of patients with irritable bowel syndrome. *Nutr. Metab.* **2016**, *13*, 10. [CrossRef] [PubMed]
73. Saadi, M.; McCallum, R.W. Rifaximin in irritable bowel syndrome: Rationale, evidence and clinical use. *Ther. Adv. Chronic. Dis.* **2013**, *4*, 71–75. [CrossRef] [PubMed]
74. Distrutti, E.; Monaldi, L.; Ricci, P.; Fiorucci, S. Gut microbiota role in irritable bowel syndrome: New therapeutic strategies. *World J. Gastroenterol.* **2016**, *22*, 2219–2241. [CrossRef] [PubMed]
75. Menees, S.B.; Maneerattannaporn, M.; Kim, H.M.; Chey, W.D. The efficacy and safety of rifaximin for the irritable bowel syndrome: A systematic review and meta-analysis. *Am. J. Gastroenterol.* **2012**, *107*, 28–35. [CrossRef] [PubMed]
76. Lembo, A.; Pimentel, M.; Rao, S.S.; Schoenfeld, P.; Cash, B.; Weinstock, L.B.; Paterson, C.; Bortey, E.; Forbes, W.P. Repeat Treatment With Rifaximin Is Safe and Effective in Patients With Diarrhea-Predominant Irritable Bowel Syndrome. *Gastroenterology* **2016**, *151*, 1113–1121. [CrossRef]
77. Konig, J.; Siebenhaar, A.; Hogenauer, C.; Arkkila, P.; Nieuwdorp, M.; Noren, T.; Ponsioen, C.Y.; Rosien, U.; Rossen, N.G.; Satokari, R.; et al. Consensus report: Faecal microbiota transfer—Clinical applications and procedures. *Aliment. Pharmacol. Ther.* **2017**, *45*, 222–239. [CrossRef]

78. Vaughn, B.P.; Rank, K.M.; Khoruts, A. Fecal Microbiota Transplantation: Current Status in Treatment of GI and Liver Disease. *Clin. Gastroenterol. Hepatol.* **2019**, *17*, 353–361. [CrossRef]
79. Jiang, Z.D.; Ajami, N.J.; Petrosino, J.F.; Jun, G.; Hanis, C.L.; Shah, M.; Hochman, L.; Ankoma-Sey, V.; DuPont, A.W.; Wong, M.C.; et al. Randomised clinical trial: Faecal microbiota transplantation for recurrent Clostridum difficile infection—Fresh, or frozen, or lyophilised microbiota from a small pool of healthy donors delivered by colonoscopy. *Aliment. Pharmacol. Ther.* **2017**, *45*, 899–908. [CrossRef]
80. Kassinen, A.; Krogius-Kurikka, L.; Makivuokko, H.; Rinttila, T.; Paulin, L.; Corander, J.; Malinen, E.; Apajalahti, J.; Palva, A. The fecal microbiota of irritable bowel syndrome patients differs significantly from that of healthy subjects. *Gastroenterology* **2007**, *133*, 24–33. [CrossRef]
81. Holvoet, T.; Joossens, M.; Wang, J.; Boelens, J.; Verhasselt, B.; Laukens, D.; van Vlierberghe, H.; Hindryckx, P.; De Vos, M.; De Looze, D.; et al. Assessment of faecal microbial transfer in irritable bowel syndrome with severe bloating. *Gut* **2017**, *66*, 980–982. [CrossRef] [PubMed]
82. Mazzawi, T.; Lied, G.A.; Sangnes, D.A.; El-Salhy, M.; Hov, J.R.; Gilja, O.H.; Hatlebakk, J.G.; Hausken, T. The kinetics of gut microbial community composition in patients with irritable bowel syndrome following fecal microbiota transplantation. *PLoS ONE* **2018**, *13*, e0194904. [CrossRef] [PubMed]
83. Halkjaer, S.I.; Christensen, A.H.; Lo, B.Z.S.; Browne, P.D.; Gunther, S.; Hansen, L.H.; Petersen, A.M. Faecal microbiota transplantation alters gut microbiota in patients with irritable bowel syndrome: Results from a randomised, double-blind placebo-controlled study. *Gut* **2018**, *67*, 2107–2115. [CrossRef] [PubMed]
84. Myneedu, K.; Deoker, A.; Schmulson, M.J.; Bashashati, M. Fecal microbiota transplantation in irritable bowel syndrome: A systematic review and meta-analysis. *United Eur. Gastroenterol. J.* **2019**, *7*, 1033–1041. [CrossRef] [PubMed]
85. Paramsothy, S.; Walsh, A.J.; Borody, T.; Samuel, D.; van den Bogaerde, J.; Leong, R.W.; Connor, S.; Ng, W.; Mitchell, H.M.; Kaakoush, N.O.; et al. Gastroenterologist perceptions of faecal microbiota transplantation. *World J. Gastroenterol.* **2015**, *21*, 10907–10914. [CrossRef]
86. Cammarota, G.; Ianiro, G.; Kelly, C.R.; Mullish, B.H.; Allegretti, J.R.; Kassam, Z.; Putignani, L.; Fischer, M.; Keller, J.J.; Costello, S.P.; et al. International consensus conference on stool banking for faecal microbiota transplantation in clinical practice. *Gut* **2019**, *68*, 2111–2121. [CrossRef]
87. Clevers, E.; Tran, M.; Van Oudenhove, L.; Storsrud, S.; Bohn, L.; Tornblom, H.; Simren, M. Adherence to diet low in fermentable carbohydrates and traditional diet for irritable bowel syndrome. *Nutrition* **2020**, *73*, 110719. [CrossRef]
88. Harper, A.; Naghibi, M.M.; Garcha, D. The Role of Bacteria, Probiotics and Diet in Irritable Bowel Syndrome. *Foods* **2018**, *7*, 13. [CrossRef]
89. Rao, S.S.; Yu, S.; Fedewa, A. Systematic review: Dietary fibre and FODMAP-restricted diet in the management of constipation and irritable bowel syndrome. *Aliment. Pharmacol. Ther.* **2015**, *41*, 1256–1270. [CrossRef]
90. Eswaran, S.L.; Chey, W.D.; Han-Markey, T.; Ball, S.; Jackson, K. A Randomized Controlled Trial Comparing the Low FODMAP Diet vs. Modified NICE Guidelines in US Adults with IBS-D. *Am. J. Gastroenterol.* **2016**, *111*, 1824–1832. [CrossRef]
91. Zahedi, M.J.; Behrouz, V.; Azimi, M. Low fermentable oligo-di-mono-saccharides and polyols diet versus general dietary advice in patients with diarrhea-predominant irritable bowel syndrome: A randomized controlled trial. *J. Gastroenterol. Hepatol.* **2018**, *33*, 1192–1199. [CrossRef] [PubMed]
92. Schumann, D.; Langhorst, J.; Dobos, G.; Cramer, H. Randomised clinical trial: Yoga vs. a low-FODMAP diet in patients with irritable bowel syndrome. *Aliment. Pharmacol. Ther.* **2018**, *47*, 203–211. [CrossRef] [PubMed]
93. Eswaran, S.; Dolan, R.D.; Ball, S.C.; Jackson, K.; Chey, W. The Impact of a 4-Week Low-FODMAP and mNICE Diet on Nutrient Intake in a Sample of US Adults with Irritable Bowel Syndrome with Diarrhea. *J. Acad. Nutr. Diet.* **2019**. [CrossRef] [PubMed]
94. Dolan, R.; Chey, W.D.; Eswaran, S. The role of diet in the management of irritable bowel syndrome: A focus on FODMAPs. *Expert Rev. Gastroenterol. Hepatol.* **2018**, *12*, 607–615. [CrossRef] [PubMed]
95. O'Keeffe, M.; Jansen, C.; Martin, L.; Williams, M.; Seamark, L.; Staudacher, H.M.; Irving, P.M.; Whelan, K.; Lomer, M.C. Long-term impact of the low-FODMAP diet on gastrointestinal symptoms, dietary intake, patient acceptability, and healthcare utilization in irritable bowel syndrome. *Neurogastroenterol. Motil.* **2018**, *30*. [CrossRef] [PubMed]
96. Staudacher, H.M. Nutritional, microbiological and psychosocial implications of the low FODMAP diet. *J. Gastroenterol. Hepatol.* **2017**, *32*, 16–19. [CrossRef]

97. Singh, R.K.; Chang, H.W.; Yan, D.; Lee, K.M.; Ucmak, D.; Wong, K.; Abrouk, M.; Farahnik, B.; Nakamura, M.; Zhu, T.H.; et al. Influence of diet on the gut microbiome and implications for human health. *J. Transl. Med.* **2017**, *15*, 73. [CrossRef]
98. Staudacher, H.M.; Whelan, K. The low FODMAP diet: Recent advances in understanding its mechanisms and efficacy in IBS. *Gut* **2017**, *66*, 1517–1527. [CrossRef]
99. Biesiekierski, J.R.; Newnham, E.D.; Irving, P.M.; Barrett, J.S.; Haines, M.; Doecke, J.D.; Shepherd, S.J.; Muir, J.G.; Gibson, P.R. Gluten causes gastrointestinal symptoms in subjects without celiac disease: A double-blind randomized placebo-controlled trial. *Am. J. Gastroenterol.* **2011**, *106*, 508–514. [CrossRef]
100. Rej, A.; Sanders, D.S. Gluten-Free Diet and Its 'Cousins' in Irritable Bowel Syndrome. *Nutrients* **2018**, *10*, 1727. [CrossRef]
101. Skodje, G.I.; Sarna, V.K.; Minelle, I.H.; Rolfsen, K.L.; Muir, J.G.; Gibson, P.R.; Veierod, M.B.; Henriksen, C.; Lundin, K.E. Fructan, Rather Than Gluten, Induces Symptoms in Patients With Self-Reported Non-Celiac Gluten Sensitivity. *Gastroenterology* **2018**, *154*, 529–539. [CrossRef] [PubMed]
102. Liang, D.; Longgui, N.; Guoqiang, X. Efficacy of different probiotic protocols in irritable bowel syndrome: A network meta-analysis. *Medicine* **2019**, *98*, e16068. [CrossRef] [PubMed]
103. McFarland, L.V.; Dublin, S. Meta-analysis of probiotics for the treatment of irritable bowel syndrome. *World J. Gastroenterol.* **2008**, *14*, 2650–2661. [CrossRef] [PubMed]
104. Connell, M.; Shin, A.; James-Stevenson, T.; Xu, H.; Imperiale, T.F.; Herron, J. Systematic review and meta-analysis: Efficacy of patented probiotic, VSL#3, in irritable bowel syndrome. *Neurogastroenterol. Motil.* **2018**, *30*, e13427. [CrossRef] [PubMed]
105. Tiequn, B.; Guanqun, C.; Shuo, Z. Therapeutic effects of Lactobacillus in treating irritable bowel syndrome: A meta-analysis. *Intern. Med.* **2015**, *54*, 243–249. [CrossRef]
106. Ritchie, M.L.; Romanuk, T.N. A meta-analysis of probiotic efficacy for gastrointestinal diseases. *PLoS ONE* **2012**, *7*, e34938. [CrossRef]
107. Horvath, A.; Dziechciarz, P.; Szajewska, H. Meta-analysis: Lactobacillus rhamnosus GG for abdominal pain-related functional gastrointestinal disorders in childhood. *Aliment. Pharmacol. Ther.* **2011**, *33*, 1302–1310. [CrossRef]
108. Hoveyda, N.; Heneghan, C.; Mahtani, K.R.; Perera, R.; Roberts, N.; Glasziou, P. A systematic review and meta-analysis: Probiotics in the treatment of irritable bowel syndrome. *BMC Gastroenterol.* **2009**, *9*, 15. [CrossRef]
109. Moayyedi, P.; Ford, A.C.; Talley, N.J.; Cremonini, F.; Foxx-Orenstein, A.E.; Brandt, L.J.; Quigley, E.M. The efficacy of probiotics in the treatment of irritable bowel syndrome: A systematic review. *Gut* **2010**, *59*, 325–332. [CrossRef]
110. Nikfar, S.; Rahimi, R.; Rahimi, F.; Derakhshani, S.; Abdollahi, M. Efficacy of probiotics in irritable bowel syndrome: A meta-analysis of randomized, controlled trials. *Dis. Colon. Rectum.* **2008**, *51*, 1775–1780. [CrossRef]
111. Xu, D.; Chen, V.L.; Steiner, C.A.; Berinstein, J.A.; Eswaran, S.; Waljee, A.K.; Higgins, P.D.R.; Owyang, C. Efficacy of Fecal Microbiota Transplantation in Irritable Bowel Syndrome: A Systematic Review and Meta-Analysis. *Am. J. Gastroenterol.* **2019**, *114*, 1043–1050. [CrossRef] [PubMed]
112. Ianiro, G.; Eusebi, L.H.; Black, C.J.; Gasbarrini, A.; Cammarota, G.; Ford, A.C. Systematic review with meta-analysis: Efficacy of faecal microbiota transplantation for the treatment of irritable bowel syndrome. *Aliment. Pharmacol. Ther.* **2019**, *50*, 240–248. [CrossRef] [PubMed]
113. Li, J.; Zhu, W.; Liu, W.; Wu, Y.; Wu, B. Rifaximin for Irritable Bowel Syndrome: A Meta-Analysis of Randomized Placebo-Controlled Trials. *Medicine* **2016**, *95*, e2534. [CrossRef] [PubMed]

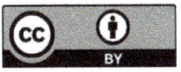

© 2020 by the authors. Licensee MDPI, Basel, Switzerland. This article is an open access article distributed under the terms and conditions of the Creative Commons Attribution (CC BY) license (http://creativecommons.org/licenses/by/4.0/).

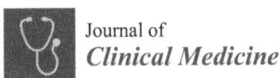

Article

Clinical Response and Changes of Cytokines and Zonulin Levels in Patients with Diarrhoea-Predominant Irritable Bowel Syndrome Treated with *Bifidobacterium Longum* ES1 for 8 or 12 Weeks: A Preliminary Report

Gian Paolo Caviglia [1],* Alessandra Tucci [2] Rinaldo Pellicano [2] Sharmila Fagoonee [3]
Chiara Rosso [1], Maria Lorena Abate [1], Antonella Olivero [1] Angelo Armandi [2], Ester Vanni [2],
Giorgio Maria Saracco [1] Elisabetta Bugianesi [1], Marco Astegiano [2] and
Davide Giuseppe Ribaldone [1],*

[1] Department of Medical Sciences, University of Turin, 10124 Turin, Italy; chiara.rosso@unito.it (C.R.); marialorena.abate@unito.it (M.L.A.); antonella.olivero@unito.it (A.O.); giorgiomaria.saracco@unito.it (G.M.S.); elisabetta.bugianesi@unito.it (E.B.)
[2] Unit of Gastroenterology, Città della Salute e della Scienza di Torino—Molinette Hospital, 10126 Turin, Italy; alessandra.tucci@outlook.com (A.T.); rinaldo_pellican@hotmail.com (R.P.); armandiangelo91@gmail.com (A.A.); evanni@cittadellasalute.to.it (E.V.); marcoastegiano58@gmail.com (M.A.)
[3] Institute of Biostructure and Bioimaging, CNR c/o Molecular Biotechnology Centre, 10126 Turin, Italy; sharmila.fagoonee@unito.it
* Correspondence: gianpaolo.caviglia@unito.it (G.P.C.); davidegiuseppe.ribaldone@unito.it (D.G.R.); Tel.: +39-011-633-3918 (G.P.C. & D.G.R.); Fax: +39-011-633-3623 (G.P.C. & D.G.R.)

Received: 16 June 2020; Accepted: 22 July 2020; Published: 23 July 2020

Abstract: *Bifidobacterium longum* (*B. longum*) ES1 is a probiotic strain capable of modulating microbiome composition, anti-inflammatory activity and intestinal barrier function. We investigated the use of *B. Longum* ES1 in the treatment of patients with diarrhoea-predominant irritable bowel syndrome (IBS-D). Sixteen patients were treated for 8 or 12 weeks with *B. Longum* ES1 (1×10^9 CFU/day). Serum zonulin and cytokines were measured at baseline (T0) and at the end of therapy (T1). Clinical response to therapy was assessed by IBS Severity Scoring System. Interleukin (IL)-6, IL-8, IL-12p70 and tumor necrosis factor (TNF) α levels decreased from T0 to T1, irrespective of treatment duration ($p < 0.05$), while zonulin levels diminished only in patients treated for 12 weeks ($p = 0.036$). Clinical response was observed in 5/16 patients (31%): 4/8 (50%) treated for 12 weeks and 1/8 (13%) treated for 8 weeks. Abdominal pain improved only in patients treated for 12 weeks (5/8 vs. 0/8, $p = 0.025$), while stool consistency improved regardless of therapy duration ($p < 0.001$). In conclusion, the results of this pilot study showed, in IBS-D patients treated for 12 weeks with *B. longum* ES1, a reduction in the levels of pro-inflammatory cytokines, and intestinal permeability as well as an improvement in gastrointestinal symptoms, but further studies including a placebo-control group are necessary to prove a causal link.

Keywords: IBS; IL-6; IL-8; IL-12p70; intestinal permeability; zonulin

1. Introduction

Irritable bowel syndrome (IBS) is a functional gastrointestinal (GI) disorder affecting approximately 15–25% of the population, with higher prevalence in the female gender [1]. The pathophysiological mechanisms underlying IBS are not completely known. Different factors may participate in disease onset and perpetuation, including genetics, intestinal microbiota and low-grade inflammation [2]. In addition, the role of the intestinal barrier in the pathogenesis of IBS is being increasingly recognised [3]. The loss of barrier integrity allows an increased passage of luminal antigens into the intestinal mucosa, hence stimulating the immune response and sensitizing the afferent nerve fibres [4].

Zonulin is a 47-kDa protein involved in the regulation of tight junctions (TJs), the primary determinants of paracellular permeability [5]. Serum zonulin is increased in various diseases in which alteration of intestinal permeability is central, including coeliac disease (CD), inflammatory bowel diseases (IBDs) and type 1 diabetes mellitus [6–8]. Moreover, higher serum zonulin levels were seen in patients with IBS compared to controls. Importantly, zonulin levels were directly correlated with the severity of bowel habits in patients with diarrhoea-predominant irritable bowel syndrome (IBS-D) [9].

Many studies have reported the presence of moderate immuno-inflammatory activity in both large and small intestine of patients with IBS [10]. Accordingly, patients with IBS showed increased levels of pro-inflammatory cytokines including interleukin (IL)-1b, tumour necrosis factor-alpha (TNFα), IL-6 and IL-8, and reduced levels of anti-inflammatory cytokines such as IL-10 [11], IL-5 and IL-13 [10]. Through the release of inflammatory cytokines such as TNFα and interferon-gamma (IFNγ), T lymphocytes contribute to TJ dysfunction [12,13].

Emerging literature data support a pathophysiological role of microbiome in IBS. The dysbiosis observed in subjects with IBS is characterized by reduced biodiversity, an increase in Bacteroides and Clostridia, and a reduction in Bifidobacteria [14,15]. There is also evidence of the ability of microbiome to regulate the intestinal barrier. The alteration of the commensal microbiota entails the presence of a morphologically aberrant intestinal mucosa, characterized by shorter ileal villi and smaller intestinal crypts, as demonstrated in germ-free mice [16]. In vitro studies showed that eubiotic microbiome favoured cell renewal process and expression of junctional proteins and mucins [17]. The reduced concentration in Bifidobacteria was associated with the severity of abdominal pain and number of bowel movements. Thus, targeting Bifidobacteria in the intestinal tract may alleviate microbiota-related diseases [18].

The rationale for the use of *Bifidobacterium longum* (*B. longum*) ES1 [19] in patients with IBS-D lies in its ability to modulate the microbiome improving intestinal dysbiosis [20], exert anti-inflammatory activity through the down-regulation of TNF-alpha and the up-regulation of IL-10 [21], and restore the integrity of the intestinal barrier, inducing the synthesis of TJ proteins [22,23].

Several meta-analyses have reported on the effectiveness and safety of probiotics in patients with IBS, especially for products containing Bifidobacteria and Lactobacilli. However, there was significant inter-study heterogeneity, warranting cautious interpretation of the findings. The heterogeneity mainly regarded differences in subgroup analyses of probiotics type, combination and dose, IBS subtype, symptomatic assessment scores and treatment duration [24,25]. Finally, not only probiotics but also prebiotics, such as inositol and beta-glucan, have been shown to improve symptoms in patients with IBS and in patients with concurrent IBD and IBS [26,27].

The aim of this pilot study was (1) to assess the use of *B. longum* ES1 treatment in a homogeneous group of patients with IBS-D, by evaluating clinical response, through the use of validated questionnaires for IBS, and serological response, by the determination of serum levels of inflammatory cytokines and zonulin, in order to analyse potential effects on immune modulation and restoration of the intestinal barrier, respectively, and (2) to evaluate differences in response depending on the treatment duration. The results of this pilot study will allow us to define the optimal duration of probiotic therapy and to calculate the necessary sample size to conduct a subsequent randomized, double-blind, placebo-controlled clinical trial.

2. Materials and Methods

2.1. Patients

We carried out a prospective study at the Gastroenterology Unit of "A.O.U. Città della Salute e della Scienza di Torino" hospital, Italy from April 2019 to October 2019.

Patients affected by IBS-D were recruited and treated with a strain-specific probiotic therapy for 8 or 12 weeks. Probiotic therapy consisted of daily administration of 1×10^9 colony-forming unit (CFU) of *B. longum* ES1 away from meals. Inclusion criteria were: age between 16 and 65 years old, diagnosis of IBS-D according to the Rome IV criteria and Bristol stool scale [28], body mass index (BMI) < 30 kg/m^2, willingness to sign the informed consent to participate to the study. Exclusion criteria were: history of GI surgery, diagnosis of IBD or CD, thyroid diseases, diverticular disease, small intestine bacterial overgrowth (SIBO), colorectal cancer, other clinically relevant diseases, treatment with drugs that alter intestinal function (e.g., opiates, anticholinergics and laxatives), treatment with antibiotics (any previous antibiotic therapy should have been discontinued at least 4 weeks before the start of probiotic therapy) and other pre/probiotics (other pre/probiotics therapy should have been discontinued at least 2 weeks before starting therapy), pregnancy/breastfeeding.

Clinical history, data on physical examination, recent biochemical examinations and signed informed consent were collected. Disease severity was assessed at baseline with the Functional Bowel Disorder Severity Index (FBDSI) questionnaire [29]. At baseline (T0) and after 8 or 12 weeks of probiotic therapy (T1), patients were evaluated with Irritable Bowel Syndrome Severity Scoring System (IBS-SSS) questionnaire for the clinical evaluation of disease [30] and Irritable Bowel Syndrome Quality of Life (IBS-QoL) questionnaire for life quality assessment [31]. IBS-QoL consists of 34 items and 8 domains; for the purpose of analysis, we considered the overall questionnaire score. The final raw scores of IBS-QoL were presented on a scale between 0 (poor quality of life) and 100 (maximum quality of life).

All patients underwent baseline venous sampling (T0) and after 8 or 12 weeks of therapy (T1); serum was collected in polypropylene 2 mL tubes labelled with the study participant identification code and stored at −80 °C until analysis.

The study followed the principles of the Declaration of Helsinki and was approved by the local ethics committee (Comitato Etico Interaziendale A.O.U. Città della Salute e della Scienza di Torino—A.O. Ordine Mauriziano—A.S.L. Città di Torino) (approval code 0056924).

2.2. Measurement of Serum Zonulin and Cytokines

Serum zonulin was assessed by competitive enzyme-linked immunosorbent assay (ELISA) (IDK® Zonulin ELISA Kit, Immunodiagnostik AG, Bensheim, Germany) according to the manufacturer's instructions. Concentrations were calculated using a four-parameter algorithm, and the results were given in ng/mL, as previously reported [8]. The cytokine panel, including IL-6, IL-8, IL-10, IL-12p70, IL-23, IL-33, IFNγ and TNFα, was measured in serum samples by Bio-Plex® Multiplex Immunoassay (Bio-rad Laboratories, Hercules, CA, USA) on a Luminex® 200 system (Luminex Corporation, Austin, TX, USA). Individual standard curves were generated for each cytokine; the results are given in pg/mL [32]. Personnel performing laboratory investigations were blind to all the characteristics of the patients included in the study.

2.3. Outcomes

Clinical and serological outcomes were considered in the study. The clinical outcomes included an IBS-SSS score decrease of ≥50 points, reduction of at least 30% in abdominal pain [33] and bloating by a visual analogic scale (VAS), normalization of stool shape by Bristol Stool Scale and IBS-QoL overall score increase ≥14 points [34,35]. The serological outcomes included the variation in inflammatory cytokines and zonulin levels during the follow-up period to assess potential changing of immune-inflammatory activity and of intestinal permeability, respectively. Both clinical and serological outcomes were evaluated in the overall study population and according to treatment duration.

2.4. Statistical Analysis

Continuous variables were expressed as median and 95% confidence interval (CI) or as mean ± standard deviation (SD). The normality of data distribution was tested by D'Agostino-Pearson test. The comparison between quantitative variables was carried out using the Student *t*-test; for the comparison between values at T0 and at T1, the Student *t*-test for paired measurements was used. The comparison between qualitative variables was carried out by Fisher exact test or chi-squared test for trend where appropriate. Nonparametric variables were analysed with the Wilcoxon test for paired samples and with the Mann-Whitney test for independent samples. The correlation between quantitative variables was carried out by non-parametric Spearman test. The results of all analyses were considered significant for *p* values < 0.05. All statistical analyses were performed using MedCalc software version 18.9.1 (MedCalc Software bvba, Ostend, Belgium; http://www.medcalc.org; 2018).

3. Results

Sixteen patients aged between 16 and 59 years were enrolled. Basal characteristics of the included cohort are reported in Table 1. Most patients were female (*n* = 10/16, 38%). Patients mainly had normal weight (BMI < 25 kg/m^2) and all of them consumed a Mediterranean diet [36]. No dietary changes were made prior to study initiation. According to FBDSI score, severity of IBS was mild in 1 patient (6%), moderate in 8 patients (50%), and severe in 7 patients (44%). Anamnestic collection showed that 4 of the 16 enrolled patients (25%) had lactose intolerance confirmed by hydrogen breath test (HBT). All affected patients had reported little or no benefit after the elimination of lactose from diet in the previous years, and no changes in the diet were performed during the study period.

Table 1. Baseline characteristics of the included patients.

Characteristics	*n* (%)
Patients, *n*	16
Female gender, *n* (%)	10 (62)
Age (mean years ± SD)	37.6 ± 15.6
BMI (mean kg/m^2 ± SD)	21.3 ± 3.4
Married/in a relationship, *n* (%)	4 (25)
Caesarean childbirth, *n* (%)	5 (31)
History of breastfeeding, *n* (%)	7 (44)
Current smokers, *n* (%)	0, (0)
Lactose intolerance, *n* (%)	4 (25)
Atopy, *n* (%)	5 (31)
FBDSI (mean ± SD)	101 ± 52
IBS-SSS (mean ± SD)	289 ± 91
Abdominal pain (mean ± SD)	57 ± 28
IBS-QoL overall score (mean ± SD)	71 ± 16
Bristol Stool Scale (mean ± SD)	6 ± 1
Zonulin (ng/mL, mean ± SD)	42.5 ± 9.3
IL-6 (pg/mL, median, 95% CI)	4.22, 2.87–7.06
IL-8 (pg/mL, median, 95% CI)	3.47, 1.96–5.32
IL-12p70 (pg/mL, median, 95% CI)	1.77, 0.57–2.16
TNFα (pg/mL, median, 95% CI)	5.69, 2.23–11.09

Abbreviations: body mass index (BMI), confidence interval (CI), Functional Bowel Disorder Severity Index (FBDSI), interleukin (IL), Irritable Bowel Syndrome Quality of Life (IBS-QoL), Irritable Bowel Syndrome Severity Scoring System (IBS-SSS), *n* (number), standard deviation (SD), tumour necrosis factor-alpha (TNFα).

As expected, we observed a positive correlation between FBDSI and IBS-SSS (r_s = 0.658, 95% CI 0.241–0.870, *p* = 0.006) and an inverse correlation between IBS-SSS and overall IBS-QoL score (r_s = −0.550, 95% CI −0.822–−0.074, *p* = 0.027). Age positively correlated with serum zonulin levels (r_s = 0.558, 95% CI 0.086–0.825, *p* = 0.025) and negatively correlated with FBDSI (r_s = −0.570, 95% CI −0.831–−0.104, *p* = 0.021). A significant positive correlation was also observed between abdominal pain intensity and TNFα levels (r_s = 0.585, 95% CI 0.126–0.838, *p* = 0.017). Only a slight positive trend was observed regarding the correlation between serum zonulin and BMI (r_s = 0.459, 95% CI −0.047–0.778, *p* = 0.074), between serum zonulin and IL-6 values (r_s = 0.453, 95% CI −0.055–0.775, *p* = 0.078) and between IL-8 and TNFα values (r_s = 0.439, 95% CI −0.072–0.768, *p* = 0.089). No other significant correlations were observed between serum zonulin or cytokines levels and other demographic and clinical characteristics of the study population (Figure 1).

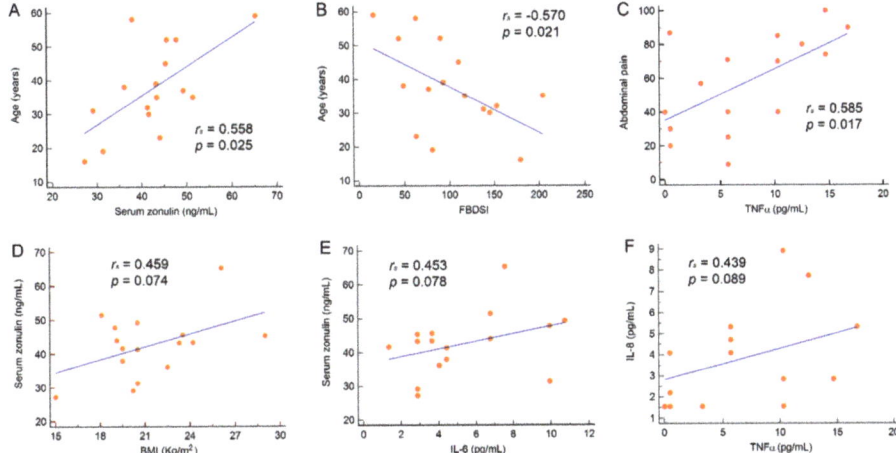

Figure 1. Correlation between age and serum zonulin levels (**A**), age and FBDSI (**B**), abdominal pain intensity and TNFα values (**C**), serum zonulin levels and BMI (**D**), serum zonulin and IL-6 values (**E**) and IL-8 and TNFα values (**F**). Abbreviations: Body Mass Index (BMI), Functional Bowel Disorder Severity Index (FBDSI), interleukin (IL), tumour necrosis factor-alpha (TNFα).

At baseline, no significant difference was observed between patients undergoing 8 weeks and 12 weeks of treatment regarding severity of disease, serum zonulin levels and cytokines values (Table 2).

Table 2. Comparison of disease severity, IBS-QoL overall score, Bristol Stool Chart, serum zonulin levels and cytokines values, assessed at baseline (T0), between the two groups of patients treated with *B. Longum* ES1 for 8 or 12 weeks.

Parameters	T0 (8w)	T0 (12w)	p Values
Patients (*n*)	8	8	
Disease severity (mild/moderate/severe)	1/2/5	0/6/2	0.248
IBS-QoL overall score (mean ± SD)	65 ± 17	78 ± 13	0.118
Bristol Stool Scale (mean ± SD)	6 ± 1	7 ± 1	0.150
Zonulin (ng/mL, mean ± SD)	41.1 ± 11.60	43.8 ± 6.8	0.570
IL-6 (pg/mL, median, 95% CI)	3.26, 2.58–5.01	6.77, 3.50–10.09	0.060
IL-8 (pg/mL, median, 95% CI)	3.46, 1.55–5.77	3.78, 1.55–5.99	0.670
IL-12p70 (pg/mL, median, 95% CI)	1.37, 0.57–3.68	1.77, 0.57–2.16	0.830
TNFα (pg/mL, median, 95% CI)	5.69, 0.47–10.70	7.99, 0.38–15.06	0.460

Abbreviations: interleukin (IL), confidence interval (CI), number (*n*), non-responder (NR), responder (R), standard deviation (SD), tumour necrosis factor-alpha (TNFα), week (w).

The changes of clinical parameters, serum zonulin and cytokines levels from baseline to end of therapy in the overall population of patients with IBS-D treated with *B. longum* ES1 are reported in Table 3.

Table 3. Changes of questionnaires scores, serum zonulin levels and cytokines values from T0 to T1 in the overall study population.

Parameters	T0	T1	p Values
Patients (n)	16	16	
IBS-SSS (mean ± SD)	289 ± 91	263 ± 118	0.103
Pain intensity (mean ± SD)	57 ± 28	47 ± 31	0.216
Bloating (mean ± SD)	39 ± 30	44 ± 32	0.340
IBS-QoL overall score (mean ± SD)	71 ± 16	73 ± 17	0.299
Bristol Stool Scale (mean ± SD)	6 ± 1	4 ± 1	<0.001 *
Zonulin (ng/mL, mean ± SD)	42.5 ± 9.3	40.5 ± 6.8	0.179
IL-6 (pg/mL, median, 95% CI)	4.22, 2.87–7.06	0.01, 0.01–3.65	<0.001 *
IL-8 (pg/mL, median, 95% CI)	3.47, 1.96–5.32	0.01, 0.01–1.12	0.011 *
IL-12p70 (pg/mL, median, 95% CI)	1.77, 0.57–2.16	0.01, 0.01–0.21	0.001 *
TNFα (pg/mL, median, 95% CI)	5.69, 2.23–11.09	0.01, 0.01–5.69	0.034 *

Abbreviations: confidence interval (CI), interleukin (IL), Irritable Bowel Syndrome Quality of Life (IBS-QoL), Irritable Bowel Syndrome Severity Scoring System (IBS-SSS), number (n), standard deviation (SD), tumour necrosis factor-alpha (TNFα), statistically significant (*).

The clinical response to probiotic therapy, in terms of IBS-SSS score decrease of ≥50 points, was observed in 5/16 patients (31%), of whom 4/8 (50%) were treated for 12 weeks and 1/8 (13%) was treated for 8 weeks ($p = 0.282$); indeed, a trend towards IBS-SSS score reduction from T0 to T1 was found only in patients treated for 12 weeks (236 ± 67 vs. 189 ± 80, $p = 0.072$). An improvement ≥30% of the abdominal pain intensity was found in 5/16 (31%) patients, all of them treated for 12 weeks (5/8; 63%); consistently, patients treated for 12 weeks showed a significant reduction in the intensity of abdominal pain compared to those treated for 8 weeks (from 63 ± 28 to 34 ± 28, $p = 0.020$ and from 52 ± 30 to 62 ± 24, $p = 0.132$, respectively). Conversely, no significant improvement in bloating was reported ($p = 0.340$), independent of therapy duration. An overall IBS-QoL score increase of ≥14 points was obtained only in 1/16 (6%), who was treated for 12 weeks. Stool consistency improved regardless of the duration of therapy ($p < 0.001$). Nine out of 16 (56%) patients normalized stool consistency (type 3 or 4 according to Bristol Stool Scale): 5/8 (63%) were treated for 12 weeks, whereas 4/8 (50%) were treated for 8 weeks ($p = 0.626$). None of the patients reported adverse events during or after treatment.

Finally, we observed a significant decrease in IL-6, IL-8, IL-12 and TNFα values from baseline to end of therapy, irrespective of treatment duration. Conversely, no significant reduction was found in serum zonulin levels in the overall study population; however, in patients treated for 12 weeks, serum zonulin decreased significantly from 43.8 ± 6.8 ng/mL at T0 to 40.8 ± 5.0 ng/mL at T1 ($p = 0.036$) (Figure 2).

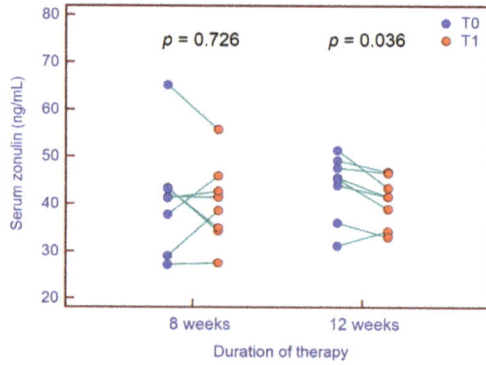

Figure 2. Variation of serum zonulin levels from baseline (T0) to end of therapy (T1) in patients with IBS-D treated with *B. longum* ES1 for 8 weeks or 12 weeks.

4. Discussion

In this pilot study, we found an improvement in overall symptoms of IBS and an improvement in the immune-inflammatory state and integrity of intestinal barrier. These aspects were especially significant in patients treated with *B. longum* ES1 for 12 weeks versus 8 weeks.

Accumulating evidence suggests that commensal bacteria may play a role in IBS and that specific probiotic therapy is able to improve GI symptoms in such patients [37]. Indeed, a recent systematic review showed that patients with IBS had lower microbial α-diversity in both stool and intestinal mucosal samples, with an overall microbial profile characterized by increased levels of Firmicutes and decreased levels of Bacteroidetes compared to healthy subjects [38]. On the other hand, there is a lack of consistency among the gut microbiota fingerprints reported in different studies, probably due to different study designs, different methods used for bacterial profiling (including samples storage, DNA extraction and sequencing) and different statistical approaches [39]. In 48% of patients with IBS-D, it has been shown that probiotic therapy provided adequate relief of overall IBS symptoms, amelioration of stool consistency and a trend towards improved quality of life [40]. More recently, Giannetti et al. reported that the administration of a probiotic mixture of *Bifidobacterium infantis* M-63, *breve* M-16V, and *longum* BB536 in patients with IBS decreased abdominal pain frequency and improved QoL in a significantly higher proportion of patients, when compared with placebo [41]. Moreover, Pinto-Sanchez et al. showed that probiotic therapy (*B. longum* NCC3001) improved psychiatric comorbidities and increased quality of life in patients with IBS [42]. Consistently, we observed an improvement in IBS symptoms especially after 12 weeks of therapy with *B. longum* ES1. However, compared to previous studies, we did not observe an amelioration in the quality of life of our population. Likely, the probiotic mixture or specific strain beneficial for each patient remains to be determined.

Human and animal studies support the concept that a low-grade inflammation may perturb GI reflexes and activate the visceral sensory system contributing to the altered GI physiology and hypersensitivity underlying IBS [43,44]. Moreover, a recent study on murine model demonstrated the important role of neuron-glial communication mediated by TNFα and glial activation in visceral inflammatory hypersensitivity [45]. Consistently, we found a significant positive correlation between abdominal pain intensity and TNFα levels. Several studies have reported an imbalance in pro-inflammatory cytokines, such as IL-6, IL-8 and TNFα, in patients with IBS compared to controls [46–49]. Unfortunately, in the present study, we were not able to substantiate this data due to the lack of a healthy control population. Lastly, we found a positive correlation between IL-8 and TNFα, in accordance with the chemotactic and activation function performed by IL-8 against neutrophils, which in turn produce TNFα. Treatment with *B. longum* ES1 led to a significant reduction in cytokine levels from baseline to the end of therapy, contributing to the clinical improvement observed in our population. Taken together, these results confirm both the low-grade inflammation described in patients with IBS [36] and the anti-inflammatory effect of *B. longum* ES1 and, overall, support probiotic therapy as a valid treatment option in patients with IBS.

Finally, in the intricate puzzle of IBS pathophysiology, it has been shown that altered intestinal permeability plays an essential role, particularly in its diarrhoea-predominant variant. Indeed, several case-control studies showed that intestinal permeability measured by multi-sugar absorption test increased in patients with IBS-D compared to healthy controls [50,51]. Moreover, Linsalata et al. identified two different IBS-D subtypes that showed different inflammatory status according to intestinal permeability function, further supporting the concept that an impaired GI barrier may allow easier passage of luminal antigens that, in turn, may elicit an inflammatory response influencing the course of the disease [52]. In support of this issue, we found a positive correlation between serum zonulin, a marker of intestinal permeability, and IL-6, secreted by macrophages as a result of the Pathogen Associated Molecular Patterns (PAMPs) binding to the Toll-like receptors. Moreover, we observed a positive correlation between age and zonulin levels. A likely explanation for these findings could lie in a prolonged period of exposure to PAMPs. More recently, it has been reported that treatment with *B. longum* BB536 and *Lactobacillus rhamnosus* HN001 with vitamin B6, compared to placebo, significantly improved GI symptoms and restored intestinal permeability in patients with IBS, as deduced by the improved percentage of sucralose recovery [53]. To date, very few studies have investigated serum zonulin concentration in patients with IBS. Singh et al. showed that serum zonulin levels in patients with IBS were higher compared with healthy controls and comparable to those with active coeliac disease [9]. Taking into account the results on serum zonulin concentration from previous studies conducted at our Center on IBD patients, we observed that serum zonulin concentration in patients with IBS-D was comparable to that found in patients with IBD (43.3 (95% CI 37.3–46.4) vs. 45.3 (95% CI 43.5–47.8) ng/mL, respectively) [30] and higher than those found in healthy controls (8.6 (95% CI 7.2–10.5) ng/mL) [8]. In the present study, a significant reduction in serum zonulin concentration was observed in patients who received probiotic therapy for 12 weeks and not in those treated for 8 weeks. These findings suggest the presence of an altered intestinal permeability in IBS-D patients, and we observed an improvement of the barrier integrity in patients treated for 12 weeks.

The main limitations of the current study are the limited sample size and the lack of a placebo-treated control group, to provide definitive conclusions on the real efficacy of *B. longum* ES1 treatment in our population. We observed a significant improvement of inflammatory status and stool consistency, irrespective of the treatment duration. None of the clinical outcomes allow any inference on the effect on IBS natural history in view of duration of therapy, nature of IBS symptoms (waxing and waning), and marginal differences. Since this was a pilot study, its aim was to evaluate whether our hypothesis could be sufficiently supported to justify a detailed investigation. Such data are promising and set the basis for controlled clinical trials with broader case studies.

5. Conclusions

In conclusion, our preliminary results showed a reduction in the levels of pro-inflammatory cytokines in the overall study cohort and possibly an improvement in intestinal permeability and gastrointestinal symptoms in a subgroup of patients with IBS-D. Further randomized, double-blind, placebo-controlled studies are fundamental to validating the results of this pilot study on larger groups of patients with IBS-D.

Author Contributions: Conceptualization, A.T. and M.A.; Data curation, A.T. and R.P.; Formal analysis, D.G.R., and G.P.C.; Investigation, G.P.C., C.R., M.L.A., E.V., A.A. and A.O.; Methodology, A.T., M.A., D.G.R., R.P., E.V., A.A. and G.P.C.; Project administration, E.B., E.V., G.M.S. and M.A.; Software, D.G.R. and G.P.C.; Supervision, E.B. and G.M.S.; Validation, R.P. and S.F.; Visualization, E.V., R.P. and S.F.; Writing—original draft, A.T., G.P.C. and D.G.R.; Writing—review & editing, M.A., R.P. and S.F. All authors have read and agreed to the published version of the manuscript.

Funding: This research received no external funding.

Acknowledgments: The authors thank PharmExtracta S.p.a. for providing reagents for the measurement of serum cytokines and zonulin.

Conflicts of Interest: The authors declare no conflict of interest.

References

1. Adriani, A.; Ribaldone, D.G.; Astegiano, M.; Durazzo, M.; Saracco, G.M.; Pellicano, R. Irritable bowel syndrome: The clinical approach. *Panminerva Med.* **2018**, *60*, 213–222. [CrossRef]
2. González-Castro, A.M.; Martínez, C.; Salvo-Romero, E.; Fortea, M.; Pardo-Camacho, C.; Pérez-Berezo, T.; Alonso-Cotoner, C.; Santos, J.; Vicario, M. Mucosal pathobiology and molecular signature of epithelial barrier dysfunction in the small intestine in irritable bowel syndrome. *J. Gastroenterol. Hepatol.* **2017**, *32*, 53–63. [CrossRef] [PubMed]
3. Martínez, C.; González-Castro, A.; Vicario, M.; Santos, J. Cellular and molecular basis of intestinal barrier dysfunction in the irritable bowel syndrome. *Gut Liver* **2012**, *6*, 305–315. [CrossRef] [PubMed]
4. Barbara, G.; Wang, B.; Stanghellini, V.; de Giorgio, R.; Cremon, C.; Di Nardo, G.; Trevisani, M.; Campi, B.; Geppetti, P.; Tonini, M.; et al. Mast cell-dependent excitation of visceral-nociceptive sensory neurons in irritable bowel syndrome. *Gastroenterology* **2007**, *132*, 26–37. [CrossRef] [PubMed]

5. Sturgeon, C.; Fasano, A. Zonulin, a regulator of epithelial and endothelial barrier functions, and its involvement in chronic inflammatory diseases. *Tissue Barriers* **2016**, *4*, e1251384. [CrossRef]
6. Caviglia, G.P.; Rosso, C.; Ribaldone, D.G.; Dughera, F.; Fagoonee, S.; Asteigano, M.; Pellicano, R. Physiopathology of intestinal barrier and the role of zonulin. *Minerva Biotecnol.* **2019**, *31*, 83–92. [CrossRef]
7. Fasano, A. All disease begins in the (leaky) gut: Role of zonulin-mediated gut permeability in the pathogenesis of some chronic inflammatory diseases. *F1000 Res.* **2020**, *9*. [CrossRef]
8. Caviglia, G.P.; Dughera, F.; Ribaldone, D.G.; Rosso, C.; Abate, M.L.; Pellicano, R.; Bresso, F.; Smedile, A.; Saracco, G.M.; Astegiano, M. Serum zonulin in patients with inflammatory bowel disease: A pilot study. *Minerva Med.* **2019**, *110*, 95–100. [CrossRef]
9. Singh, P.; Silvester, J.; Chen, X.; Xu, H.; Sawhney, V.; Rangan, V.; Iturrino, J.; Nee, J.; Duerksen, D.R.; Lembo, A. Serum zonulin is elevated in IBS and correlates with stool frequency in IBS-D. *United Eur. Gastroenterol. J.* **2019**, *7*, 709–715. [CrossRef]
10. Barbara, G.; Cremon, C.; Carini, G.; Bellacosa, L.; Zecchi, L.; De Giorgio, R.; Corinaldesi, R.; Stanghellini, V. The immune system in irritable bowel syndrome. *J. Neurogastroenterol. Motil.* **2011**, *17*, 349–359. [CrossRef]
11. Barbara, G.; Grover, M.; Bercik, P.; Corsetti, M.; Ghoshal, U.C.; Ohman, L.; Rajilić-Stojanović, M. Rome Foundation Working Team Report on Post-Infection Irritable Bowel Syndrome. *Gastroenterology* **2019**, *156*, 46–58. [CrossRef] [PubMed]
12. Musch, M.W.; Clarke, L.L.; Mamah, D.; Gawenis, L.R.; Zhang, Z.; Ellsworth, W.; Shalowitz, D.; Mittal, N.; Efthimiou, P.; Alnadjim, Z.; et al. T cell activation causes diarrhea by increasing intestinal permeability and inhibiting epithelial Na+/K+-ATPase. *J. Clin. Invest.* **2002**, *110*, 1739–1747. [CrossRef] [PubMed]
13. Wang, F.; Graham, W.V.; Wang, Y.; Witkowski, E.D.; Schwarz, B.T.; Turner, J.R. Interferon-γ and tumor necrosis factor-α synergize to induce intestinal epithelial barrier dysfunction by up-regulating myosin light chain kinase expression. *Am. J. Pathol.* **2005**, *166*, 409–419. [CrossRef]
14. Parkes, G.C.; Rayment, N.B.; Hudspith, B.N.; Petrovska, L.; Lomer, M.C.; Brostoff, J.; Whelan, K.; Sanderson, J.D. Distinct microbial populations exist in the mucosa-associated microbiota of sub-groups of irritable bowel syndrome. *Neurogastroenterol. Motil.* **2012**, *24*, 31–39. [CrossRef] [PubMed]
15. Carroll, I.M.; Ringel-Kulka, T.; Siddle, J.P.; Ringel, Y. Alterations in composition and diversity of the intestinal microbiota in patients with diarrhea-predominant irritable bowel syndrome. *Neurogastroenterol. Motil.* **2012**, *24*, 521–530. [CrossRef] [PubMed]
16. Abrams, G.D.; Bauer, H.; Sprinz, H. Influence of the normal flora on mucosal morphology and cellular renewal in the ileum. A comparison of germ-free and conventional mice. *Lab. Invest.* **1963**, *12*, 355–364.
17. Fan, W.T.; Ding, C.; Xu, N.N.; Zong, S.; Ma, P.; Gu, B. Close association between intestinal microbiota and irritable bowel syndrome. *Eur. J. Clin. Microbiol. Infect. Dis.* **2017**, *36*, 2303–2317. [CrossRef]
18. Tojo, R.; Suárez, A.; Clemente, M.G.; De Los Reyes-Gavilán, C.G.; Margolles, A.; Gueimonde, M.; Ruas-Madiedo, P. Intestinal microbiota in health and disease: Role of bifidobacteria in gut homeostasis. *World J. Gastroenterol.* **2014**, *20*, 15163–15176. [CrossRef]
19. Chenoll, E.; Codoñer, F.; Silva, A.; Ibáñez, A.; Martinez-Blanch, J.; Bollati-Fogolín, M.; Crispo, M.; Ramírez, S.; Sanz, Y.; Ramón, D.; et al. Genomic Sequence and Pre-Clinical Safety Assessment of Bifidobacterium longum CECT 7347, a Probiotic able to Reduce the Toxicity and Inflammatory Potential of Gliadin-Derived Peptides. *J. Probiotics Heal.* **2013**, *01*, 1–6.
20. Izquierdo, E.; Medina, M.; Ennahar, S.; Marchioni, E.; Sanz, Y. Resistance to simulated gastrointestinal conditions and adhesion to mucus as probiotic criteria for Bifidobacterium longum strains. *Curr. Microbiol.* **2008**, *56*, 613–618. [CrossRef]
21. Olivares, M.; Castillejo, G.; Varea, V.; Sanz, Y. Double-blind, randomised, placebo-controlled intervention trial to evaluate the effects of Bifidobacterium longum CECT 7347 in children with newly diagnosed coeliac disease. *Br. J. Nutr.* **2014**, *112*, 30–40. [CrossRef] [PubMed]
22. Sultana, R.; McBain, A.J.; O'Neill, C.A. Strain-dependent augmentation of tight-junction barrier function in human primary epidermal keratinocytes by Lactobacillus and Bifidobacterium lysates. *Appl. Environ. Microbiol.* **2013**, *79*, 4887–4894. [CrossRef] [PubMed]
23. Takeda, Y.; Nakase, H.; Namba, K.; Inoue, S.; Ueno, S.; Uza, N.; Chiba, T. Upregulation of T-bet and tight junction molecules by Bifidobactrium longum improves colonic inflammation of ulcerative colitis. *Inflamm. Bowel Dis.* **2009**, *15*, 1617–1618. [CrossRef] [PubMed]

24. Zhang, Y.; Li, L.; Guo, C.; Mu, D.; Feng, B.; Zuo, X.; Li, Y. Effects of probiotic type, dose and treatmenty duration on irritable bowel syndrome diagnosed by Rome III criteria: A meta-analysis. *BMC Gastroenterol.* **2016**, *16*, 62. [CrossRef]
25. Ford, A.C.; Harris, L.A.; Lucy, B.E.; Quigley, E.M.M.; Moayyedi, P. Systematic review with meta-analysis: The efficacy of prebiotics, probiotics, synbiotics and antibiotics in irritable bowel syndrome. *Aliment. Pharmacol. Ther.* **2018**, *48*, 1044–1060. [CrossRef]
26. Ciacci, C.; Franceschi, F.; Purchiaroni, F.; Capone, P.; Buccelletti, F.; Iacomini, P.; Ranaudo, A.; Andreozzi, P.; Tondi, P.; Gentiloni Silveri, N.; et al. Effect of beta-glucan, inositol and digestive enzymes in GI symptoms of patients with IBS. *Eur. Rev. Med. Pharmacol. Sci.* **2011**, *15*, 637–643.
27. Spaguolo, R.; Cosco, C.; Mancina, R.M.; Ruggiero, G.; Garieri, P.; Cosco, V.; Doldo, P. Beta-glucan, inositol and digestive enzymes improve quality of life of patients with inflammatory bowel disease and irritable bowel syndrome. *Eur. Rev. Med. Pharmacol. Sci.* **2017**, *21*, 102–107.
28. Drossman, D.A.; Hasler, W.L. Rome IV-Functional GI Disorders: Disorders of Gut-Brain Interaction. *Gastroenterology* **2016**, *150*, 1257–1261. [CrossRef]
29. Drossman, D.A.; Li, Z.; Toner, B.B.; Diamant, N.E.; Creed, F.H.; Thompson, D.; Read, N.W.; Babbs, C.; Barreiro, M.; Bank, L.; et al. Functional bowel disorders. A multicenter comparison of health status and development of illness severity index. *Dig. Dis. Sci.* **1995**, *40*, 986–995. [CrossRef]
30. Francis, C.Y.; Morris, J.; Whorwell, P.J. The irritable bowel severity scoring system: A simple method of monitoring irritable bowel syndrome and its progress. *Aliment. Pharmacol. Ther.* **1997**, *11*, 395–402. [CrossRef]
31. Patrick, D.L.; Drossman, D.A.; Frederick, I.O.; Di Cesare, J.; Puder, K.L. Quality of life in persons with irritable bowel syndrome: Development and validation of a new measure. *Dig. Dis. Sci.* **1998**, *43*, 400–411. [CrossRef] [PubMed]
32. Caviglia, G.P.; Rosso, C.; Stalla, F.; Rizzo, M.; Massano, A.; Abate, M.L.; Olivero, A.; Armandi, A.; Vanni, E.; Younes, R.; et al. On-Treatment Decrease of Serum Interleukin-6 as a Predictor of Clinical Response to Biologic Therapy in Patients with Inflammatory Bowel Dis. *J. Clin. Med.* **2020**, *9*, 800. [CrossRef] [PubMed]
33. Andresen, V.; Gschossmann, J.; Layer, P. Heat-inactivated Bifidobacterium bifidum MIMBb75 (SYN-HI-001) in the treatment of irritable bowel syndrome: A multicentre, randomised, double-blind, placebo-controlled clinical trial. *Lancet Gastroenterol. Hepatol.* **2020**, *5*, 658–666. [CrossRef]
34. Lewis, S.J.; Heaton, K.W. Stool form scale as a useful guide to intestinal transit time. *Scand. J. Gastroenterol.* **1997**, *32*, 920–924. [CrossRef] [PubMed]
35. Drossman, D.; Morris, C.B.; Hu, Y.; Toner, B.B.; Diamant, N.; Whitehead, W.E.; Dalton, C.B.; Leserman, J.; Patrick, D.L.; Bangdiwala, S.I. Characterization of health related quality of life (HRQOL) for patients with functional bowel disorder (FBD) and its response to treatment. *Am. J. Gastroenterol.* **2007**, *102*, 1442–1453. [CrossRef]
36. Davis, C.; Bryan, J.; Hodgson, J.; Murphy, K. Definition of the Mediterranean Diet; a Literature Review. *Nutrients* **2015**, *7*, 9139–9153. [CrossRef]
37. Ford, A.C.; Quigley, E.M.; Lacy, B.E.; Lembo, A.J.; Saito, Y.A.; Schiller, L.R.; Soffer, E.E.; Spiegel, B.M.; Moayyedi, P. Efficacy of prebiotics, probiotics, and synbiotics in irritable bowel syndrome and chronic idiopathic constipation: Systematic review and meta-analysis. *Am. J. Gastroenterol.* **2014**, *109*, 1547–1561. [CrossRef]
38. Duan, R.; Zhu, S.; Wang, B.; Duan, L. Alterations of gut microbiota in patients with irritable bowel syndrome based on 16 rRNA-targeted sequencing: A systemic review. *Clin. Gasteroenterol. Hepatol.* **2019**, *10*, e00012. [CrossRef]
39. Pittayanon, R.; Lau, J.T.; Yuan, Y.; Leontiadis, G.I.; Tse, F.; Surette, M.; Moayyedi, P. Gut microbiota in patients with irritable bowel syndrome—A systematic review. *Gastroenterology* **2019**, *157*, 97–108. [CrossRef]
40. Ki Cha, B.; Mun Jung, S.; Hwan Choi, C.; Song, I.D.; Woong Lee, H.; Joon Kim, H.; Hyuk, J.; Kyung Chang, S.; Kim, K.; Chung, W.S.; et al. The effect of a multispecies probiotic mixture on the symptoms and fecal microbiota in diarrhea-dominant irritable bowel syndrome: A randomized, double-blind, placebo-controlled trial. *J. Clin. Gastroenterol.* **2012**, *46*, 220–227. [CrossRef]
41. Giannetti, E.; Maglione, M.; Alessandrella, A.; Strisciuglio, C.; De Giovanni, D.; Campanozzi, A.; Miele, E.; Staiano, A. A Mixture of 3 Bifidobacteria Decreases Abdominal Pain and Improves the Quality of Life in Children With Irritable Bowel Syndrome: A Multicenter, Randomized, Double-Blind, Placebo-Controlled, Crossover Trial. *J. Clin. Gastroenterol.* **2017**, *51*, e5–e10. [CrossRef] [PubMed]

42. Pinto-Sanchez, M.I.; Hall, G.B.; Ghajar, K.; Nardelli, A.; Bolino, C.; Lau, J.T.; Martin, F.P.; Cominetti, O.; Welsh, C.; Rieder, A.; et al. Probiotic Bifidobacterium longum NCC3001 Reduces Depression Scores and Alters Brain Activity: A Pilot Study in Patients With Irritable Bowel Syndrome. *Gastroenterology* **2017**, *153*, 448–459. [CrossRef]
43. Barbara, G.; De Giorgio, R.; Stanghellini, V.; Cremon, C.; Corinaldesi, R. A role for inflammation in irritable bowel syndrome? *Gut* **2002**, *51*, i41–i44. [CrossRef] [PubMed]
44. Farzaei, M.H.; Bahramsoltani, R.; Abdollahi, M.; Rahimi, R. The Role of Visceral Hypersensitivity in Irritable Bowel Syndrome: Pharmacological Targets and Novel Treatments. *J. Neurogastroenterol. Motil.* **2016**, *22*, 558–574. [CrossRef] [PubMed]
45. Song, D.D.; Li, Y.; Tang, D.; Huang, L.Y.; Yuan, Y.Z. Neuron-glial communication mediated by TNF-alfa and glial activation in dorsal root ganglia in visceral inflammatory hypersensitivity. *Am. J. Physiol. Gastrointest. Liver Physiol.* **2014**, *306*, G788–G795. [CrossRef]
46. Bashashati, M.; Moradi, M.; Sarosiek, I. Interleukin-6 in irritable bowel syndrome: A systematic review and meta-analysis of IL-(-G174C) and circulating IL-6 levels. *Cytokine* **2017**, *99*, 132–138. [CrossRef]
47. Patel, S.R.; Singh, A.; Misra, V.; Misra, S.P.; Dwivedi, M.; Trivedi, P. Levels of interleukins 2, 6, 8, and 10 in patients with irritable bowel syndrome. *Indian J. Pathol. Microbiol.* **2017**, *60*, 385–389.
48. Bashashati, M.; Rezaei, N.; Shafieyoun, A.; McKernan, D.P.; Chang, L.; Öhman, L.; Quigley, E.M.; Schmulson, M.; Sharkey, K.A.; Simrén, M. Cytokine imbalance in irritable bowel syndrome: A systematic review and meta-analysis. *Neurogastroenterol. Motil.* **2014**, *26*, 1036–1048. [CrossRef]
49. Ng, Q.X.; Soh, A.Y.S.; Loke, W.; Lim, D.Y.; Yeo, W.S. The role of inflammation in irritable bowel syndrome (IBS). *J. Inflamm. Res.* **2018**, *11*, 345–349. [CrossRef]
50. Mujagic, Z.; Ludidi, S.; Keszthelyi, D.; Hesselink, M.A.; Kruimel, J.W.; Lenaerts, K.; Hanssen, N.M.; Conchillo, J.M.; Jonkers, D.M.; Masclee, A.A. Small intestinal permeability is increased in diarrhoea predominant IBS, while alterations in gastroduodenal permeability in all IBS subtypes are largely attributable to confounders. *Aliment. Pharmacol. Ther.* **2014**, *40*, 288–297. [CrossRef]
51. Rao, A.S.; Camilleri, M.; Eckert, D.J.; Busciglio, I.; Burton, D.D.; Ryks, M.; Wong, B.S.; Lamsam, J.; Singh, R.; Zinsmeister, A.R. Urine sugars for in vivo gut permeability: Validation and comparisons in irritable bowel syndrome-diarrhea and controls. *Am. J. Physiol. Gastrointest. Liver. Physiol.* **2011**, *301*, 919–928. [CrossRef] [PubMed]
52. Linsalata, M.; Riezzo, G.; D'Attoma, B.; Clemente, C.; Orlando, A.; Russo, F. Noninvasive biomarkers of gut barrier function identify two subtypes of patients suffering from diarrhoea predominant-IBS: A case-control study. *BMC Gastroenterol.* **2018**, *18*, 167. [CrossRef] [PubMed]
53. Bonfrate, L.; Di Palo, D.M.; Celano, G.; Albert, A.; Vitellio, P.; De Angelis, M.; Gobbetti, M.; Portincasa, P. Effects of Bifidobacterium longum BB536 and Lactobacillus rhamnosus HN001 in IBS patients. *Eur. J. Clin. Invest.* **2020**, *50*, e13201. [CrossRef] [PubMed]

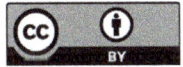

© 2020 by the authors. Licensee MDPI, Basel, Switzerland. This article is an open access article distributed under the terms and conditions of the Creative Commons Attribution (CC BY) license (http://creativecommons.org/licenses/by/4.0/).

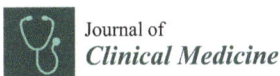 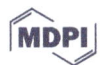

Article

Evolution of Gut Microbiome and Metabolome in Suspected Necrotizing Enterocolitis: A Case-Control Study

Camille Brehin [1,2], Damien Dubois [2,3], Odile Dicky [4], Sophie Breinig [5], Eric Oswald [2,3] and Matteo Serino [2,*]

1. General Pediatrics Department, Children Hospital, Toulouse University Hospital, 31300 Toulouse, France; brehin.c@chu-toulouse.fr
2. IRSD, Université de Toulouse, INSERM, INRAE, ENVT, UPS, 31024 Toulouse, France; dubois.d@chu-toulouse.fr (D.D.); eric.oswald@inserm.fr (E.O.)
3. Service of Bacteriology-Hygiene, Toulouse University Hospital, 31300 Toulouse, France
4. Department of Neonatology, Children Hospital, University Hospital, UMR 1027, INSERM, Paul Sabatier University, 31000 Toulouse, France; dicky.o@chu-toulouse.fr
5. Neonatal and Pediatric Intensive Care Unit, Toulouse University Hospital, 31300 Toulouse, France; breinig.s@chu-toulouse.fr
* Correspondence: matteo.serino@inserm.fr; Tel.: +33-(0)5-6274-4525

Received: 2 June 2020; Accepted: 15 July 2020; Published: 17 July 2020

Abstract: Background: Necrotizing enterocolitis (NEC) is a devastating condition in preterm infants due to multiple factors, including gut microbiota dysbiosis. NEC development is poorly understood, due to the focus on severe NEC (NEC-2/3). Methods: We studied the gut microbiota, microbiome and metabolome of children with suspected NEC (NEC-1). Results: NEC-1 gut microbiota had a higher abundance of the Streptococcus (second 10-days of life) and Staphylococcus (third 10-days of life) species. NEC-1 children showed a microbiome evolution in the third 10-days of life being the most divergent, and were associated with a different metabolomic signature than in healthy children. The NEC-1 microbiome had increased glycosaminoglycan degradation and lysosome activity by the first 10-days of life, and was more sensitive to childbirth, low birth weight and gestational age, than healthy microbiome. NEC-1 fecal metabolome was more divergent by the second month of life. Conclusions: NEC-1 gut microbiota and microbiome modifications appear more distinguishable by the third 10-days of life, compared to healthy children. These data identify a precise window of time (i.e., the third 10-days of life) and provide microbial targets to fight/blunt NEC-1 progression.

Keywords: necrotizing enterocolitis; intestinal microbiology; microbiome; infant gut; metabolomics

1. Introduction

Necrotizing enterocolitis (NEC), defined by the Bell classification [1–3], is the most severe intestinal disease in preterm infants, with a mortality score of 25% and long-term neurological morbidity [4]. Yet, a precise initiating factor of this pathology is missing. In the last decade, gut microbiota was identified and recognized as a specific organ with functions widely beyond digestion [5]. Both its taxonomic (relative abundance) and functional (microbial pathway) alterations, named dysbiosis, were described in several pathologies, in particular, metabolic diseases such as type 2 diabetes and obesity [6–8], and intestinal inflammatory diseases [9,10]. Importantly, a dysbiotic gut microbiota associated with a very high inflammatory status of the gut [11,12] may trigger NEC development, since germ-free mice do not develop NEC [13].

From a clinical and microbiological point of view, studies of NEC were focused only on established and severe phenotypes, such as NEC-2 and NEC-3. Based on the French study Etude épidémiologique sur les petits âges gestationnels (EPIPAGE 2), the incidence of proved NEC-2 and NEC-3 is 1–5% in preterm infants born at less than 32 weeks of gestation [14].

By contrast, NEC suspicions such as lethargy, bradycardia, thermic instability associated with biliary gastric residues, vomiting, abdominal distension with or without rectal bleeding, with a normal abdominal x-ray image or a simple dilatation, which identifies suspected NEC (NEC-1), have not been studied yet. In fact, enteropathies are frequent in the first weeks of life in preterm infants, though no data are available about NEC-1 incidence. This induces the end of alimentation, a prolonged (sometime life-lasting) parenteral nutrition, with a delayed gut maturation and failure to thrive [15]. Therefore, to study the evolution of gut microbiota and microbiome during the early onset of NEC, we focused on NEC-1 children within the first two months of life. We studied the fecal metabolome, to understand how a change in gut microbiota may drive alterations in intestinal metabolites. To further understand which factor of mother and child may affect the evolution of gut microbiota, microbiome and fecal metabolome during NEC-1, we analyzed: the presence of neonatal antibiotherapy (ABx), ABx treatment on the mother, childbirth (Cesarean-section (C-sec) vs. vaginal birth (VB)), very low birth weight (VLBW), extreme low birth weight (ELBW) and gestational age (GA) > or ≤ 28 weeks.

2. Research Design and Methods

2.1. Cohort Constitution

We conducted a prospective monocentric case-control cohort study. This study was approved (number of the approval: DC 2016-2804) by Neonatal and Pediatric Intensive Care Unit and Neonatology Department of Purpan Hospital in Toulouse, France. The parents of the children involved in this study gave their approval by written consent. The inclusion criteria regarding all of the children hospitalized into the Neonatal and Pediatric Intensive Care Unit or Neonatology Departments of the Purpan Hospital, were:

− Newborn of gestational age under 34 weeks of gestation;
− Diagnosis of suspected necrotizing enterocolitis (NEC-1) made by a neonatologist;
− Obtainment of the non-opposition from parents or their legal representative.

Following the inclusion of every case, we conducted in parallel a search for two controls, according to the following matching criteria, listed in decreasing priority:

− Gestational age (±1 week of gestation, priority to matched age);
− Body weight;
− Neonatal antibiotherapy;
− Childbirth (C-section vs. vaginal);
− Maternal antibiotherapy.

Inclusion criteria for controls were:

− Newborn of gestational age under 34 weeks of gestation;
− Respect of the matching according to the priority order of the established criteria;
− Obtainment of the oral non-opposition from parents or their legal representative.

Children with complex congenital cardiopathy or with spontaneous intestinal perforation without a radiological evidence of NEC were excluded from the study.

Based on these criteria, we included 11 NEC-1 children, with 27 feces collection (4 fecal samples for time-point 1–10 days (d); 10 fecal samples for time-point 11–20 d; 7 fecal samples for time-point 21–30 d; 6 fecal samples for time-point > 30 d) and 21 healthy children, with 53 feces collection (15 fecal samples for time-point 1–10 d; 14 fecal samples for time-point 11–20 d; 13 fecal samples for time-point 21–30 d; 11 fecal samples for time-point > 30 d). Hence, a total of 80 fecal samples was analyzed in our study. The period of collection was day 1 to day 68 of life of the newborn.

2.2. Taxonomic and Functional Analysis of Gut Microbiota

Feces analyzed in this study were collected by nurses in the related department in the first week of life and once a week till the end of the hospitalization. Feces were firstly kept at 4 °C in a 5 mL Eppendorf tube with 20% glycerol/Lysogeny Broth and then stored at −80 °C. Total DNA was extracted from feces as previously described [16], with a modification: a thermic shock of 30 seconds was performed between each bead-shaking step (3 bead-shaking steps of 30 seconds each at maximum speed). The 16S bacterial DNA V3–V4 regions were targeted by 357wf-785R primers and analyzed by MiSeq (RTLGenomics, Texas, USA). An average of 68,669 sequences was generated per sample. Bioinformatic filters applied as already described [17]. Cladogram and LDA scores were drawn via the LEfSe algorithm [18]. Diversity indices were calculated using the software Past 4.02 (Hammer, Ø., Harper, D.A.T., and P. D. Ryan, 2001. PAST: Paleontological Statistics Software Package for Education and Data Analysis. Palaeontologia Electronica 4(1): 9pp). The predictive functional analysis of the gut microbiota was performed via PICRUSt [19]. Diseases and host genetic variation linked to NEC-1_21–30 d-associated gut microbiota were identified via MicrobiomeAnalyst [20], with the Taxon Set Enrichment Analysis module.

2.3. Fecal Metabolome Analysis

The metabolome (total metabolites) analysis of the feces was performed as previously described [17]. Fecal samples have been prepared as it follows: 50 mg of feces were homogenized for 30 seconds in 500 μL of a pH 7.0 phosphate buffer, prepared in D_2O. Then, the homogenate was chilled into ice for 1 minute and centrifuged at 12,000 RPM for 10 minutes at 4 °C. The supernatant was then recovered, and the pellet was re-homogenized again at the same conditions of 12,000 RPM for 10 minutes at 4 °C. All the supernatants were then pooled and centrifuged at 18,000 RPM for 30 minutes at 4 °C. The supernatant was recovered and centrifuged again at the same conditions of 18,000 RPM for 30 minutes at 4 °C. A total of 600 μL of the final supernatant was then analyzed into nuclear magnetic resonance (NMR) tubes of 5 mm of diameter. The conformity criterium to validate the final sample was the aspect, to be crystal clear.

Pathway-associated metabolite sets and SNP-associated metabolite sets (Supplementary Figure S3 C,D, Supplementary Figure S4 B,C and Supplementary Figure S6 G) were analyzed via MetaboAnalyst 4.0 [21], with the enrichment analysis module.

2.4. Statistical Analysis

The results are presented as mean ± SEM for histograms and box and whiskers graphs. Statistical analyses were performed by two-way analysis of variance (ANOVA) followed by a two-stage linear step-up procedure of Benjamini, Krieger and Yekutieli to correct for multiple comparisons by controlling the false discovery rate (<0.05) (for histograms) or the Mann-Whitney test (for box and whiskers), as indicated in the figure legend, by using GraphPad Prism version 7.05 for Windows Vista (GraphPad Software, San Diego, CA, USA). For Table 1, results are presented as median or as indicated and P value was calculated using Fisher's exact test. Significant values were considered starting at $P < 0.05$. For the taxonomical and predictive functional analysis of gut microbiota, significant values were considered, starting at $P < 0.05$ or $P < 0.01$ when indicated. Principal component analysis (PCA) graphs were drawn by using Past 4.02.

Table 1. Cohorts characteristics.

Variables, Description	NEC-1 $n = 11$	Healthy $n = 21$	P (Fisher's Exact Test)
Birth weight, median, inter-quartile (IQ)	1150 (845–1815)	1360 (700–2105)	Not significant (ns) (> 0.05)
Gestational age, median (weeks) (IQ)	28.4 (26–31)	30 (26, 4–32)	ns
Gender			
Girls, number (%)	2 (18)	8 (38)	ns
Boys, number	9	13	-
Patent Ductus arteriosus, number (%)	3 (27)	6 (28)	ns
Parity, number (%)	3 (27)	3 (10)	ns
Antenatal corticosteroids, number (%)	11 (100)	19 (90)	ns
Hypertension, eclampsia, number (%)	2 (18)	3 (14)	ns
Multiple births, number (%)	2 (18)	4 (19)	ns
Antenatal antibiotics, number (%)	4 (36)	5 (24)	ns
Chorioamniotitis, number (%)	2 (18)	1 (5)	ns
Apgar Score, 1 min (IQ)	8 (1–10)	7 (1–10)	ns
5 min (IQ)	10 (4–10)	8 (1–10)	ns
Cordon pH (IQ)	7.23 (6.8–7.4)	7.31 (7.04–7.43)	ns
Cordon lactates (IQ)	5.7 (2.9–9.6)	3 (1–7.2)	0.04 * (<0.05)
Mean arterial pressure at hospital admission (IQ)	29 (20–47)	29.5 (17–43)	ns
Hospital Admission T (°C) (IQ)	36.5 (35.1–37.8)	36.8 (35.8–37.5)	ns
Antibiotics in the first week of life (%)	10 (90)	18 (85)	ns
Days under antibiotics (IQ)	7.5 (2–17)	3 (0–18)	ns
Days under antibiotics (Third-Generation-Cephalosporin (3GC) ± Penicillin A, ±aminoglycoside) in the first week of life (IQ)	3 (0–7)	3 (0–7)	ns
Children under glycopeptides number (%)	8 (72)	3 (14)	0.0018 ** (<0.01)
Bacteremia, number (%)	5 (45)	1 (5)	0.01 * (<0.05)
Exposition to mother milk, number (%)	11 (100)	21 (100)	ns
Age of enteropathy (days) (IQ)	12 (4–60)	-	-
Exposition to inotropes, number (%)	1 (9)	0 (0)	ns
Blood transfusion, number (%)	2 (18)	4 (19)	ns
Full enteral feeding (days) (IQ)	23 (14–39)	11 (3–29)	0.0002 *** (<0.001)
Median fasting time (median in days) (IQ)	1 (1–4)	-	-

3. Results

3.1. Analysis of Gut Microbiota, Microbiome and Fecal Metabolome During NEC-1

To understand the microbial and metabolomic evolution during the early onset of necrotizing enterocolitis (NEC), we studied clinical profile suspected NEC (NEC-1) preterm infants. NEC-1 children underwent more glycopeptides treatment, showed significantly higher cordon lactates, bacteremia and a longer full enteral feeding, when compared to age-matched healthy children (Table 1). NEC-1 children also displayed a lower plasma pH and enteral milk volume at day 7 (Supplementary Figure S1A,B) and a higher abundance of *Streptoccoccus* species (Supplementary Figure S2A) compared to healthy children. Both populations of children showed a high intragroup variance in terms of gut microbiota (Supplementary Figure S2B) and overall microbial diversity (Supplementary Figure S2C). NEC-1 microbiome showed increased activity for pathway related to transcription, glycosaminoglycan degradation and lysosome, compared to healthy children (Supplementary Figure S2D). Then, we analyzed the fecal metabolome to appreciate NEC-1-induced changes in gut microbial metabolic activity. NEC-1 children displayed a reduced intragroup variation and significantly lower levels of ethanol (Supplementary Figure S2E). Overall, these data show that NEC-1 is characterized by a precise gut microbiota, microbiome and gut microbial metabolites profile.

3.2. Analysis of Gut Microbiota, Microbiome and Fecal Metabolome During the Evolution of NEC-1 over the First Two Months of Life

Given the presence of a NEC-1-specific gut microbiota and microbiome profile, we aimed to identify at what time these profiles establish. We divided both NEC-1 and healthy children populations in subgroups according to periods of ten days of life as it follows: 1–10 d (d stands for "days"), 11–20 d, 21–30 d for the first month of life and > 30 d for the second one. In the first 10 days, NEC-1 children displayed a divergent and more homogenous gut microbiota compared to healthy children, with the latter characterized by a higher abundance of *Klebsiella* species (Figure 1A,B). At this stage of life, gut microbiota in NEC-1 had a lower diversity based on Chao-1 index (Figure 1C) and a different microbial activity related to replication, recombination and repair proteins, lysosome and glycosaminoglycan degradation (Figure 1D). No significant changes were observed in fecal metabolites (Figure 1E). Overall, these data show that gut microbiome starts to diverge at the early onset of NEC-1.

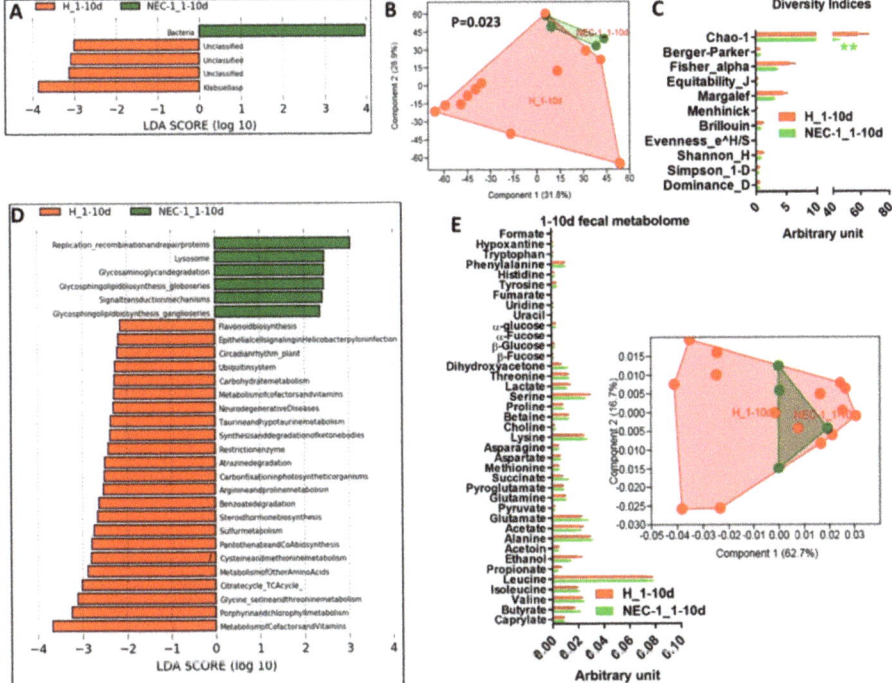

Figure 1. Analysis of gut microbiota, microbiome and metabolome in the first 10-days of life in healthy vs. necrotizing enterocolitis (NEC)-1 children. (**A**) Gut microbiota analysis via linear discriminant analysis (LDA) score between healthy (H) vs. NEC-1 children, in the first 10-days of life, 1 to 10 days; (**B**) principal component analysis (PCA) of the gut microbiota; (**C**) indices of gut microbiota diversity; (**D**) LDA score for microbial pathways; (**E**) histogram of the overall fecal metabolites and PCA as inset. **P < 0.01. Two-way ANOVA, followed by a two-stage linear step-up procedure of Benjamini, Krieger and Yekutieli to correct for multiple comparisons, by controlling the false discovery rate (<0.05); $N = 15$ for H and $N = 4$ for NEC-1.

In the second 10-days of life, NEC-1 gut microbiota was characterized again by a higher abundance of *Streptococcus* species and bacteria from the Micrococcales order (Figure 2A), with a high intragroup variance (Figure 2B). At this stage of life, NEC-1 gut microbiota also showed a higher diversity based on Chao-1 index (Figure 2C), but no microbial pathway differently regulated (Figure 2D). As for the fecal metabolome, NEC-1 children displayed significant lower levels of serine (Figure 2E). Overall, these data show a stronger evolution of gut microbiota than gut microbiome in the second 10-days of life, between NEC-1 and healthy children.

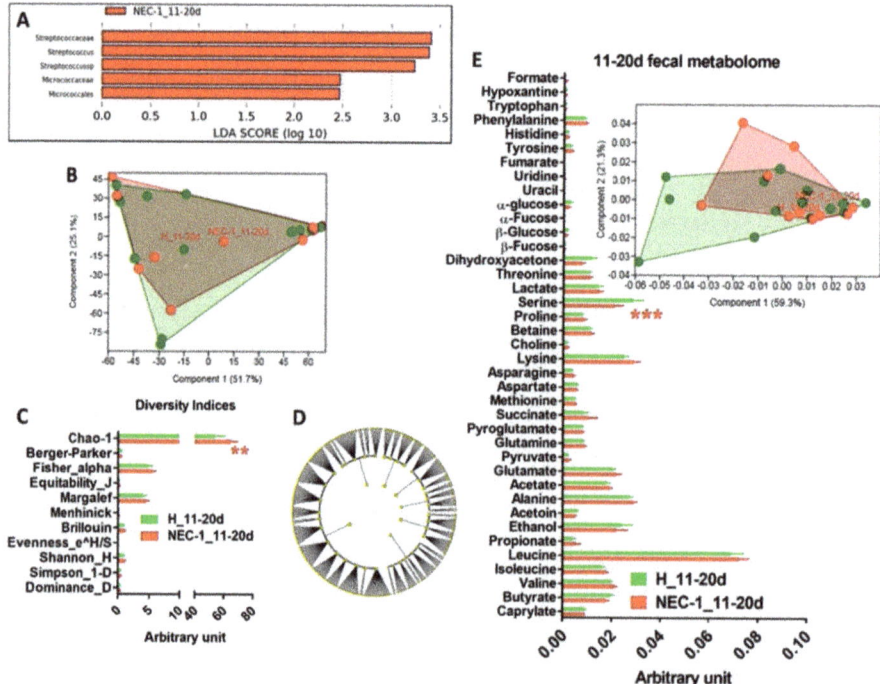

Figure 2. Analysis of gut microbiota, microbiome and metabolome in the second 10-days of life in healthy vs. NEC-1 children. (**A**) Gut microbiota analysis via LDA score between healthy (H) vs. NEC-1 children, in the second 10-days of life, 11 to 20 days (d) (the LDA score is only shown for NEC-1 children meaning that no bacteria are significantly higher in the H group vs. NEC-1); (**B**) PCA of the gut microbiota; (**C**) indices of gut microbiota diversity; (**D**) null cladogram for microbial pathways; (**E**) histogram of the overall fecal metabolites and PCA as inset. **$P < 0.01$. ***$P < 0.001$. Two-way ANOVA, followed by a two-stage linear step-up procedure of Benjamini, Krieger and Yekutieli to correct for multiple comparisons by controlling the false discovery rate (<0.05); $N = 14$ for H and $N = 10$ for NEC-1.

In the third 10-days of life, changes in NEC-1 gut microbiota compared to healthy children occurred to a bigger extent and were related to increased *Staphylococcus* and *Streptococcus* species (Figure 3A,B), together with a high intragroup variance (Figure 3C) and no change in the overall diversity indices (Figure 3D). We also observed a NEC-1 microbiome profile, mainly based on thiamine and seleno-compound metabolism (Figure 3E). The NEC-1 gut microbiota profile of the third 10-days of life was associated with: (i) multiple diseases and found significantly increased in ulcerative colitis (Figure 4A); (ii) host genetic variation and significantly related to ANP32E, a gene involved in ulcerative colitis [22], in line with previous reports. In terms of fecal metabolome, we observed no significant changes in NEC-1 vs. healthy children (Figure 4C). Then, we studied feces collected in the second month of life. In this period of life, the taxonomical differences in the gut microbiota of NEC-1 vs. healthy children were related to the increase in *Raoultella* species in NEC-1 gut microbiota (Figure 5A), with a still high intragroup variance (Figure 5B), and no change in the overall microbial diversity indices (Figure 5C). We also observed microbial functions related to DNA repair increased in the NEC-1 gut microbiome (Figure 5D). This period of life was characterized by the highest separation in terms of fecal metabolome, with significant lower levels of ethanol and leucine in NEC-1 children (Figure 5E).

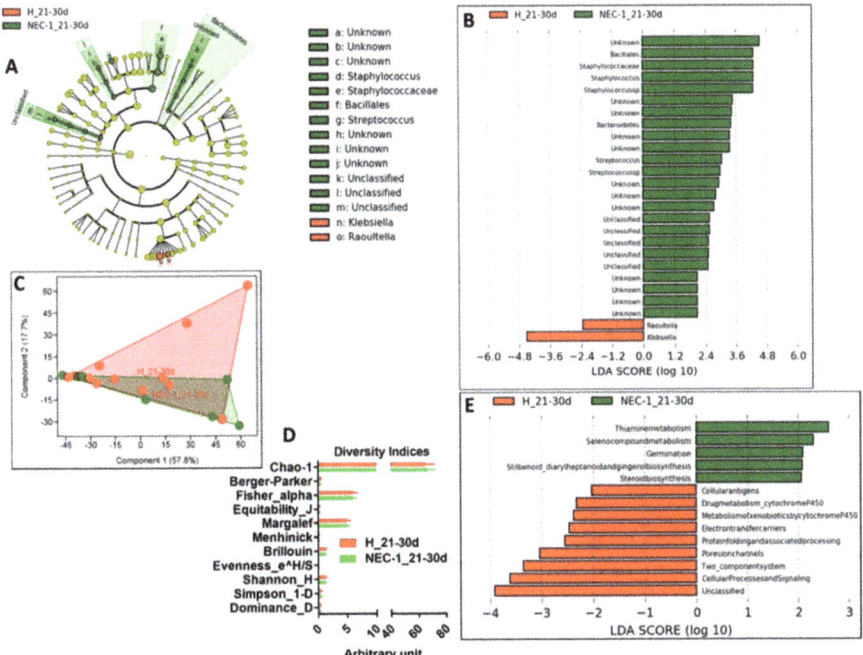

Figure 3. A specific gut microbiota and microbiome exist in the third 10-days of life in healthy vs. NEC-1 children. (**A**) Comparative analysis of the gut microbiota by LDA effect size (LEfSe): the cladogram shows bacterial taxa significantly higher in the group of children of the same color, in the fecal microbiota between healthy (H) vs. NEC-1 children, in the third 10-days of life, 21 to 30 days (**D**) (the cladogram shows the taxonomic levels represented by rings with phyla at the innermost and genera at the outermost ring and each circle is a bacterial member within that level); (**B**) LDA score used to build the cladogram in (A); (**C**) PCA of the gut microbiota; (**D**) indices of gut microbiota diversity; (**E**) LDA score for microbial pathways. $N = 13$ for H and $N = 7$ for NEC-1.

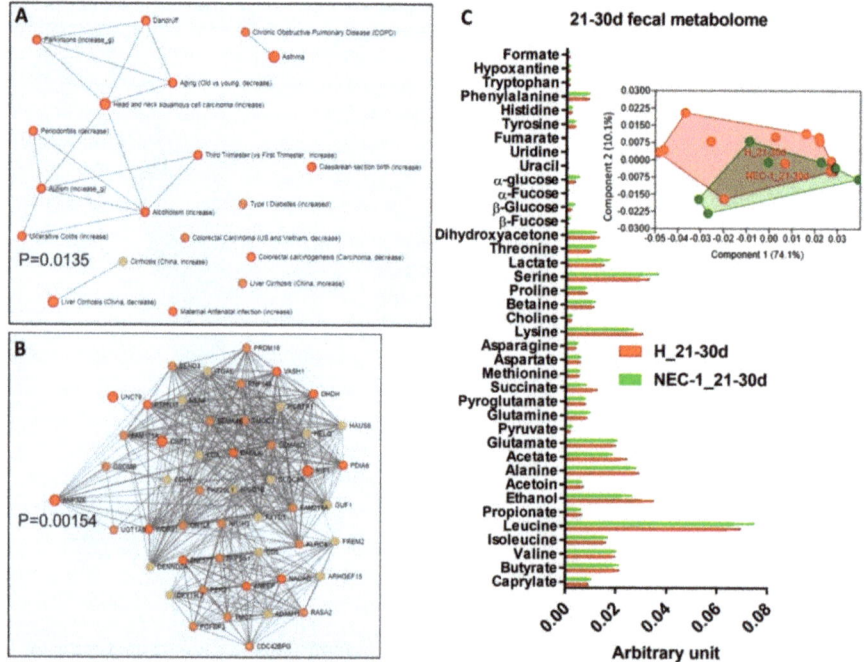

Figure 4. Diseases, host genetic variation and metabolome analysis in the third 10-days of life during NEC-1. (**A**) Diseases and (**B**) host genetic variation linked to NEC-1_21–30d associated gut microbiota; (**C**) histogram of the overall fecal metabolites and PCA, as inset. $N = 13$ for H and $N = 7$ for NEC-1.

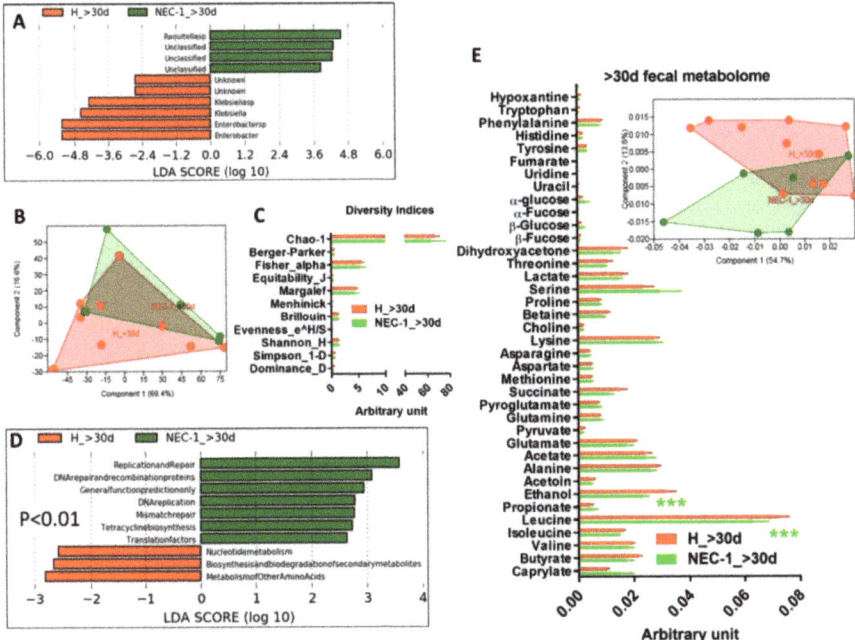

Figure 5. Analysis of gut microbiota, microbiome and metabolome in the second month of life in healthy vs. NEC-1 children. (**A**) Gut microbiota analysis via LDA score between healthy (H) vs. NEC-1 children, in the second month of life > 30 days (d); (**B**) principal component analysis (PCA) of the gut microbiota; (**C**) indices of gut microbiota diversity; (**D**) LDA score for predictive microbial pathways ($P < 0.01$); (**E**) histogram of the overall fecal metabolites and PCA, as inset. ***$P < 0.001$. Two-way ANOVA, followed by a two-stage linear step-up procedure of Benjamini, Krieger and Yekutiel,i to correct for multiple comparisons by controlling the false discovery rate (<0.05); $N = 11$ for H and $N = 6$ for NEC-1.

3.3. Specific Impact of NEC-1 on the Evolution of Gut Microbiota. Microbiome and Fecal Metabolome over the First Two Months of Life, Compared to Healthy Children

To investigate the evolution of gut microbiota, microbiome and fecal metabolome over the first two months of life, we conducted an intra-group study in both NEC-1 and healthy children, according to the four groups reported above: 1–10 d, 11–20 d, 21–30 d and > 30 d. We did not observe any taxonomic significant change in the gut microbiota of NEC-1 children. However, the group NEC-1_21–30 d had a specific gut microbiome with an increased restriction enzyme activity, among others (Supplementary Figure S3A). The four NEC-1 groups also differed in terms of fecal metabolome, with regard to leucine, ethanol and serine amounts (Supplementary Figure S3B). Based on these results, we performed a metabolomic enrichment analysis on two levels: (i) pathway-associated metabolite sets (Supplementary Figure S3C) and (ii) single nucleotide polymorphism (SNP)-associated metabolite sets (Supplementary Figure S3D). NEC-1 metabolomic profile (increased ethanol and serine) was significantly associated with both homocysteine degradation and phosphatidylethanolamine biosynthesis (Supplementary Figure S3C), with serine being the metabolite the most linked to NEC-1-associated SNP (Supplementary Figure S3D). By contrast, in healthy children, the four groups reported above did not differ in terms of both gut microbiota and microbiome, but only with regard to fecal metabolome (Supplementary Figure S4A). Healthy metabolomic profile (increased leucine, ethanol and dihydroxyacetone) was significantly associated with valine, leucine and isoleucine degradation and to ketone body metabolism (Supplementary Figure S4B), with leucine being the metabolite the most linked to healthy-associated SNP (Supplementary Figure S4C). Overall, these data suggest that: (i) a different intragroup evolution exists between NEC-1 and healthy children, with regard to gut microbiota and microbiome; and (ii) the NEC-1 microbiome appears to be more sensitive to mother-related factors.

3.4. Maternal and Child Factors Influencing the Gut Microbiota, Microbiome and Fecal Metabolome During NEC-1

Next, we asked which factor related to both mother and child may affect the most the above reported parameters. We analyzed six conditions: neonatal antibiotherapy (ABx), ABx treatment on mother, childbirth (C-section (C-sec) vs. vaginal birth (VB)), very low birth weight (VLBW), extreme low birth weight (ELBW) and gestational age (GA) > or ≤ 28 weeks.

Only neonatal ABx treatment affected the gut microbiota in both NEC-1 and healthy children (Supplementary Figure S5A). By contrast, all the above factors, except the VLBW, affected the gut microbiome (Supplementary Figure S5B–F). Note that childbirth modality, ELBW and GA affected the gut microbiome only in NEC-1 children (Supplementary Figure S5D–F). Moreover, all the above factors, except the neonatal ABx treatment and ELBW, affected the fecal metabolome between NEC-1 and healthy children (Supplementary Figure S6A–F). Then, we performed a metabolomic enrichment analysis on the pathway-associated metabolite sets, based on Supplementary Figure S6F, in which there is an increase in ethanol and succinate within in the NEC-1_GA ≤ 28 w. Ketone body and butyrate metabolism were the most significantly associated with this metabolomic set (Supplementary Figure S6G).

4. Discussion

In this prospective study, we focused on suspected necrotizing enterocolitis NEC-1 preterm infants. NEC-1 phenotype has been poorly clinically investigated, with no data available on gut microbiota, microbiome and fecal metabolome. By contrast, NEC-2 and NEC-3, more severe and established phenotypes, have been more characterized. As for clinical parameters, the increased cordon lactate levels we found in NEC-1 has been recently positively correlated to the development of enteropathy [23]. Hence, the hypothesis of hypoxic lesions in utero or during birth may not be excluded, and could even be predictive of neonatal morbidity. Importantly, the observed reduced enteral nutrition volume in NEC-1 is not a protective factor during the development of severe NEC (NEC-2 and NEC-3), but rather, it may lengthen hospitalization and infections risk [24]. Moreover, a recent multicentric study showed that a slow rate enteral feeding is associated with an increased risk of developing NEC-2 and NEC-3 [14].

NEC-1 children showed a high general variance for gut microbiota and fecal metabolome, which is in line with a personalized microbiota and fecal metabolome profiles of preterm infant [25]. This is evident from PCA analyses in Figure 4 C and Figure 5 E, where the metabolome profiles of the healthy vs. NEC-1 children appear to diverge, but are still presenting some overlap, due to high intragroup variance. Both this evidence and the delayed intestinal colonization of preterm infants [26,27] may explain the lack of NEC-1-specific microbial group in the first 10-days of life. The analysis by periods of ten days of life revealed a divergence for both gut microbiota and microbiome in NEC-1 by the third 10-days of life. In particular, the higher abundance of *Staphylococcus* in NEC-1 is in accordance with the early colonization by *Staphylococcus* bacteria of the intestine of preterm infants [28]. This datum suggests the third 10-days as an optimal time window to be targeted by antibiotics directed against bacterial species higher in NEC-1, such as *Staphylococcus*. However, in our study NEC-1 children who underwent glycopeptide and aminoglycoside therapy were more numerous than healthy children. Therefore, this evidence suggests that NEC-1 may be associated with glycopeptide and/or aminoglycoside-resistance, since NEC-1 gut microbiota was characterized by an increase, and not a decrease, of *Staphylococcus*. Since aminoglycosides are active antibiotics against enterobacteria, their administration could delay intestinal colonization by Proteobacteria, and thus promote the implantation of resistant genera, such as *Staphylococcus* and *Streptococcus*. Based on this evidence, our data suggest not to prolong antibiotic therapy beyond the first week of life in preterm infants, if inflammatory parameters have been normalized. Furthermore, NEC-1 gut microbiota profile was associated with ulcerative colitis and host genetic variation in the ANP32E gene, encoding a protein implicated in cortico-resistance during ulcerative colitis [22]. NEC-1 children showed increased exposition to antenatal corticosteroids compared to healthy children, even though a study has not identified antenatal corticosteroids as a NEC-inducing factor [29]. Despite Anp32e-deficient mice display no sign of disease [30], it has not to be excluded the role of Anp32e in a model of gut inflammation mimicking ulcerative colitis. Hence, further studies are warranted on genetic factors of NEC. In terms of microbial functions, the intragroup analysis showed in the third 10-days of life a higher restriction enzyme activity in the NEC-1 gut microbiome. This bacterial activity, directed against bacteriophages and enriched in the newborn intestine [31], suggests an increased virus activity and, hence, a virome dysbiosis, beyond a microbiota dysbiosis, during NEC-1 evolution. Notably, with regard to the time-point > 30 days, microbiota and microbiome changes are still present and, most importantly, different from those observed at earlier time-points. This suggests that NEC-1 onset may have influenced the evolution of gut microbiota. All these microbial data are associated with our observation about a change in fecal amino-acids, such as leucine and serine, confirming the association between gut microbiota dysbiosis and a change in amino-acids metabolism [32].

Finally, several factors may affect the gut microbiota of preterm infants, e.g., hospital regimens, even with regard to the putative use of probiotics to blunt NEC. In a very recent publication, Kurath-Koller et al. showed the efficacy of some probiotics in improving the gut microbiome of very low birth weight infants during the first two weeks of age, in a triple-center cohort study [33]. In our mono-centric study, the very low birth weight had an impact on the fecal metabolome of both healthy and NEC-1 children, but not on their gut microbiota nor on their microbiome. This evidence underlines the importance of the hospital environment for the evolution of both an eubiotic and a dysbiotic, e.g., during NEC-1, gut microbiota.

5. Conclusions

The small cohort represents a limitation of our work, due to the difficulty to investigate NEC at its early onset. However, our data may provide neonatal departments with immediate indications to blunt NEC-1 evolution such as: i) increasing the enteral volume of nutrition, especially in the first days of life; ii) revising and reducing antibiotic therapy up to the first week of life in preterm infants.

Availability of data and materials: All data are available in the main text or the supplementary materials and via the following repositories: Sequence Read Archive (SRA) database with the assigned identifier PRJNA579480.

Ethics approval and consent to participate: This study was approved (number of the approval: DC 2016-2804) by Neonatal and Pediatric Intensive Care Unit and Neonatology Department of Purpan Hospital in Toulouse, France. The parents of the children involved in this study gave their approval by written consensus.

Supplementary Materials: The following are available online at http://www.mdpi.com/2077-0383/9/7/2278/s1, Figure S1: Baseline plasma characteristics in healthy vs. NEC-1 children, Figure S2: Analysis of gut microbiota, microbiome and metabolome during NEC-1 over the first two months of life, Figure S3: A specific microbiome and metabolome exist in healthy vs. NEC-1 children over the first two months of life, Figure S4: Fecal metabolome progression over the first two months of life in healthy children, Figure S5: Maternal and child factors shaping gut microbiota and microbiome in healthy vs. NEC-1 children, Figure S6: Maternal and child factors shaping fecal metabolome in healthy vs. NEC-1 children.

Author Contributions: Conceptualization, C.B. and M.S.; Data curation, C.B. and M.S.; Formal analysis, C.B. and M.S.; Funding acquisition, M.S.; Investigation, M.S.; Methodology, C.B., D.D. and M.S.; Project administration, M.S.; Resources, C.B., O.D. and S.B.; Supervision, M.S. and E.O.; Validation, M.S.; Writing—original draft, C.B. and M.S.; Writing—review & editing, C.B. and M.S. All authors have read and agreed to the published version of the manuscript.

Funding: This research was funded by LONGEVIE SA, grant to M.S.

Acknowledgments: We thank the departments of Neonatal and Pediatric Intensive Care Unit and Neonatology of the Purpan Hospital, Toulouse, France. We also thank Cecile Canlet and the Platform MetaToul-AXIOM for the metabolomic NMR analysis.

Conflicts of Interest: The authors declare no conflict of interest. The funders had no role in the design of the study; in the collection, analyses, or interpretation of data; in the writing of the manuscript, or in the decision to publish the results.

References

1. Bell, R.S. Neonatal necrotizing enterocolitis. *N. Engl. J. Med.* **1970**, *283*, 153–154. [CrossRef] [PubMed]
2. Bell, M.J. Neonatal necrotizing enterocolitis. *N. Engl. J. Med.* **1978**, *298*, 281–282. [CrossRef]
3. Kliegman, R.M.; Walsh, M.C. Neonatal necrotizing enterocolitis: Pathogenesis, classification, and spectrum of illness. *Curr. Probl. pediatr.* **1987**, *17*, 213–288. [CrossRef]
4. Ancel, P.Y.; Goffinet, F.; Group, E.-W.; Kuhn, P.; Langer, B.; Matis, J.; Hernandorena, X.; Chabanier, P.; Joly-Pedespan, L.; Lecomte, B.; et al. Survival and morbidity of preterm children born at 22 through 34 weeks' gestation in France in 2011: Results of the EPIPAGE-2 cohort study. *JAMA Pediatr.* **2015**, *169*, 230–238. [CrossRef] [PubMed]
5. Durazzo, M.; Ferro, A.; Gruden, G. Gastrointestinal Microbiota and Type 1 Diabetes Mellitus: The State of Art. *J. Clin. Med.* **2019**, *8*, 1843. [CrossRef] [PubMed]
6. Serino, M.; Blasco-Baque, V.; Nicolas, S.; Burcelin, R. Managing the manager: Gut microbes, stem cells and metabolism. *Diabetes Metab.* **2014**, *40*, 186–190. [CrossRef]
7. Serino, M.; Chabo, C.; Burcelin, R. Intestinal MicrobiOMICS to define health and disease in human and mice. *Curr. Pharm. Biotechnol.* **2012**, *13*, 746–758. [CrossRef]
8. Serino, M.; Luche, E.; Chabo, C.; Amar, J.; Burcelin, R. Intestinal microflora and metabolic diseases. *Diabetes Metab.* **2009**, *35*, 262–272. [CrossRef]
9. Bertani, L.; Caviglia, G.P.; Antonioli, L.; Pellicano, R.; Fagoonee, S.; Astegiano, M.; Saracco, G.M.; Bugianesi, E.; Blandizzi, C.; Costa, F.; et al. Serum Interleukin-6 and -8 as Predictors of Response to Vedolizumab in Inflammatory Bowel Diseases. *J. Clin. Med.* **2020**, *9*, 1323. [CrossRef]
10. Ni, J.; Wu, G.D.; Albenberg, L.; Tomov, V.T. Gut microbiota and IBD: Causation or correlation? *Nat. Rev. Gastroenterol. Hepatol.* **2017**, *14*, 573–584. [CrossRef]
11. Claud, E.C.; Walker, W.A. Bacterial colonization, probiotics, and necrotizing enterocolitis. *J. Clin. Gastroenterol.* **2008**, *42* (Suppl. S2), S46–S52. [CrossRef]
12. Pammi, M.; Cope, J.; Tarr, P.I.; Warner, B.B.; Morrow, A.L.; Mai, V.; Gregory, K.E.; Kroll, J.S.; McMurtry, V.; Ferris, M.J.; et al. Intestinal dysbiosis in preterm infants preceding necrotizing enterocolitis: A systematic review and meta-analysis. *Microbiome* **2017**, *5*, 31. [CrossRef] [PubMed]
13. Musemeche, C.A.; Kosloske, A.M.; Bartow, S.A.; Umland, E.T. Comparative effects of ischemia, bacteria, and substrate on the pathogenesis of intestinal necrosis. *J. Pediatr. Surg.* **1986**, *21*, 536–538. [CrossRef]
14. Roze, J.C.; Ancel, P.Y.; Lepage, P.; Martin-Marchand, L.; Al Nabhani, Z.; Delannoy, J.; Picaud, J.C.; Lapillonne, A.; Aires, J.; Durox, M.; et al. Nutritional strategies and gut microbiota composition as risk factors for necrotizing enterocolitis in very-preterm infants. *Am. J. Clin. Nutr.* **2017**, *106*, 821–830. [CrossRef]
15. Bazacliu, C.; Neu, J. Necrotizing Enterocolitis: Long Term Complications. *Curr. Pediatr. Rev.* **2019**, *15*, 115–124. [CrossRef] [PubMed]
16. Serino, M.; Luche, E.; Gres, S.; Baylac, A.; Berge, M.; Cenac, C.; Waget, A.; Klopp, P.; Iacovoni, J.; Klopp, C.; et al. Metabolic adaptation to a high-fat diet is associated with a change in the gut microbiota. *Gut* **2012**, *61*, 543–553. [CrossRef] [PubMed]
17. Nicolas, S.; Blasco-Baque, V.; Fournel, A.; Gilleron, J.; Klopp, P.; Waget, A.; Ceppo, F.; Marlin, A.; Padmanabhan, R.; Iacovoni, J.S.; et al. Transfer of dysbiotic gut microbiota has beneficial effects on host liver metabolism. *Mol. Syst. Biol.* **2017**, *13*, 921. [CrossRef]
18. Segata, N.; Izard, J.; Waldron, L.; Gevers, D.; Miropolsky, L.; Garrett, W.S.; Huttenhower, C. Metagenomic biomarker discovery and explanation. *Genome. Biol.* **2011**, *12*, R60. [CrossRef]
19. Langille, M.G.; Zaneveld, J.; Caporaso, J.G.; McDonald, D.; Knights, D.; Reyes, J.A.; Clemente, J.C.; Burkepile, D.E.; Vega Thurber, R.L.; Knight, R.; et al. Predictive functional profiling of microbial communities using 16S rRNA marker gene sequences. *Nat. Biotechnol.* **2013**, *31*, 814–821. [CrossRef] [PubMed]

20. Dhariwal, A.; Chong, J.; Habib, S.; King, I.L.; Agellon, L.B.; Xia, J. MicrobiomeAnalyst: A web-based tool for comprehensive statistical, visual and meta-analysis of microbiome data. *Nucleic Acids Res.* **2017**, *45*, W180–W188. [CrossRef]
21. Xia, J.; Psychogios, N.; Young, N.; Wishart, D.S. MetaboAnalyst: A web server for metabolomic data analysis and interpretation. *Nucleic Acids Res.* **2009**, *37*, W652–W660. [CrossRef] [PubMed]
22. Loren, V.; Garcia-Jaraquemada, A.; Naves, J.E.; Carmona, X.; Manosa, M.; Aransay, A.M.; Lavin, J.L.; Sanchez, I.; Cabre, E.; Manye, J.; et al. ANP32E, a Protein Involved in Steroid-Refractoriness in Ulcerative Colitis, Identified by a Systems Biology Approach. *J. Crohns Colitis* **2019**, *13*, 351–361. [CrossRef] [PubMed]
23. Tuuli, M.G.; Stout, M.J.; Shanks, A.; Odibo, A.O.; Macones, G.A.; Cahill, A.G. Umbilical cord arterial lactate compared with pH for predicting neonatal morbidity at term. *Obstet. Gynecol.* **2014**, *124*, 756–761. [CrossRef] [PubMed]
24. Oddie, S.J.; Young, L.; McGuire, W. Slow advancement of enteral feed volumes to prevent necrotising enterocolitis in very low birth weight infants. *Cochrane Database Syst. Rev.* **2017**, *8*, CD001241. [CrossRef]
25. Wandro, S.; Osborne, S.; Enriquez, C.; Bixby, C.; Arrieta, A.; Whiteson, K. The Microbiome and Metabolome of Preterm Infant Stool Are Personalized and Not Driven by Health Outcomes, Including Necrotizing Enterocolitis and Late-Onset Sepsis. *Msphere* **2018**, *3*. [CrossRef]
26. Groer, M.W.; Luciano, A.A.; Dishaw, L.J.; Ashmeade, T.L.; Miller, E.; Gilbert, J.A. Development of the preterm infant gut microbiome: A research priority. *Microbiome* **2014**, *2*, 38. [CrossRef]
27. Ho, T.T.B.; Groer, M.W.; Kane, B.; Yee, A.L.; Torres, B.A.; Gilbert, J.A.; Maheshwari, A. Dichotomous development of the gut microbiome in preterm infants. *Microbiome* **2018**, *6*, 157. [CrossRef]
28. Gibson, M.K.; Wang, B.; Ahmadi, S.; Burnham, C.A.; Tarr, P.I.; Warner, B.B.; Dantas, G. Developmental dynamics of the preterm infant gut microbiota and antibiotic resistome. *Nat. Microbiol.* **2016**, *1*, 16024. [CrossRef]
29. Travers, C.P.; Clark, R.H.; Spitzer, A.R.; Das, A.; Garite, T.J.; Carlo, W.A. Exposure to any antenatal corticosteroids and outcomes in preterm infants by gestational age: Prospective cohort study. *BMJ* **2017**, *356*, j1039. [CrossRef]
30. Reilly, P.T.; Afzal, S.; Wakeham, A.; Haight, J.; You-Ten, A.; Zaugg, K.; Dembowy, J.; Young, A.; Mak, T.W. Generation and characterization of the Anp32e-deficient mouse. *PLoS ONE* **2010**, *5*, e13597. [CrossRef]
31. Lim, E.S.; Zhou, Y.; Zhao, G.; Bauer, I.K.; Droit, L.; Ndao, I.M.; Warner, B.B.; Tarr, P.I.; Wang, D.; Holtz, L.R. Early life dynamics of the human gut virome and bacterial microbiome in infants. *Nat. Med.* **2015**, *21*, 1228–1234. [CrossRef] [PubMed]
32. Mardinoglu, A.; Shoaie, S.; Bergentall, M.; Ghaffari, P.; Zhang, C.; Larsson, E.; Backhed, F.; Nielsen, J. The gut microbiota modulates host amino acid and glutathione metabolism in mice. *Mol. Syst. Biol.* **2015**, *11*, 834. [CrossRef] [PubMed]
33. Kurath-Koller, S.; Neumann, C.; Moissl-Eichinger, C.; Kraschl, R.; Kanduth, C.; Hopfer, B.; Pausan, M.R.; Urlesberger, B.; Resch, B. Hospital Regimens Including Probiotics Guide the Individual Development of the Gut Microbiome of Very Low Birth Weight Infants in the First Two Weeks of Life. *Nutrients* **2020**, *12*, 1256. [CrossRef] [PubMed]

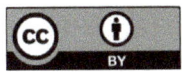

© 2020 by the authors. Licensee MDPI, Basel, Switzerland. This article is an open access article distributed under the terms and conditions of the Creative Commons Attribution (CC BY) license (http://creativecommons.org/licenses/by/4.0/).

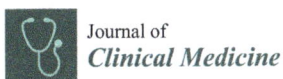

Article

Adalimumab Therapy Improves Intestinal Dysbiosis in Crohn's Disease

Davide Giuseppe Ribaldone [1,*], Gian Paolo Caviglia [2,*], Amina Abdulle [2], Rinaldo Pellicano [3], Maria Chiara Ditto [4], Mario Morino [1], Enrico Fusaro [4], Giorgio Maria Saracco [2], Elisabetta Bugianesi [2] and Marco Astegiano [3]

1. Department of Surgical Sciences, University of Turin, 10124 Turin, Italy; mario.morino@unito.it
2. Department of Medical Sciences, University of Turin, 10124 Turin, Italy; amina.abdulle@edu.unito.it (A.A.); giorgiomaria.saracco@unito.it (G.M.S.); ebugianesi@yahoo.it (E.B.)
3. Unit of Gastroenterology, Molinette Hospital, 10126 Turin, Italy; rinaldo_pellican@hotmail.com (R.P.); marcoastegiano58@gmail.com (M.A.)
4. S.C. Reumatologia, Città della Salute e della Scienza di Torino, 10126 Turin, Italy; mariachiaraditto@gmail.com (M.C.D.); fusaro.reumatorino@gmail.com (E.F.)
* Correspondence: davrib_1998@yahoo.com (D.G.R.); caviglia.giampi@libero.it (G.P.C.); Tel.: +39-011-6333918 (D.G.R.)

Received: 17 September 2019; Accepted: 8 October 2019; Published: 9 October 2019

Abstract: The response to treatment with biologic drugs, in patients with Crohn's disease, could be associated with changes in gut microbiota composition. The aim of our study was to analyse the modification of microbiota during adalimumab therapy in patients with Crohn's disease. We performed a prospective study in patients with Crohn's disease analysing gut microbiota before start of adalimumab therapy (T0) and after six months of therapy (T1). Among the 20 included patients, the phylum *Proteobacteria* fell from 15.7 ± 3.5% at T0 to 10.3 ± 3.4% at T1 ($p = 0.038$). Furthermore, the trend in relation to therapeutic success was analysed. Regarding bacterial phyla, *Proteobacteria* decreased in patients in whom therapeutic success was obtained, passing from a value of 15.8% (± 4.6%) to 6.8 ± 3.1% ($p = 0.049$), while in non-responder patients, percentages did not change (T0 = 15.6 ± 5.7%, T1 = 16.8 ± 7.6%, $p = 0.890$). Regarding the *Lachnospiraceae* family, in patients with normalization of C reactive protein six 6 months of adalimumab therapy, it increased from 16.6 ± 3.1% at T0 to 23.9 ± 2.6% at T1 ($p = 0.049$). In conclusion, in patients who respond to Adalimumab therapy by decreasing inflammation, there is a trend of intestinal eubiosis being restored.

Keywords: *Bacteroides ovatus*; *Bifidobacterium adolescentis*; Dysbiosis; *Faecalibacterium prausnitzii*; *Ruminococcus gnavus*

1. Introduction

Inflammatory bowel diseases (IBD) are chronic diseases that share immune-mediated pathogenesis and relapsing course [1]. Crohn's disease (CD) and ulcerative colitis (UC) are the two main IBD types. The exact pathogenesis of IBD remains unknown. The most recent studies agree in identifying an individual genetic susceptibility strongly conditioned by environmental factors and by the interaction between intestinal microbiota and the body's immune response [2,3]. Changes in the epidemiology of IBD over time and in different geographical areas suggest that environmental factors play an important role in inducing or modifying the expression of the disease [4]. Considering that IBD emerged in Western countries around the middle of the 20th century and the increased incidence of IBD in developing countries over the last 25 years, this epidemiological evolution is supposed to be linked to both the Westernization of the lifestyle and industrialization. Urbanization is associated with dietary changes, antibiotic use, hygienic status, microbial exposure and pollution, all implicated as potential environmental risk factors for IBD [5]. A consequence of Westernization of the lifestyle seems to be dysbiosis, defined as a loss of diversity of composition of microbiome in an individual. Microbial diversity decreases in patients with CD compared to subjects without CD [6].

Biological drugs, first of all anti-tumor necrosis factor (TNF), are able to modify the natural history of numerous inflammatory diseases [7], in part by acting directly on inflammation and partly indirectly with mechanisms not yet fully understood. Few studies have analysed the effect of adalimumab therapy on specific bacteria of intestinal microbiota in adult IBD patients [8].

The aim of our study was to analyse microbiome modifications and the association of microbiome characteristics with inflammatory parameters during the first six months of adalimumab therapy in adult patients with CD.

2. Materials and Methods

We performed a prospective study at the Gastroenterology Unit of "City of Health and Science of Turin", Italy. From May 2018 to March 2019 we recruited patients: (1) affected by CD with indications to treatment with adalimumab; (2) naive to anti-TNF drugs or other biological drugs; (3) older than or equal to 18 years; (4) on a typical Mediterranean diet; (5) who agreed to sign the informed consent to participate in the study. Exclusion criteria were: (1) recent (in the last month) use of probiotic therapy; (2) recent (in the last month) use of antibiotic therapy.

2.1. Screening Procedures

The selected patients underwent an infectious screening (HBsAg, HBcAb, HBsAb; HCV-Ab; quantiferon-TB gold assay, chest X-ray, HIV-Ab, HPV test, VZV-Ab, EBV-Ab) before starting adalimumab therapy. Clinical history, data on physical examination, instrumental examinations, recent biochemical examinations and signed informed consent for the purpose of enrolment in the study were collected. Before starting adalimumab therapy, a faecal sample from the patients was taken, collected in the previous 24 h, in a sterile container, with the caution to reduce as much as possible contaminating contacts of the sample. The faecal samples were associated with a numerical identification code and stored frozen at −80 °C. Two faecal samples were collected from each CD patient; the first before the start of adalimumab therapy and the second after six months of treatment. The samples underwent metagenomic NGS (next generation sequencing or sequencing in parallel) sequencing with the use of the Illumina MiSeq platform (San Diego, CA, USA) following the amplification of the V3-V4 regions of the 16s-rRNA gene (ribosomal 16-S gene) using a 2×300 bp-end approach [9–11].

2.2. Outcomes

The primary outcome was to evaluate a possible modification of the microbiota at six months of therapy. The secondary outcomes were to evaluate: (1) the possible association of the microbiome characteristics with C-reactive protein (CRP) levels at six months of therapy; (2) the possible predictive role of the microbiome on the response to anti-TNF therapy. Response to adalimumab therapy was defined as a decrease in the Harvey-Bradshaw index (HBI) score greater than or equal to 2 (or HBI ≤ 4 at six months), in the absence of corticosteroid therapy and with adalimumab still in therapy, in agreement with the literature [12]. The study followed the principles of the Declaration of Helsinki and was approved by the local ethical committee (Comitato Etico Interaziendale A.O.U. Città della Salute e della Scienza di Torino-A.O. Ordine Mauriziano-A.S.L. Città di Torino) (approval code 0056924).

2.3. Statistical Analysis

Continuous variables were reported as mean ± standard error of the mean (SEM) or as median (range) depending on data distribution. The normality of the data was evaluated by D'Agostino-Pearson test. The comparison of continuous variables between independent groups was done by employing the Mann-Whitney test. The comparison of paired measurements was carried out by t-student test for paired measurements or by Wilcoxon test, depending on the distribution of the data. For dichotomous qualitative variables, the Chi-square test was performed. A logistic regression was performed in order to derive the odds ratio (OR), with its 95% confidence interval, as a measure of the strength of association of the two variables. A p value of less than 0.05 was considered significant. The statistical analysis was performed with MedCalc Statistical Software version 18.9.1 (MedCalc Software bvba, Ostend, Belgium; http://www.medcalc.org; 2018).

3. Results

The cohort included 20 patients. The epidemiological characteristics of the recruited patients are reported in Table 1.

Table 1. Features of the study population.

General Characteristics (n = 20)	
Sex (M/F), n (%)	12/8 (60%)
Age (years), median (range)	52.5 (26–69)
Prior ileocecal resection (yes/no), n (%)	9/11 (45%)
Smoke (current/no), n (%)	4/16 (20%)
Localization (colon/ileum only), n (%)	12/8 (60%)
Years of illness (years), median (range)	14.5 (1–38)

Abbreviations: female (F), male (M).

Upon initiation of adalimumab therapy, 90% of patients received in combination mesalazine, 60% of patients took systemic corticosteroids and 20% took an immunosuppressant (azathioprine). Clinical, biochemical and endoscopic activity, before starting adalimumab therapy, is reported in Table 2.

Table 2. Activity according to Harvey-Bradshaw index (HBI) score, biochemical activity and endoscopic activity according to simple endoscopic score for Crohn's disease (SES-CD) at baseline.

Total Patients (n = 20)	
Clinical activity	
Remission or mild, n (%)	14 (70%)
Moderate or severe, n (%)	6 (30%)
Biochemical activity	
CRP (mg/L), median (range)	6.5 (0.7–45.5)
ESR (mm/h), median (range)	22 (1–94)
FC (µg/g), median (range)	262 (35–726)
Endoscopic activity	
Mild, n (%)	2 (10%)
Moderate, n (%)	13 (65%)
Severe, n (%)	5 (25%)

Abbreviations: C-reactive protein (CRP), erythrocyte sedimentation rate (ESR), faecal calprotectin (FC).

3.1. Clinical Outcomes

After six months of therapy, no patient discontinued adalimumab due to adverse effects and 100% of the patients achieved clinical remission, but the success of the therapy was only achieved in 65% of patients (13 out of 20), namely the remaining seven on corticosteroid therapy. CRP decreased from a median value of 6.5 mg/L (0.7–45.5 mg/L) at T0 to a median value of 2.9 mg/L (0.1–16.5 mg/L) at T1 (p = 0.010). Similarly, erythrocyte sedimentation rate (ESR) decreased from the median value of 22 mm/h (1–94 mm/h) at T0 to 9 mm/h (4–60 mm/h) at T1 (p = 0.020). Calprotectin decreased from a median value of 262 ug/g (35–726 ug/g) at T0 to a median value of 80 ug/g (39–969 ug/g) at T1 (p = 0.035) (Figure 1).

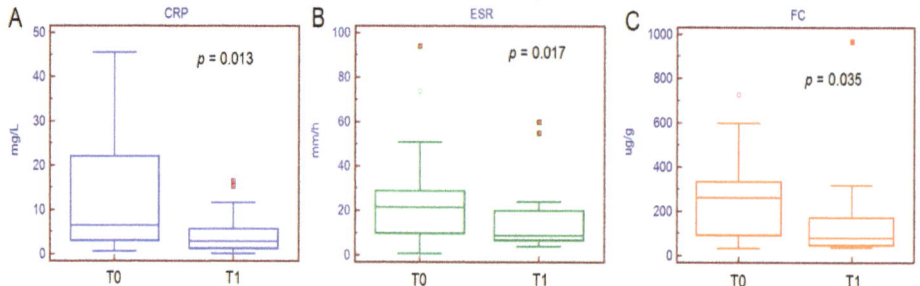

Figure 1. Serum and faecal inflammatory biomarkers trend after six months of adalimumab therapy.

3.2. Trend of Microbiota During Therapy

Focusing on the temporal trend, regarding the phyla, *Firmicutes* rose from 45.5 ± 5.1% at T0 to 48.9 ± 3.0% at T1 ($p = 0.523$), *Bacteroidetes* from 33.5 ± 4.7% at T0 to 37.1 ± 4.0% at T1 ($p = 0.411$), *Proteobacteria* fell from 15.7% ± 3.5% at T0 to 10.3 ± 3.4% at T1 ($p = 0.038$). Finally, the *Actinobacteria* increased from 2.6% ± 0.7% at T0 to 3.0% ± 0.7% at T1 ($p = 0.928$) (Figure 2).

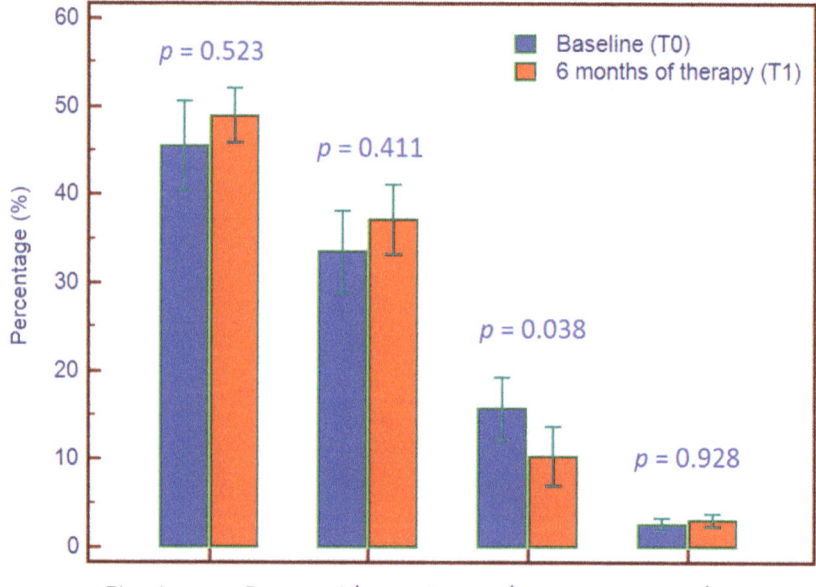

Figure 2. Per cent composition of phyla of bacterial microbiome at baseline and six months after starting adalimumab therapy.

Regarding the bacterial families, that of *Lachnospiraceae* was the most represented both at T0 (18.2 ± 2.6%), and at T1 (23.6 ± 2.2%), without statistical difference between these two periods ($p = 0.100$). Regarding the species, *Ruminococcus gnavus* decreased from 3.3 ± 1.8% at T0 to 1.6 ± 0.3% at T1 ($p = 0.350$); *Bacteroides ovatus* rose from 2.9 ± 0.9% to 2.4 ± 0.6% ($p = 0.540$); *Faecalibacterium prausnitzii* rose from 3.7 ± 1.2% to 2.2 ± 0.8% ($p = 0.130$), *Bifidobacterium adolescentis* decreased from 1.3 ± 0.5% to 1.2 ± 0.5% ($p = 0.260$); *Escherichia coli* did not change (11.4%, $p = 0.998$).

Baseline microbiota changes in relation to success or therapeutic failure are reported in Table 3.

Table 3. Relationship between bacterial populations of phyla, family and species and therapeutic success.

	Success = Yes (%)	Success = No (%)	p Value
Phyla			
Firmicutes	45.6 ± 6.7	45.2 ± 8.4	0.960
Bacteroidetes	34.7 ± 5.3	31.1 ± 9.6	0.320
Proteobacteria	15.8 ± 4.6	15.6 ± 5.7	0.980
Actinobacteria	2.6 ± 0.8	2.6 ± 1.4	0.980
Family			
Lachnospiraceae	17.8 ± 3.3	18.8 ± 4.8	0.860
Species			
Bifidobacterium adolescentis	1.1 ± 0.5	1.6 ± 1.2	0.650
Ruminococcus gnavus	2.2 ± 1.0	5.5 ± 4.9	0.390
Bacteroides ovatus	3.9 ± 1.4	1.0 ± 0.5	0.150
Faecalibacterium prausnitzii	3.6 ± 1.6	3.8 ± 2.0	0.940
Escherichia coli	11.4 ± 4.5	11.4 ± 4.9	0.998

We also analysed the trend in composition of microbiome in relation to therapeutic success. Regarding bacterial phyla, Proteobacteria decreased in patients in whom therapeutic success was obtained, passing from a value of 15.8 ± 4.6% to 6.8 ± 3.1% (p = 0.049), while in non-responders, their percentage did not change (T0 = 15.6 ± 5.7% vs. T1 = 16.8 ± 7.6%, p = 0.890). The data regarding changes in composition of the microbiome in responders and in non-responders to adalimumab therapy are shown in Table 4.

Table 4. Trend in phyla, family and bacterial species according to pharmacological success or failure.

	Pharmacological Success			Pharmacological Failure		
	T0 (%)	T1 (%)	p Value	T0 (%)	T1 (%)	p Value
Phyla						
Firmicutes	45.6 ± 6.7	51.4 ± 3.4	0.470	45.2 ± 8.4	44.4 ± 5.8	0.900
Bacteroidetes	34.7 ± 5.3	38.2 ± 3.7	0.510	31.1 ± 9.6	35.2 ± 9.5	0.650
Actinobacteria	2.6 ± 0.8	3.2 ± 0.9	0.540	2.6 ± 1.4	2.6 ± 1.3	0.980
Proteobacteria	15.8 ± 4.6	6.8 ± 3.1	0.049	15.6 ± 5.7	16.8 ± 7.6	0.890
Family						
Lachnospiraceae	17.8 ± 3.3	25.4 ± 3.2	0.100	18.8 ± 4.8	20.4 ± 1.8	0.730
Species						
Bifidobacterium adolescentis	1.1 ± 0.5	1.4 ± 0.6	0.700	1.6 ± 1.2	0.7 ± 0.7	0.150
Ruminococcus gnavus	2.2 ± 1.0	1.8 ± 0.4	0.710	5.5 ± 4.9	1.3 ± 0.5	0.420
Bacteroides ovatus	3.9 ± 1.4	2.6 ± 0.6	0.240	1.0 ± 0.5	1.9 ± 1.4	0.470
Faecalibacterium prausnitzii	3.6 ± 1.6	2.1 ± 1.2	0.080	3.8 ± 2.0	2.2 ± 1.2	0.540
Escherichia coli	11.4 ± 4.5	4.3 ± 3.1	0.078	11.4 ± 4.9	13.1 ± 7.7	0.812

In Table 5, the microbiome trend is reported according to CRP values after six months of adalimumab therapy.

With regards to the Lachnospiraceae family in patients with normalization of CRP levels after six months of adalimumab therapy, at T0 it showed a mean value of 16.6 ± 3.1% and at T1 this increased to 23.9 ± 2.6% among bacterial families (p = 0.049).

According to disease localization, the phylum Actinobacteria was more represented if the colon was inflamed (3.9 ± 1.0%) compared to an ileal CD (0.7 ± 0.5%); the differences among the other phyla were not statistically significant (Table S1). The changes in phyla according to disease localization were not statistically significant (Table S2).

Table 5. Trend of the intestinal microbiome between T0 and T1 according to C-reactive protein levels at six months.

	Normalization of CRP			Positive CRP		
	T0 (%)	T1 (%)	*p* Value	T0 (%)	T1 (%)	*p* Value
Phyla						
Firmicutes	43.7 ± 4.7	48.4 ± 3.2	0.290	42.2 ± 14.8	41.6 ± 8.1	0.970
Bacteroidetes	34.8 ± 5.9	36.9 ± 4.7	0.700	39.3 ± 10.6	48.8 ± 6.3	0.460
Actinobacteria	3.1 ± 1.0	3.2 ± 1.0	0.940	2.4 ± 1.4	2.4 ± 1.0	0.990
Proteobacteria	14.5 ± 4.4	11.4 ± 4.9	0.510	16.1 ± 7.3	2.5 ± 4.9	0.250
Family						
Lachnospiraceae	16.6 ± 3.1	23.9 ± 2.6	0.049	15.1 ± 1.9	16.6 ± 4.0	0.810
Species						
Bifidobacterium adolescentis	1.5 ± 0.7	1.0 ± 0.6	0.560	1.5 ± 0.8	0.9 ± 0.5	0.610
Ruminococcus gnavus	1.7 ± 0.9	1.3 ± 0.4	0.660	1.0 ± 0.5	1.9 ± 0.4	0.320
Bacteroides ovatus	3.2 ± 1.4	2.3 ± 0.7	0.290	1.6 ± 0.6	4.2 ± 1.9	0.260
Faecalibacterium prausnitzii	3.6 ± 1.4	3.0 ± 1.2	0.520	6.9 ± 3.7	1.0 ± 1.0	0.170
Escherichia coli	12.2 ± 4.3	8.0 ± 4.4	0.349	9.0 ± 4.0	5.4 ± 4.0	0.490

According to disease severity, the phylum Bacteroidetes was much more represented in patients with mild or moderate endoscopic activity (41.4 ± 4.5%), compared to patients with severe endoscopic activity (15.0 ± 7.5%) ($p = 0.006$); the phylum Proteobacteria was more represented in patients with severe endoscopic activity (25.2 ± 8.6%) compared to patients with mild or moderate endoscopic activity (11.7 ± 3.0%) ($p = 0.076$) (Table S3). The changes in phyla according to endoscopic disease activity were not statistically significant (Table S4).

4. Discussion

It is now known that intestinal microbiota is one of the main elements capable of influencing immunity, health status, susceptibility to various diseases including chronic and autoimmune inflammatory diseases [13].

In literature, it has been reported that 25% fewer bacterial genes are detected in faecal samples of patients with IBD compared to the control groups. Furthermore, this reduction in diversity has been shown to occur early in the course of CD in a paediatric population, suggesting that dysbiosis may not only be an effect of CD, but also can contribute to the pathogenesis [14]. Further studies have shown that patients with IBD have fewer bacteria with anti-inflammatory properties and more bacteria with pro-inflammatory properties. Joossens et al. have identified stool samples containing microbiota from patients with CD with a reduced abundance of *Faecalibacterium prausnitzii*, *Bifidobacterium adolescentis* and *Dialister invisus* and a greater abundance of *Ruminococcus gnavus*, a potentially inflammatory bacterium [15]. The decrease in both biodiversity and in phyla *Bacteroidetes* and *Firmicutes* was observed in faecal and bioptic samples of patients with CD. Furthermore, many kinds of potentially protective bacteria, such as *Bacteroides*, *Eubacterium* and *Lactobacillus*, were significantly reduced in patients with active or inactive CD. *Roseburia*, a genus producing butyrate and *Phascolarctobacterium faecium* that produces propionate, have been found to be significantly reduced in patients with CD [16]. A study analysed faecal samples from a prospective cohort of patients with paediatric CD that underwent anti-TNF therapy. Regarding the dynamics of the microbiome (including viroma and micoma) with respect to therapy and diet, the dysbiosis decreased in concomitance with the reduction of the intestinal inflammation [17]. To characterise the intestinal microbiota associated with paediatric CD, Wang et al. recruited 11 children diagnosed with CD and healthy control subjects. A total of 32 samples of patients with CD were included: eight at baseline (before treatment with infliximab) and 24 at various times during therapy. Analysis of alpha diversity revealed that both wealth and diversity were lower in paediatric patients with CD before infliximab therapy compared to healthy controls.

In particular, in the pre-infliximab samples a lower relative abundance of *Bacteroidetes* and a greater abundance of *Proteobacteria* were observed in patients compared to controls. After treatment, both the richness and the diversity of the intestinal microbiota improved in patients with paediatric CD. The community of bacteria in the post-infliximab samples was more similar to the control group, suggesting that the diversity between CD cases and healthy controls was reduced after treatment [18].

Changes in the composition of the faecal microbial community could therefore prove useful as biomarkers, in particular for monitoring disease activity, assessing the response to treatments [19] and as predictor of response to therapy [20,21].

In our study, we examined the relative percentage abundances of the four main bacterial phyla, namely *Firmicutes*, *Proteobacteria*, *Actinobacteria* and *Bacteroidetes*, of the family *Lachnospiraceae* and of the species *Bifidobacterium adolescentis*, *Faecalibacterium prausnitzii*, *Bacteroides Ovatus*, *Escherichia coli* and *Ruminococcus gnavus*. We focused on these taxa because each of them seems to have an interesting role in the pathophysiology of IBD: the *Lachnospiraceae* family (including several genera of *Clostridia* cluster XIVa, XIVb, IV and *Faecalibacterium prausnitzii*) is composed mainly of anti-inflammatory butyrogenic species and is reduced in patients with IBD, increasing proportionally to the remission of the disease [22]. *Ruminococcus gnavus* is a mucolytic bacterium found increased in IBD compared to healthy controls and is considered a possible biomarker of mucosal damage [19]. *Bifidobacteria* play a positive role in preserving intestinal barrier functions [23] and in the production of short-chain fatty acids (SCFA) [24]; of note, the analysis of the faecal microbiome of patients with IBD has shown an attenuation of *Bifidobacterium adolescentis* [25]. High antibody titres have been found targeting the antigens of *Bacteroides ovatus* [26], a bacterium that appears to be involved in the pathogenesis of IBD [27].

We assessed whether the taxa examined between the first faecal sampling and the second after six months of adalimumab therapy showed changes in terms of percentage abundance. It is interesting to note the course of the phylum *Proteobacteria* and of the family *Lachnospiraceae*. The former decreased significantly ($p = 0.038$), from 15.7 ± 3.5% to 10.3 ± 3.4%, while *Lachnospiraceae* increased from 18.2 ± 2.6% to 23.6 ± 2.2% ($p = 0.100$).

Bacterial concentrations before starting adalimumab therapy were considered in relation to achievement of therapeutic response. Although a predictive value of Firmicutes on response to therapy has been highlighted in the literature [28], and in particular of anti-inflammatory bacteria such as *Faecalibacterium prausnitzii* [20,28–31], this trend was not found in our study. Responder and non-responder patients had non-significant concentration differences of all taxa.

Then, we compared the trend of bacterial populations between T0 and T1 in those who responded versus those in whom the therapy failed. We found interesting modifications of both the phylum *Proteobacteria* and the family *Lachnospiraceae*: in those who responded to the therapy, the former decreased from T0 (15.8 ± 4.6%) to T1 (6.8 ± 3.1%) in a significant manner ($p = 0.049$). In those who did not respond to therapy, the trend was T0 = 15.6 ± 5.7%, T1 = 16.8 ± 7.6% ($p = 0.890$). With regards to the bacteria belonging to the *Lachnospiraceae* family, they increased more in responders (from 17.8 ± 3.3% to 25.4 ± 3.2%, $p = 0.100$) compared to those who did not respond (T0 = 18.8 ± 4.8%, T1 = 20.4 ± 1.8%, $p = 0.730$). With regards to the bacteria belonging to Proteobacteria phylum, *Escherichia coli* decreased from 11.4% to 4.3% ($p = 0.078$) in responders, while it remained substantially stable in those who did not respond (from 11.4% to 13.1, $p = 0.81$). Considering the trend of the intestinal microbiota during biologic therapy and the CRP values at the sixth month, there was an increase in the *Lachnospiraceae* family from T0 (16.6 ± 11%) to T1 (23.9 ± 9.6%) in patients who showed a normalization of CRP (significant: $p = 0.049$), while in those with persistent high CRP, it remained stable. The increasing trend of phylum Firmicutes and Lachnospiraceae family in patients with normalization of CRP is coherent (from 43.7–48.4% and from 16.6–23.9%, respectively): our explanation of the fact that in Lachnospiraceae family this trend is more evident is that, probably, Lachnospiraceae family, among the families belonging to phylum Firmicutes, is a species more represented in an "eubiotic" microbiota.

The decrease of *Proteobacteria* and the increase of *Lachnospiraceae* is consistent with the hypothesis that adalimumab therapy, by decreasing inflammation, tends to restore the intestinal eubiosis [8,18,32].

The higher prevalence of the phylum Bacteroidetes in patients with mild or moderate endoscopic activity and the higher prevalence of the phylum Proteobacteria in patients with severe endoscopic activity confirm the potential role as protective bacteria of the former and as bacteria correlated to the inflammation of the latter.

Some limitations of our study must be discussed. The sample size of our population is not very large, although the prospective design contributes to reducing the possible biases. In all patients, diagnosis, treatment and follow-up of CD followed International Guidelines [33]. Another limit is that we focused only on some components of the human intestinal microbiota (according to literature data), even though viroma and micoma should add precious information on this topic.

5. Conclusions

In conclusion, in patients with CD who respond to adalimumab therapy, there is a shift of intestinal microbiome from dysbiosis closer to eubiosis. Further studies about the products of microbiota (metabolomic), and about micoma and viroma, should be performed to better understand the relationship between CD and microbiota.

Supplementary Materials: The following are available online at http://www.mdpi.com/2077-0383/8/10/1646/s1, Table S1: Relationship between bacterial populations of phyla and disease localization, Table S2: Changes in phyla according to disease localization, Table S3: Relationship between bacterial populations of phyla and disease severity, Table S4: Changes in phyla according to disease severity.

Author Contributions: Conceptualization, R.P., M.M., E.F., G.M.S., E.B. and M.A.; Data curation, D.G.R., G.P.C., A.A. and M.C.D.; Formal analysis, A.A.; Investigation, A.A. and M.C.D.; Methodology, D.G.R. and G.P.C.; Project administration, E.F.; Software, G.P.C.; Supervision, M.M., E.F., G.M.S. and E.B.; Validation, R.P., M.M., E.F., G.M.S. and M.A.; Visualization, E.F., E.B. and M.A.; Writing—original draft, D.G.R., G.P.C. and A.A.; Writing—review and editing, R.P.

Funding: This research received no external funding.

Conflicts of Interest: The authors declare no conflict of interest.

References

1. Torres, J.; Mehandru, S.; Colombel, J.F.; Peyrin-Biroulet, L. Crohn's disease. *Lancet* **2017**, *389*, 1741–1755. [CrossRef]
2. Khan, I.; Ullah, N.; Zha, L.; Bai, Y.; Khan, A.; Zhao, T.; Che, T.; Zhang, C. Alteration of Gut Microbiota in Inflammatory Bowel Disease (IBD): Cause or Consequence? IBD Treatment Targeting the Gut Microbiome. *Pathogens* **2019**, *8*, 126. [CrossRef] [PubMed]
3. Caviglia, G.P.; Rosso, C.; Ribaldone, D.G.; Dughera, F.; Fagoonee, S.; Astegiano, M.; Pellicano, R. Physiopathology of intestinal barrier and the role of zonulin. *Minerva Biotecnol.* **2019**, *31*, 83–92. [CrossRef]
4. Ribaldone, D.G.; Pellicano, R.; Actis, G.C. Inflammation in gastrointestinal disorders: Prevalent socioeconomic factors. *Clin. Exp. Gastroenterol.* **2019**, *12*, 321–329. [CrossRef] [PubMed]
5. Ribaldone, D.G.; Pellicano, R.; Actis, G.C. Pathogenesis of Inflammatory Bowel Disease: Basic Science in the Light of Real-World Epidemiology. *Gastrointest. Disord.* **2019**, *1*, 129–146. [CrossRef]
6. Mirsepasi-Lauridsen, H.C.; Vrankx, K.; Engberg, J.; Friis-Møller, A.; Brynskov, J.; Nordgaard-Lassen, I.; Petersen, A.M.; Krogfelt, K.A. Disease-Specific Enteric Microbiome Dysbiosis in Inflammatory Bowel Disease. *Front. Med.* **2018**, *5*, 304. [CrossRef] [PubMed]
7. Monaco, C.; Nanchahal, J.; Taylor, P.; Feldmann, M. Anti-TNF therapy: Past, present and future. *Int. Immunol.* **2015**, *27*, 55–62. [CrossRef] [PubMed]
8. Busquets, D.; Mas-de-Xaxars, T.; López-Siles, M.; Martínez-Medina, M.; Bahí, A.; Sàbat, M.; Louvriex, R.; Miquel-Cusachs, J.O.; Garcia-Gil, J.L.; Aldeguer, X. Anti-tumour Necrosis Factor Treatment with Adalimumab Induces Changes in the Microbiota of Crohn's Disease. *J. Crohns Colitis.* **2015**, *9*, 899–906. [CrossRef]
9. Dubourg, G.; Baron, S.; Cadoret, F.; Couderc, C.; Fournier, P.E.; Lagier, J.C.; Raoult, D. From Culturomics to Clinical Microbiology and Forward. *Emerg. Infect. Dis.* **2018**, *24*, 1683–1690. [CrossRef]

10. Voelkerding, K.V.; Dames, S.A.; Durtschi, J.D. Next-generation sequencing: From basic research to diagnostics. *Clin. Chem.* **2009**, *55*, 641–658. [CrossRef]
11. Sattin, E.; Andreani, N.A.; Carraro, L.; Lucchini, R.; Fasolato, L.; Telatin, A.; Balzan, S.; Novelli, E.; Simionati, B.; Cardazzo, B. A multi-omics approach to evaluate the quality of milk whey used in ricotta cheese production. *Front. Microbiol.* **2016**, *7*, 1272. [CrossRef] [PubMed]
12. Sprakes, M.B.; Hamlin, P.J.; Warren, L.; Greer, D.; Ford, A.C. Adalimumab as second line anti-tumour necrosis factor alpha therapy for Crohn's disease: A single centre experience. *J. Crohns Colitis* **2011**, *5*, 324–331. [CrossRef]
13. Kho, Z.Y.; Lal, S.K. The Human Gut Microbiome-A Potential Controller of Wellness and Disease. *Front. Microbiol.* **2018**, *9*, 1835. [CrossRef] [PubMed]
14. Moustafa, A.; Li, W.; Anderson, E.L.; Wong, E.H.M.; Dulai, P.S.; Sandborn, W.J.; Biggs, W.; Yooseph, S.; Jones, M.B.; Venter, J.C.; et al. Genetic risk, dysbiosis, and treatment stratification using host genome and gut microbiome in inflammatory bowel disease. *Clin. Transl. Gastroenterol.* **2018**, *9*, e132. [CrossRef] [PubMed]
15. Joossens, M.; Huys, G.; Cnockaert, M.; De Preter, V.; Verbeke, K.; Rutgeerts, P.; Vandamme, P.; Vermeire, S. Dysbiosis of the faecal microbiota in patients with Crohn's disease and their unaffected relatives. *Gut* **2011**, *60*, 631–637. [CrossRef]
16. Lucas López, R.; Grande Burgos, M.J.; Gálvez, A.; Pérez Pulido, R. The human gastrointestinal tract and oral microbiota in inflammatory bowel disease: a state of the science review. *APMIS* **2017**, *125*, 3–10. [CrossRef]
17. Lewis, J.D.; Chen, E.Z.; Baldassano, R.N.; Otley, A.R.; Griffiths, A.M.; Lee, D.; Bittinger, K.; Bailey, A.; Friedman, E.S.; Hoffmann, C.; et al. Inflammation, antibiotics, and diet as environmental stressors of the gut microbiome in pediatric Crohn's disease. *Cell Host. Microbe* **2017**, *22*, 247. [CrossRef]
18. Wang, Y.; Gao, X.; Ghozlane, A.; Hu, H.; Li, X.; Xiao, Y.; Li, D.; Yu, G.; Zhang, T. Characteristics of Faecal Microbiota in Paediatric Crohn's Disease and Their Dynamic Changes During Infliximab Therapy. *J. Crohns Colitis* **2018**, *12*, 337–346. [CrossRef]
19. Berry, D.; Reinisch, W. Intestinal microbiota: A source of novel biomarkers in inflammatory bowel diseases? *Best Pract. Res. Clin. Gastroenterol.* **2013**, *27*, 47–58. [CrossRef]
20. Magnusson, M.K.; Strid, H.; Sapnara, M.; Lasson, A.; Bajor, A.; Ung, K.A.; Öhman, L. Anti-TNF therapy response in patients with ulcerative colitis is associated with colonic antimicrobial peptide expression and microbiota composition. *J. Crohns Colitis* **2016**, *10*, 943–952. [CrossRef]
21. Ananthakrishnan, A.N.; Luo, C.; Yajnik, V.; Khalili, H.; Garber, J.J.; Stevens, B.W.; Cleland, T.; Xavier, R.J. Gut Microbiome Function Predicts Response to Anti-integrin Biologic Therapy in Inflammatory Bowel Diseases. *Cell Host Microbe* **2017**, *21*, 603–610. [CrossRef] [PubMed]
22. Ribaldone, D.G.; Pellicano, R.; Actis, G.C. Inflammation: A highly conserved, Janus-like phenomenon-a gastroenterologist' perspective. *J. Mol. Med.* **2018**, *96*, 861–871. [CrossRef] [PubMed]
23. Arboleya, S.; Watkins, C.; Stanton, C.; Ross, R.P. Gut Bifidobacteria Populations in Human Health and Aging. *Front. Microbiol.* **2016**, *7*, 1204. [CrossRef] [PubMed]
24. Rios-Covian, D.; Gueimonde, M.; Duncan, S.H.; Flint, H.J.; De Los Reyes-Gavilan, C.G. Enhanced butyrate formation by cross-feeding between Faecalibacterium prausnitzii and Bifidobacterium adolescentis. *FEMS Microbiol. Lett.* **2015**, *362*. [CrossRef] [PubMed]
25. Nagao-Kitamoto, H.; Kamada, N. Host-microbial Cross-talk in Inflammatory Bowel Disease. *Immune Netw.* **2017**, *17*, 1–12. [CrossRef] [PubMed]
26. Saitoh, S.; Noda, S.; Aiba, Y.; Takagi, A.; Sakamoto, M.; Benno, Y.; Koga, Y. Bacteroides ovatus as the predominant commensal intestinal microbe causing a systemic antibody response in inflammatory bowel disease. *Clin. Diagn. Lab. Immunol.* **2002**, *9*, 54–59. [CrossRef] [PubMed]
27. Lavoie, S.; Conway, K.L.; Lassen, K.G.; Jijon, H.B.; Pan, H.; Chun, E.; Michaud, M.; Lang, J.K.; Gallini Comeau, C.A.; Dreyfuss, J.M.; et al. The Crohn's disease polymorphism, ATG16L1 T300A, alters the gut microbiota and enhances the local Th1/Th17 response. *Elife* **2019**, *8*, e39982. [CrossRef]
28. Chaput, N.; Lepage, P.; Coutzac, C.; Soularue, E.; Le Roux, K.; Monot, C.; Boselli, L.; Routier, E.; Cassard, L.; Collins, M.; et al. Baseline gut microbiota predicts clinical response and colitis in metastatic melanoma patients treated with ipilimumab. *Ann. Oncol.* **2019**, *28*, 1368–1379. [CrossRef]
29. Rajca, S.; Grondin, V.; Louis, E.; Vernier-Massouille, G.; Grimaud, J.C.; Bouhnik, Y.; Laharie, D.; Dupas, J.L.; Pillant, H.; Picon, L.; et al. Alterations in the intestinal microbiome (Dysbiosis) as a predictor of relapse after infliximab withdrawal in Crohn's disease. *Inflamm. Bowel Dis.* **2014**, *20*, 978–986.

30. Doherty, M.K.; Ding, T.; Koumpouras, C.; Telesco, S.E.; Monast, C.; Das, A.; Brodmerkel, C.; Schloss, P.D. Fecal microbiota signatures are associated with response to ustekinumab therapy among crohn's disease patients. *MBio* **2018**, *9*. [CrossRef]
31. Papa, E.; Docktor, M.; Smillie, C.; Weber, S.; Preheim, S.P.; Gevers, D.; Giannoukos, G.; Ciulla, D.; Tabbaa, D.; Ingram, J.; et al. Non-invasive mapping of the gastrointestinal microbiota identifies children with inflammatory bowel disease. *PLoS ONE* **2012**, *7*, e39242. [CrossRef] [PubMed]
32. Jones-Hall, Y.L.; Nakatsu, C.H. The Intersection of TNF, IBD and the Microbiome. *Gut Microbes* **2016**, *7*, 58–62. [CrossRef] [PubMed]
33. Gomollón, F.; Dignass, A.; Annese, V.; Tilg, H.; Van Assche, G.; Lindsay, J.O.; Peyrin-Biroulet, L.; Cullen, G.J.; Daperno, M.; Kucharzik, T.; et al. 3rd European Evidence-based Consensus on the Diagnosis and Management of Crohn's Disease 2016: Part 1: Diagnosis and Medical Management. *J. Crohns Colitis* **2017**, *11*, 3–25. [CrossRef] [PubMed]

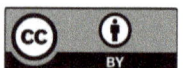

© 2019 by the authors. Licensee MDPI, Basel, Switzerland. This article is an open access article distributed under the terms and conditions of the Creative Commons Attribution (CC BY) license (http://creativecommons.org/licenses/by/4.0/).

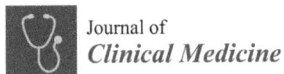

Article

Multimodal Approach to Assessment of Fecal Microbiota Donors Based on Three Complementary Methods

Jaroslaw Bilinski [1,*], Mikolaj Dziurzynski [2,*], Pawel Grzesiowski [3], Edyta Podsiadly [4], Anna Stelmaszczyk-Emmel [5], Tomasz Dzieciatkowski [6], Lukasz Dziewit [2,*] and Grzegorz W. Basak [1]

1. Department of Hematology, Oncology and Internal Medicine, Medical University of Warsaw, 02-091 Warsaw, Poland; grzegorz.basak@wum.edu.pl
2. Department of Environmental Microbiology and Biotechnology, Institute of Microbiology, Faculty of Biology, University of Warsaw, 02-096 Warsaw, Poland
3. Foundation for the Infection Prevention Institute, 02-991 Warsaw, Poland; paolo@fipz.edu.pl
4. Department of Microbiology, Institute of Medical Sciences, University of Rzeszów, 35-310 Rzeszów, Poland; edyta.podsiadly@uckwum.pl
5. Department of Laboratory Diagnostics and Clinical Immunology of Developmental Age, Medical University of Warsaw, 02-091 Warsaw, Poland; anna.stelmaszczyk-emmel@wum.edu.pl
6. Department of Medical Microbiology, Medical University of Warsaw, 02-091 Warsaw, Poland; dzieciatkowski@wp.pl
* Correspondence: jaroslaw.bilinski@gmail.com (J.B.); mikolaj.dziurzynski@biol.uw.edu.pl (M.D.); ldziewit@biol.uw.edu.pl (L.D.)

Received: 4 June 2020; Accepted: 26 June 2020; Published: 29 June 2020

Abstract: Methods of stool assessment are mostly focused on next-generation sequencing (NGS) or classical culturing, but only rarely both. We conducted a series of experiments using a multi-method approach to trace the stability of gut microbiota in various donors over time, to find the best method for the proper selection of fecal donors and to find "super-donor" indicators. Ten consecutive stools donated by each of three donors were used for the experiments (30 stools in total). The experiments assessed bacterial viability measured by flow cytometry, stool culturing on different media and in various conditions, and NGS (90 samples in total). There were no statistically significant differences between live and dead cell numbers; however, we found a group of cells classified as not-dead-not-alive, which may be possibly important in selection of "good" donors. Donor C, being a regular stool donor, was characterized by the largest number of cultivable species (64). Cultivable core microbiota (shared by all donors) was composed of only 16 species. ANCOM analysis of NGS data highlighted particular genera to be more abundant in one donor vs. the others. There was a correlation between the not-dead-not-alive group found in flow cytometry and *Anaeroplasma* found by NGS, and we could distinguish a regular stool donor from the others. In this work, we showed that combining various methods of microbiota assessment gives more information than each method separately.

Keywords: fecal microbiota transplantation; feces donor; fecal microbiota; flow cytometry; viability of bacteria; next-generation sequencing; culturing of fecal microbiota

1. Introduction

Stool suspension is commonly used as a straightforward, cheap and non-invasive material for treating several conditions and diseases. Outcomes of fecal microbiota transplantation (FMT) are encouraging in many diseases (e.g., inflammatory bowel diseases [1]) and excellent in others (e.g.,

Clostridioides difficile infection, especially as a life-saving therapy [2,3]). Not surprisingly, there are more than 250 FMT clinical trials completed or ongoing worldwide [4].

Despite the thriving of the FMT trials, our knowledge on the real composition of "healthy microbiota" is still scarce. We do not exactly know how the transplanted bacteria survive, colonize, and function in the recipient's gut or, most importantly, which methods may, or should, be used to diagnose and monitor transplanted feces to assess whether the fecal microbiota solution is appropriate for transplantation and consists of a "healthy microbiota". We also acknowledge that a healthy gut microbiota requires proper virus and fungi composition [5,6].

Analyses of human intestinal microorganisms were, until recently, mostly performed by culture-dependent methodologies, limiting the screened biodiversity only to the cultivable species, although it is known that only about 15–20% of microbes living in the human gut are cultivable as of now. The availability of novel tools, primarily next-generation sequencing (NGS), has enabled the assessment of marker taxonomical genes and even whole genomes retrieved from the complex microbial communities. The most widely used NGS method for the taxonomic and phylogenetic evaluation of bacterial community composition relies on 16S rRNA gene PCR amplicon analysis [7–9].

Currently, it can be observed that the market offering fecal microbiota suspensions and tools for FMT suspensions assessments is growing rapidly. Companies provide material from different donors, using various methodologies for testing the donors and stool processing. However, each of these methods is usually applied separately, and on these distinct analyses far-reaching conclusions are built. There are very few reports comparing different methods for the assessment of gut microbiota [10–13] and indicating how to assess the stability of fecal microbiota in the donors. There is also a need to identify "super-donor" units, i.e., persons whose microbiota contains all relevant microbes and potentially can cure the vast majority of microbiota-related diseases and conditions [14].

There is also a need for defining "super-donors" for FMT. It is postulated that there are individuals whose gut microbiome possesses certain characteristics, such as the presence or absence of specific (unfortunately not fully recognized) bacteria, phages and metabolites, which protect the donor from the vast majority of gut-related dysbiosis [14]. Furthermore, it is postulated that these individuals are the most desired donors (namely "super-donors"), and that their fecal microbiota is highly suitable for transplantation. Theoretically, such donors should be adequate for every FMT intervention. However, recent studies prove that there are some (still unknown) specific features making these (super) donors not so universal [15,16]. Therefore, an algorithm for finding perfectly matching donor–recipient couples still needs elucidation. We believe that this coupling of donor and recipient may be possible, but this requires more data and more diagnostic/analytical tools. To define what exactly "super-donor" means, we need to have more well-designed comparable clinical trials for dysbiosis-related diseases [17]. Only then will we be able to conduct a general investigation, looking for features common to all donors. Our study is in line with this general quest in medicine. Summarizing, for the purpose of this study, the term "super-donor" was used with its complex definition, including an indication that the microbiota of the "super-donor" has all the necessary beneficial components to maintain human welfare and that it will most probably cure the majority of dysbiosis. Besides, the most important conclusion must be the statement that the donor can be defined as a "super-donor" only when the majority (ideally all) clinical outcomes of FMT (from this donor) are good.

In this study, we conducted a series of experiments using a multi-method approach to trace the stability of the composition of the gut microbiota in various donors over time and to find the most suitable method for assessing the quality of the gut microbiota for the proper selection of fecal donors and to pave the way to find "super-donors". Moreover, we were looking for bacterial indicators of "good" and/or "bad" donors to simplify and parametrize the selection of suitable givers of stool samples for FMTs. We hypothesized that various methodologies of microbiota assessment to evaluate donors gives more data than each method separately.

2. Material and Methods

2.1. Stool Donors

Ten consecutive stools donated by each of three donors were used for the experiments (30 stools in total). The donors of stool were randomly selected males (donors named A and B) and an intentionally chosen male (donor C, that is, a regular stool donor registered in the Polish stool bank). They were selected according to our protocol published previously [18]. Donor C was selected with respect to criteria described by Cammarota et al. [19]. All donors were screened by a questionnaire based on international guidelines that was presented in our previous publication [18]. Briefly, one of them (donor C; male, 28 years old, healthy, with normal BMI) was a regular donor of feces, for the purpose of producing a preparation for fecal microbiota transplantation (chosen from the stool donor bank) and the other two were randomly selected males (donor A—male, 16 years old with food allergy, recurrent aphthous stomatitis and normal BMI, and donor B—male, 55 years old, a medical worker with inhaled allergy and a BMI of 27). A medical questionnaire with basic data was received from each person. Each feces sample was prepared in the same time frame and in the same way by homogenizing, diluting in normal saline, and sieving through sterile gauze or sieves to obtain a clear, homogeneous fluid being a suspension of feces. This is the regular way of producing feces for use as FMT [18]). The material prepared in this way was divided into three parts—one for assessment by flow cytometry in the LIVE/DEAD method (Molecular Probes, Eugene, OR, USA), the other for performing classical culturing, and the third for immediate isolation of DNA for V3V4 16S rDNA variable region sequencing (90 samples in total).

2.2. Flow Cytometry

Bacterial viability in samples was measured by flow cytometry using the LIVE/DEAD BacLight™ Bacterial Viability and Counting Kit (L34856, Molecular Probes) according to manufacturer instructions (Molecular Probes) [20]. Briefly, 977 µL of 0.9% NaCl, 1.5 µL of SYTO9, 1.5 µL of propidium iodide (PI) and 10 µL of diluted sample were added to a flow cytometry analysis tube. Samples were 10-fold diluted in 0.9% NaCl. The tube was incubated for 15 min in a dark at room temperature. A quantity of 10 µL of the microsphere suspension (beads) was added to the stained sample. The total volume of the sample in the flow cytometry analysis tube was 1000 µL. The samples were analyzed on a LSR Fortessa flow cytometer (Becton Dickinson, Franklin Lakes, NJ, USA) with FACS Diva v8 software (Becton Dickinson). The gating strategy is shown in Figure 1 and shows three main cell populations—alive, dead and unknown (probably alive, probably dead) with a special "double negative" group of cells (SYTO9$^-$PI$^-$). The number of bacteria per mL in each analyzed gate was counted according to the following formula taken from the manufacturer materials:

$$\frac{((\# \, of \, events \in gated \, bacteria \, region) \times (dillution \, factors))}{[(\# \, of \, events \in bead \, region) \times 10^{-6}]} = bacteria/mL$$

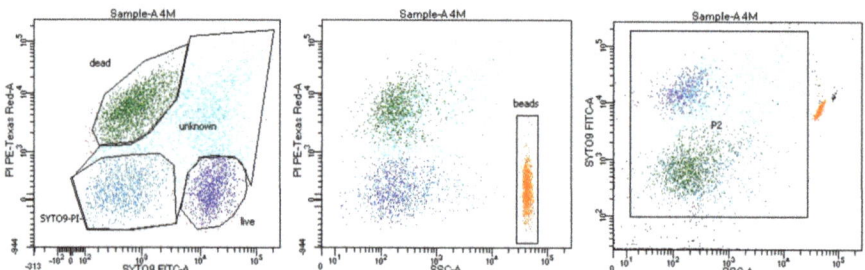

Figure 1. Gating strategy shown on one of the samples. SYTO9-positive PI-negative cells were considered alive, SYTO9-negative PI-positive cells were considered dead, other cells were considered as unknown, with special gating on SYTO9-negative PI-negative cells, which were called "double negative" cells.

2.3. Cultivation of Stool Microbiota

Samples were plated on six different agar media and incubated under conditions as follows. (i) CNA medium (colistin nalidixic acid agar; Oxoid, Basingstoke, UK) for cultivation of Gram-positive aerobes, an enriched agar medium containing sheep's blood, colistin and nalidixic acid (to inhibit the growth of Gram-negative bacteria). Culture conditions: aerobic with 5% CO_2, 37 °C, 48 h. (ii) MacConkey medium (bioMérieux, Marcy l'Etoile, France) for the isolation of Gram-negative rods, containing bile salts and crystal violet (to inhibit the growth of Gram-positive bacteria). Culture conditions: aerobic, 37 °C, 48 h. (iii) Bile and esculin (CC) medium (Oxoid)—a medium intended for the isolation and identification of bacteria belonging to the genus *Enterococcus*, which grow well in the presence of bile and have the ability to break down esculin. Culture conditions: aerobic, 37 °C, 48 h. (iv) Schaedler Anaerobe KV Selective Agar with freeze-dried horse blood and the addition of kanamycin and vancomycin (bioMérieux)—a highly nutritious medium for the selective growth and isolation of anaerobic bacteria, especially of the genus *Bacteroides* and *Prevotella*. Culture conditions: anaerobic, 37 °C, 4 days. (v) Schaedler Anaerobe KV Selective Agar with freeze-dried horse blood (bioMérieux)—a highly nutritious medium for the isolation of absolute and relative anaerobes. Culture conditions: anaerobic, 37 °C, 4 days. (vi) Sabouraud agar with gentamicin and chloramphenicol (Oxoid)—selective medium for cultivation of mold and yeast, high glucose concentration. The presence of antibiotics (chloramphenicol and gentamicin) and acidic pH inhibits bacterial growth; the presence of antibiotics is another selection factor. Culture conditions: aerobic, 37 °C, 10 days. The anaerobic incubations were carried out in anaerobic jars and atmosphere generators (Oxoid).

After the initial sample processing, colonies were selected (at least one colony per morphology) for identification using a Microflex LT mass and MBT Compass IVD Biotyper software (Bruker Daltonics, Bremen, Germany). The colonies were deposited on a MALDI-TOF (Bruker Daltonics) target microflex and extracted with 5% formic acid, air dried and then overlaid with 1 µL matrix solution of α-cyano-4-hydroxycinnamic acid in 50% acetonitrile and 2.5% trifluoroacetic acid. Two spots were examined for each colony. The Biotyper software was used to compare the protein profile of the cultured bacteria from a database of Bruker consisting of 2750 of protein profiles. A score >1.9 was considered a high-level identification of a species, a score >1.7 indicated the identification of a genus. Strains of bacteria with scores lower than 1.7 were considered unidentified.

To enumerate the number of colony-forming units (CFU) in the stool samples, 0.2 g of stool was diluted in 1 mL of phosphate-buffered saline (PBS), and 1–5 µL of watery sample was spread on each media. Bacterial counts were recorded as CFU per gram of feces for each isolated species.

2.4. DNA Sequencing

Total bacterial DNA was extracted using a Qiagen DNeasy Power Soil kit (Qiagen, Hilden, Germany) according to the manufacturer's instructions and stored at −20 °C. Using isolated

DNA as a matrix, PCR reactions were performed in triplicate (to reduce PCR bias) using a Bakt_341F 5′-CCTACGGGNGGCWGCAG-3′ and Bakt_805R 5′-GACTACHVGGGTATCTAATCC-3′ primer pair amplifying the variable V3 and V4 regions of the 16S rRNA genes [21,22]. Electrophoretic analysis was performed for each of three replicates for qualitative and quantitative evaluation of the PCR products. Then, products of three independent PCR reactions for each sample were mixed and used for the DNA sequencing as one amplicon to minimize the error due to the selectivity of the PCR reactions. The amplified PCR products were sequenced using an Illumina MiSeq instrument (Illumina, San Diego, CA, USA) in paired-end mode using a v3 chemistry kit (Illumina) at BIOBANK LAB (Chair and Department of Molecular Biophysics, University of Lodz, Łódź, Poland).

2.5. Bioinformatic Analysis

Sequencing data were subjected to NonPareil 3 [23] for sequencing depth assessment and later processed with Qiime2 (version 2018.11) package [24]. The reads were imported into Qiime2 and run through the dada2 plugin to obtain amplicon sequence variants (ASV) [25]. Taxonomy was assigned for each of the ASVs using a pre-trained naive Bayes classifier, based on the Silva 132 99% database [26], which was trimmed to include only the V3 and V4 regions of the 16S rRNA gene, bound by the Bakt_341F and Bakt_805R primer sequences. Alfa and beta diversity metrics were generated using the following Qiime2 plugins: phylogeny (including mafft aligner and FastTree tool), diversity and emperor [27–29].

2.6. Statistical Analysis

In order to identify genera that differ in abundance between samples from different donors, ANCOM analysis was used [30]. All additional statistics were generated using R (version 3.5.1) in the RStudio environment. Libraries such as ggplot2, cowplot and ggpubr were used for data visualization [31–33]. Except when otherwise stated, p-values of less than 0.05 were considered statistically significant.

2.7. Sequencing Data Availability

Next-generation sequencing data has been deposited and is available under the number PRJEB36368 and link www.ebi.ac.uk/ena/data/view/PRJEB36368.

2.8. Ethics

All subjects gave their informed consent for inclusion before they participated in the study. The investigations were carried out following the rules of the Declaration of Helsinki. According to local bioethics committee rules for non-intervention studies, no approval was needed to conduct this study.

3. Results

3.1. Analyses Applying the Flow Cytometry

The flow cytometry analysis allowed evaluation of the total number of cells in each sample as well as live versus dead cells. This analysis was used to answer the question whether the number of bacterial cells is important in the evaluation of fecal microbiota and can be used as an estimator of a "good" or "bad" donor. The performed analysis showed that there were no statistically significant differences between cell numbers in the fecal microbiota suspensions prepared from the donors' stools (see Figure 2a). The summarized average cell count of all samples was equal to 1.664×10^{10} cells/mL, ($\pm 0.913 \times 10^{10}$ cells/mL). Looking at numbers of live, dead and unknown cells each day for each donor, we noted discrete differences in the number of cells per mL of stool suspension; however, this was not statistically significant (donor A: mean 1.627×10^{10}, $\pm 1.015 \times 10^{10}$; donor B: mean 1.632×10^{10}, $\pm 0.852 \times 10^{10}$; donor C: mean 1.732×10^{10}, $\pm 0.96 \times 10^{10}$). As shown in Figure 2b (right column), the percentages of all fractions of cells, i.e., alive, dead, unknown (not stained with one of the reagents) and SYTO9-PI- (subgroup of "unknown", not stained by both reagents considered as "double negative") showed relatively stable numbers in each stool sample per day and per donor. The noticeable domination of the alive cells was observed (Figure 2b).

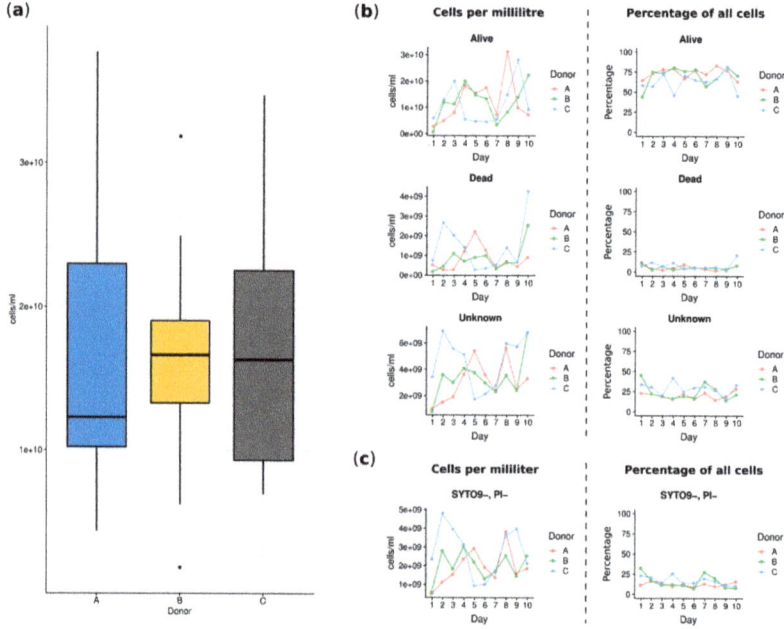

Figure 2. Cytometry cell count charts. (**a**) Total cell count per donor summed over all samples. (**b**) Charts depicting variability in collected samples per day per donor. The first column shows absolute counts of cells classified as alive, dead or unknown. The second column shows cell counts as a percentage of the total number of cells counted in a given sample. (**c**) Two charts showing the variability of cells classified as a subgroup of unknown clusters: SYTO9-, PI-. The percentage was calculated versus the unknown group cell count.

In the next step, we specifically focused on alive cells, searching for if the number of this group of bacterial cells is important for the evaluation of fecal microbiota. As we observed, there were no significant differences in the viability of cells for each donor, and alive cells accounted for similar average percentages (Table S1).

3.2. Cultivation of Stool Microbiota—Classical Microbiological Evaluation

A complex cultivation experiment was performed to evaluate whether this technique can reveal culturable bacterial indicators for "good" versus "bad" stool donors. In total, 104 species representing 36 genera were found. The summarized bacterial species composition for each donor is indicated (Figure 3). Presentation of data in the form of a Venn diagram enabled us to indicate bacterial species that were characteristic of each donor, species that were shared by two donors and, finally, species that created a core microbiota and were found in all analyzed donors (Figure 3). Clearly, we can see that donor C, being a regular stool donor, is characterized by the largest number of cultivable species (64) obtained from his stool. Samples from other donors had lower numbers of cultivable species (48 and 56, respectively). Moreover, in the stool samples collected from donor C, the largest number of unique species (29) was found. Interestingly, the cultivable core microbiota was composed of only 16 species.

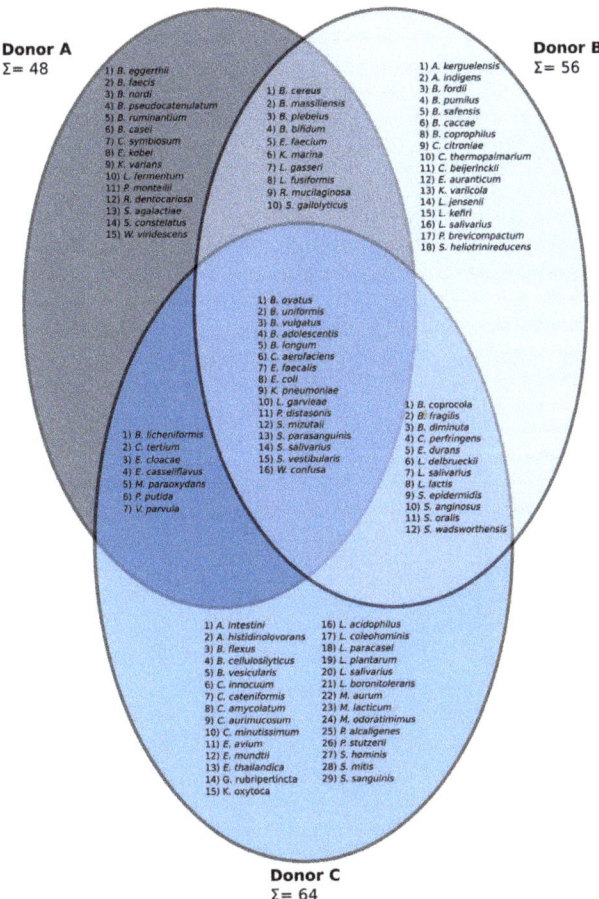

Figure 3. A three-set Venn diagram constructed based on the data from a classical microbiology approach. Identified genera are as follows: *Acidaminococcus* (*A. intestini*), *Arthrobacter* (*A. histidinolovorans*, *A. kerguelensis*), *Azoarcus* (*A. indigens*), *Bacillus* (*B. cereus*, *B. flexus*, *B. fordii*, *B. licheniformis*, *B. pumilus*, *B. safensis*), *Bacteroides* (*B. caccae*, *B. cellulosilyticus*, *B. coprocola*, *B. coprophilus*, *B. eggerthii*, *B. faecis*, *B. fragilis*, *B. massiliensis*, *B. nordi*, *B. ovatus*, *B. plebeius*, *B. uniformis*, *B. vulgatus*), *Bifidobacterium* (*B. adolescentis*, *B. bifidum*, *B. longum*, *B. pseudocatenulatum*, *B. ruminantium*), *Brevibacterium* (*B. casei*), *Brevundimonas* (*B. diminuta*, *B. vesicularis*), *Clostridium* (*C. beijerinckii*, *C. citroniae*, *C. innocuum*, *C. perfringens*, *C. symbiosum*, *C. tertium*, *C. thermopalmarium*), *Collinsella* (*C. aerofaciens*), *Coprobacillus* (*C. cateniformis*), *Corynebacterium* (*C. amycolatum*, *C. aurimucosum*, *C. minutissimum*), *Enterobacter* (*E. cloacae*, *E. kobei*), *Enterococcus* (*E. avium*, *E. casseliflavus*, *E. durans*, *E. faecalis*, *E. faecium*, *E. mundtii*, *E. thailandica*), *Escherichia* (*E. coli*), *Exiguobacterium* (*E. auranticum*), *Gordonia* (*G. rubripertincta*), *Klebsiella* (*K. oxytoca*, *K. pneumoniae*, *K. variicola*), *Kocuria* (*K. marina*, *K. varians*), *Lactobacillus* (*L. acidophilus*, *L. coleohominis*, *L. delbrueckii*, *L. fermentum*, *L. gasseri*, *L. jensenii*, *L. kefiri*, *L. paracasei*, *L. plantarum*, *L. salivarius*), *Lactococcus* (*L. garvieae*, *L. lactis*), *Lysinibacillus* (*L. boronitolerans*, *L. fusiformis*), *Microbacterium* (*M. aurum*, *M. lacticum*, *M. paraoxydans*), *Myroides* (*M. odoratimimus*), *Parabacteroides* (*P. distasonis*), *Penicillium* (*P. brevicompactum*), *Pseudomonas* (*P. alcaligenes*, *P. monteilii*, *P. putida*, *P. stutzerii*), *Rothia* (*R. dentocariosa*, *R. mucilaginosa*), *Slackia* (*S. heliotrinireducens*), *Sphingobacterium* (*S. mizutaii*), *Staphylococcus* (*S. epidermidis*, *S. hominis*), *Streptococcus* (*S. agalactiae*, *S. anginosus*, *S. constelatus*, *S. gallolyticus*, *S. mitis*, *S. oralis*, *S. parasanguinis*, *S. salivarius*, *S. vestibularis*), *Stretococcus* (*S. sanguinis*), *Sutterella* (*S. wadsworthensis*), *Veillonella* (*V. parvula*), *Weissella* (*W. confusa*, *W. viridescens*).

In the next step, we evaluated the presence of identified species over time, i.e., throughout 10 sampling days (Figure 4). It was shown that the most persistent species was *Escherichia coli*, being detected in all samples. Other species, such as *Enterococcus faecalis*, *Streprococcus parasanguinis*, *Bifidobacterium adolescentis*, *Enterococcus faecium* and *Streptococcus salivarius* were also detected in the majority of samples, yet their persistence varied greatly between donors (Figure 4). It is noticeable that a plethora of bacterial species occurred only on individual days. This may be a consequence of the bias of this method or of a simple one-time variation depending on the food consumed. Therefore, when using conventional culturing as an evaluation strategy for the assessment of the quality of stool samples, it is important to repeat sampling from particular donors for several days. Single sampling can deliver non-representative and possibly false results.

3.3. Next-Generation Sequencing

A total of 5,694,140 reads were obtained from Illumina MiSeq sequencing, with reads per sample ranging from 111,656 to 291,029. Quality control and merging of paired-end reads using the dada2 software package resulted in the retention of, on average, 47.74% ($\sigma = 2.21$) reads per sample (Table S2). Both the Nonpareil 3 and alpha rarefaction analysis (Qiime2 diversity plugin) showed sequencing depths close to 100%.

Merged reads subjected to further analyses were dereplicated into 9868 amplicon sequence variants (ASV), with the number of reads for ASV ranging from 1 to 10,098. Taxonomy assignment based on the Silva database (release 132), showed 97.75% of ASVs classified down to the genus level. Overall classification showed that 99.98% of all reads were bacterial, 0.01% archeal and less than 0.01% were unclassified. The bacterial ASVs represent 18 classes, with Bacteroidia and Clostridia in relative abundance, constituting averages of 49.9% and 40.0%, respectively. At a genus level, the most dominant taxa were *Bacteroides* and *Faecalibacterium*, with relative abundance in each sample no less than 35% and 11%, respectively. The data was not analyzed on species level because a single marker region does not allow this kind of resolution [34]. Figure 5 shows the abundances of each taxon identified in stool samples.

The Shannon diversity index along with Pielou's evenness index have been calculated for all of the samples, and the Kruskal–Wallis test was used to determine if there were any statistical differences between them. The Pielous evenness index for all of the samples was relatively high, ranging from 0.94 to 0.95, and no statistical differences between donors were detected. Interestingly, the Shannon index was similar for donors A and B, with its mean values equal to 10.11 and 10.02, while it was slightly, but significantly, higher for donor C—10.39 ($p = 0.0191$ for donor A versus C and $p = 0.0005$ for donor B versus C according to Kruskal–Wallis test, H value = 12.18; see Figure 6).

Given that the above statistical test for significant differences yielded two pairs, donor A versus C and donor B versus C, these pairs were subjected to ANCOM analysis. In the first case, ANCOM analysis highlighted two Gram-negative, obligatory anaerobe genera to be more abundant in samples from donor C; these were *Acidaminococcus* and *Paraprevotella*. The same analysis showed *Anaeroplasmatales* and *Gastranaerophilales* orders to be more abundant in samples from donor A.

An ANCOM analysis of the second pair (donor B versus C) highlighted *Anaeroplasma* as more abundant in donor B, along with *Holdermanella* genera and two, not well described, bacterial families—*Muribaculaceae* and *Puniceicoccaceae*, members of the *Bacteroidetes* and *Verrucomicrobia* phyla, respectively. As for taxa more abundant in the donor C microbiota, two members of the *Firmucutes* phylum were detected: *Lachnospiraceae* and *Dialister*.

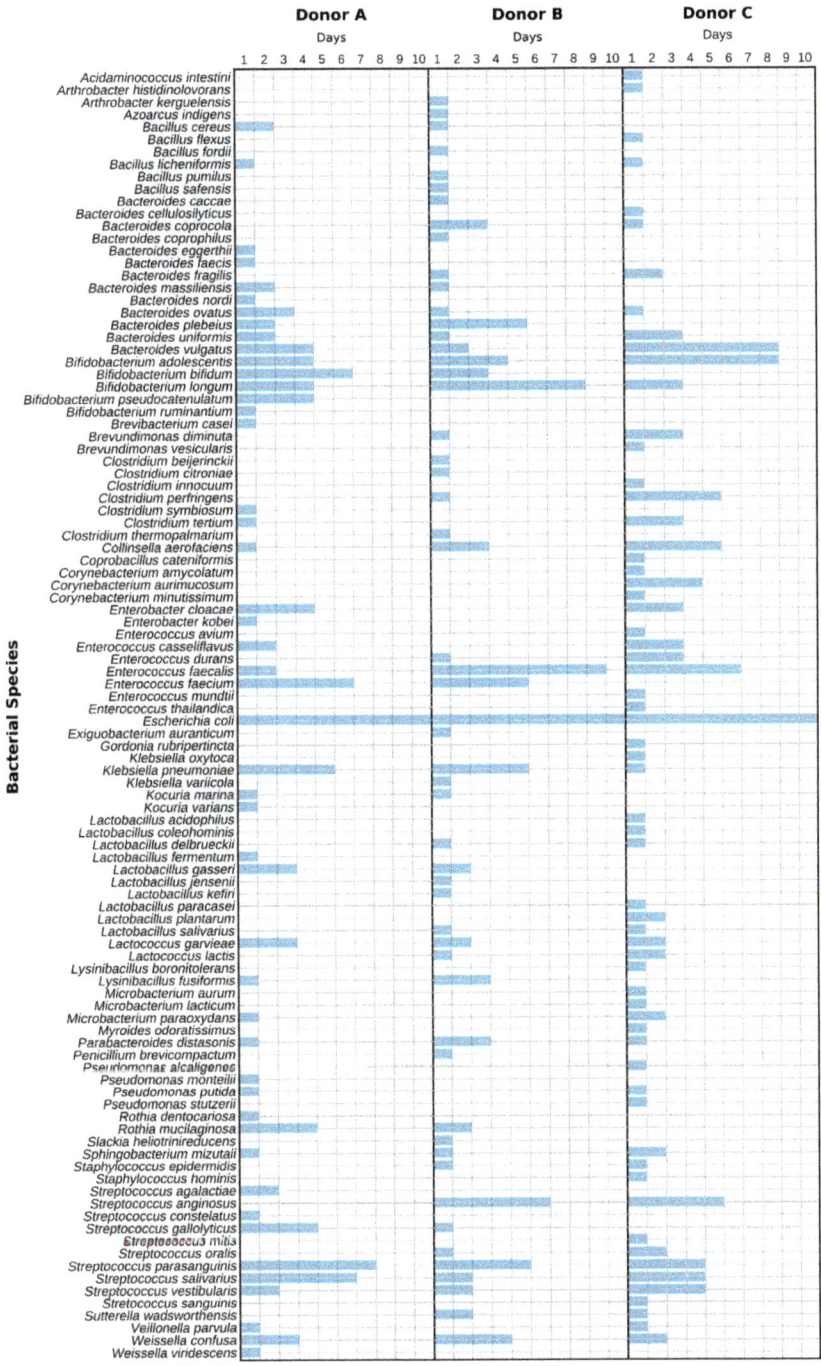

Figure 4. Diagram showing the daily presence of the particular cultivable bacterial species in stool samples.

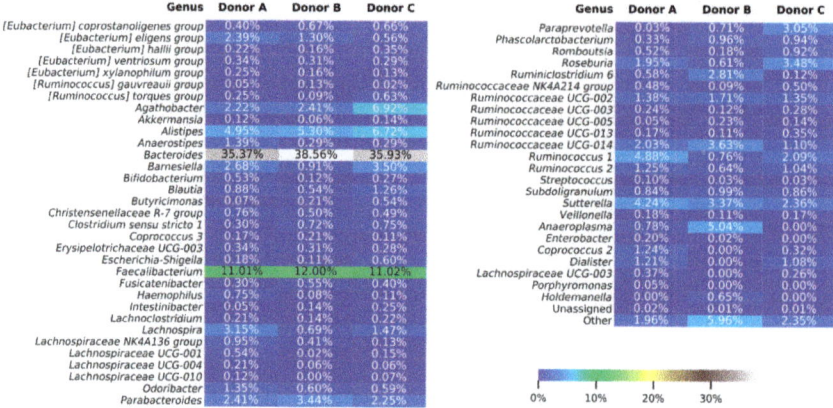

Figure 5. Heat map showing bacterial genera detected using amplicon sequencing (V3–V4 region of 16S rDNA). The summarized data for each donor are presented. The "others" group summarizes genera with individual abundances lower than 0.5% in any sample. Sequences unassigned at the genera taxonomy level were grouped and named "unassigned".

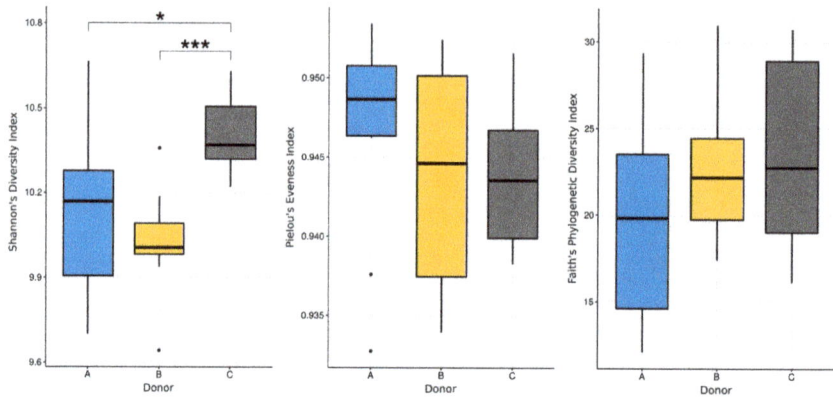

Figure 6. Boxplots showing selected biodiversity indices calculated for the data from the metabarcoding analysis. Kruskal-Wallis test was used to detect statistically significant differences. *—p-value less than 0.01; ***—p-value less than 0.001.

As was done for classical culturing experiments, the stability of the intestinal microbiota over time was assessed. Although no statistically significant differences were detected, principal coordinates analysis (PCoA) on the Bray–Curtis dissimilarity index shows that the overall internal similarity of time-resolved samples from donor C was much higher than for other donors. Clustering the bacterial composition of feces in donor C indicates the most stable composition of intestinal microbiota over time (Figure 7).

Pearson correlation coefficients between the double negative group of cells (SYTO9-, PI-) and genera-level taxonomy data showed that relative abundance of *Anaeroplasma* is positively correlated with the double negative group per sample percentage ($\rho = 0.6312$), followed by *Sanguibacteroides* ($\rho = 0.4592$).

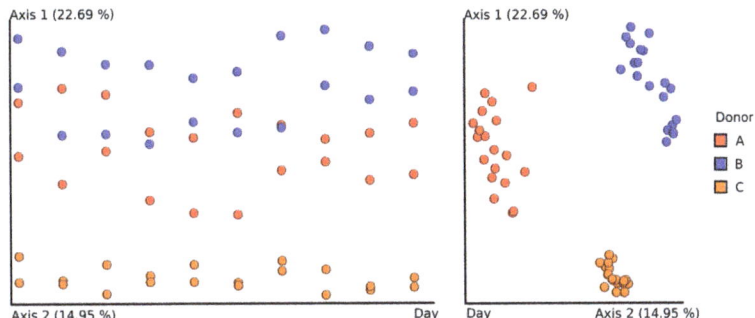

Figure 7. Principal coordinates analysis (PCoA) visualization. The PCoA was built using the Bray–Curtis dissimilarity index with day of sample collection as one axis.

4. Discussion

In this study, we used a multi-method approach to (i) test a hypothesis that each method separately may be useful in donor characterization and to (ii) try to distinguish a regular donor of feces from the stool bank (as we know his stool is beneficial for patients and he is generally healthy and meets all inclusion criteria for being a stool donor) from randomly chosen persons.

Although very complex, our analysis should be still considered as a preliminary one with several limitations. First of all, we tested only three donors in total in our study; however, our goal was to perform complex analysis with screening of multiple samples per patient in a time-resolved manner. Additionally, a relatively weak point of our analysis could also be using a limited number of media for the cultivation experiment; however, we carefully chose them to cover both aerobic and anaerobic taxa.

Taking into account all limitations, our work showed that assessment of the intestinal microbiota is very complex. Each of the applied methods separately had significant limitations, however, enabled some significant observations. Classic bacterial culturing showed that single intestinal microbiota sampling can give false, and surely not representative, results, because many bacteria are found in the feces irregularly, and the composition of fecal microbiota may, to some extent, change daily [35]. For a complete picture of the composition of the intestinal microbiota, multiple culturing should be performed, and obtained results should be analyzed together. The next applied procedure, i.e., flow cytometry, showed that live bacteria dominated the samples. However, discussion on the active component of the intestinal microbiota preparation continues. It is said that live bacteria are not necessarily responsible for the beneficial properties of intestinal microbiota, and metabolites or even individual genes should be taken into consideration [36]. Nevertheless, the prevalence of living bacteria is a positive aspect in the argument that live bacteria are the factor that restores intestinal homeostasis [37]. The last of the applied methods, i.e., next-generation sequencing, definitely brings the most abundant data, considering the bacterial diversity of the intestinal microbiota. The weakness of this method, however, is that the results are relative; we do not have absolute numbers of individual genera and the bacteria represented in a very low titer may be underrepresented in the sample [38]. Keeping in mind that this is a semi-quantitative method, not a quantitative one, and inferences based on the indicated percentages must be careful, we can see the differences that we observed between donor C and donors A and B may point to unique combinations of individual species. Possibly, the key species for health processes are present in donor C, who is a regular donor of feces. Such conclusions will always be arbitrary, but the "beneficial" species described in the literature, such as *Blautia*, *Barnesiella*, *Butiricimonas* [18] and *Roseburia*, are significantly more abundant in donor C than in others; however, other strains considered beneficial, such as *Bacteroides* and *Faecalibacterium*, occur in comparable percentages (Figure 5).

More definite conclusions can be drawn when looking collectively at the results obtained with the application of all these methods. In general, the metabarcoding analysis revealed that Shannon's biodiversity index was significantly higher for donor C than others. This is in agreement with previous results, indicating that biodiversity is one of the most important markers of a healthy microbiome [39,40]. There are no specific values of diversity indexes that particular samples of intestinal microbiota should achieve in order to be recognized as more valuable than others. However, high biodiversity indicates a richer intestinal flora and is associated, according to current knowledge, with health [14].

Regarding a microbiota composition assessed by classical culturing and NGS, we found some species and genera being unique for donor C, and it was also found that abundances of particular species may play a role. The donor C microbiota was most stable in time, which may also be an indicator of a super-donor. However, even in donor C's stool samples, we observed some day-to-day diversity. A possible lack of influence of this variability on overall microbiotal homeostasis may be explained by the hypothesis that a healthy "functional core" of the microbiome is maintained by a complement of metabolic and other molecular functions that are performed by the microbiome within a particular habitat but are not necessarily provided by the same organisms in different individuals [41]. Therefore, according this hypothesis, the microbiome as a pool of genes remains stable.

In this study, we identified genera (*Roseburia, Barnesiella, Blautia, Butiricimonas*) considered beneficial as more abundant in donor C than in the others. ANCOM analysis on samples from donor A versus C highlighted *Acidaminococcus* and *Paraprevotella* to be more abundant in samples from donor C. Both of these genera are common human gut microbiota, with the former shown to be able to use glutamic acid as the only source of energy and produce hydrogen and hydrogen sulfide from citrate [42,43]. *Paraprevotella*, on the other hand, is an opportunistic human pathogen, associated with non-alcoholic fatty liver disease [44,45]. The same analysis has shown *Anaeroplasmatales* and *Gastranaerophilales* orders to be more abundant in samples from donor A than from donor C. While not much is known about the *Gastranaerophilales* order, *Anaeroplasmatales* is a Gram-negative obligatory anaerobe, a member of Mollicutes class, which also harbors some human pathogens such as *Mycoplasma* and *Ureaplasma*.

The same analysis of the second pair (donor B versus C) also highlighted *Anaeroplasma* in this setting to be more abundant in donor B, along with the *Holdermanella* genera, a Gram-positive member of the Firmicutes phylum associated with chronic kidney disease [46]. As for taxa more abundant in the donor C microbiota, two members of the Firmucutes phylum were detected: *Lachnospiraceae* and *Dialister*. Members of the *Lachnospiraceae* family are common human gut microbiota and have been linked to protection from colon cancer (and obesity from the other side), due to their ability to produce butyric acid, which is an important factor for both microbial and host epithelial cell growth [47]. *Dialister* is a Gram-negative member of the Negativicutes class, usually associated with human dental infections [48,49]. We found that *Anaeroplasma* is more abundant in donors A and B, and positively correlates with SYTO9-, PI- cell counts (double negative, which may be considered as not-alive-not-dead). Could those be markers of "good" and "bad" donors? To answer this question, numerous population studies should be performed correlating, e.g., *C. difficile* infection remission with particular donors and particular core microbiota as well as unique bacteria present in their stool.

By comparing flow cytometry with amplicon analysis results, we found a positive correlation between the double negative cell group and *Anaeroplasma* genera. It is possible that, due to their unusual, rich in sterols, cell membrane, members of Mollicutes class, such as *Anaeroplasma*, can be attributed to high numbers of SYTO9-, PI- cells. However, they are definitely not the only ones that built this group, because the relative abundance of Mollicutes was very small in samples from donor C, while SYTO9-, PI- cells per sample percentage in this donor was comparable to others. Nonetheless, there is a possible pattern that high relative abundance of *Anaeroplasma* is more characteristic of donors A and B, being "non-donors" than of donor C, a regular stool donor. It is also possible that double negative cells are bacterial spores.

The selection of an appropriate stool donor is a key step in FMT [50]. Donors are thoroughly screened to ensure they do not harbor any transmittable pathogens or disease. Comparing the gut microbiota profiles of different donors, it is known that microbial diversity is a reliable predictor of

FMT success; however, a variety of additional factors, both genetic and environmental, are also known to influence FMT results [51]. As we showed in this work, a regular clinical questionnaire should be coupled with multiple tests results, as only together can they give reliable results, and they will definitely give more data than each method separately.

5. Conclusions

Each of the methods described in this study has its pros and cons when applied in the laboratory to characterize the gut microbiota. Classical culturing is relatively cheap and widely available, but it has been shown that culture-based methods can only detect up to 20% of all the bacterial taxa present in a given sample. Methods based on next-generation sequencing are more precise, non-dependent on the cultivation step and can describe every bacterial community with more detail. However, they are also much more expensive, laborious, may introduce PCR biases and do not discriminate between live and dead microorganisms. To tackle this problem, methods such as flow cytometry with fluorochromes (FCM) can be used, as they enable discriminating between live and dead bacteria. Based on this study and the literature searches, it is clear that there is no universal method for the assessment of human gut microbiota, and especially that some methods, such as FCM, may produce only limited results. However, when combined, the methods presented in this study may generate a detailed picture of the fecal microbiota solution for FMT.

In this study, we showed that fecal cultures are characterized by very high variability. By creating a Venn diagram, a "core cultivable microbiota" was identified, and it was composed of only 16 species. The largest number of species, mainly anaerobic, were obtained from donor C, who is a regular donor of stool for FMT. Donor C was characterized by a statistically significantly higher content of species considered beneficial (*Faecalibacterium, Bacteroides, Barnesiella, Blautia, Roseburia, Butyricimonas*). The general biodiversity of the stool microbiota of donor C was statistically significantly higher than from donors A and B. Microbiota stability over time was also transparent for donor C. In assessing the viability of bacterial cells, three groups of cells were distinguished: alive, dead and unknown. A population of "unknown" cells contained a group of double negative cells (SYTO9-, PI-). The presence of the double negative cell population correlates with the relative amount of *Anaeroplasma*, which appear more frequently in gut microbiota of "non-donors" (donors unsuitable for FMT).

Supplementary Materials: The following are available online at http://www.mdpi.com/2077-0383/9/7/2036/s1, Table S1: Table depicting raw values obtained from the flow cytometry experiment for all of the investigated samples; Table S2: Table depicting numbers of amplicon sequences remaining after each step of pre-analysis quality filtering.

Author Contributions: Conceptualization, J.B.; methodology, J.B., G.W.B., L.D., M.D., A.S.-E., E.P., T.D. and P.G.; formal analysis, M.D., L.D. and J.B.; investigation A.S.-E., E.P., J.B., L.D. and M.D.; writing—original draft preparation, J.B., M.D. and L.D.; writing—review and editing G.W.B., A.S.-E., E.P., T.D., and P.G.; funding acquisition, J.B. and G.W.B. All authors have read and agreed to the published version of the manuscript.

Funding: This research was funded by the Incubator of Innovation + program financed by the Ministry of Science and Higher Education, Poland, and financed under EU funds (SG OP), grant number 1WP/FS200/ZW2/17.

Conflicts of Interest: The authors declare no conflict of interest. The funders had no role in the design of the study; in the collection, analyses, or interpretation of data; in the writing of the manuscript; or in the decision to publish the results.

References

1. Costello, S.P.; Soo, W.; Bryant, R.V.; Jairath, V.; Hart, A.L.; Andrews, J.M. Systematic review with meta-analysis: Faecal microbiota transplantation for the induction of remission for active ulcerative colitis. *Aliment. Pharmacol. Ther.* **2017**, *46*, 213–224. [CrossRef] [PubMed]
2. Ianiro, G.; Murri, R.; Sciumè, G.D.; Impagnatiello, M.; Masucci, L.; Ford, A.C.; Law, G.R.; Tilg, H.; Sanguinetti, M.; Cauda, R.; et al. Incidence of Bloodstream Infections, Length of Hospital Stay, and Survival in Patients With Recurrent Clostridioides difficile Infection Treated With Fecal Microbiota Transplantation or Antibiotics: A Prospective Cohort Study. *Ann. Intern. Med.* **2019**, *171*, 695–702. [CrossRef] [PubMed]

3. Hocquart, M.; Lagier, J.-C.; Cassir, N.; Saidani, N.; Eldin, C.; Kerbaj, J.; Delord, M.; Valles, C.; Brouqui, P.; Raoult, D.; et al. Early Fecal Microbiota Transplantation Improves Survival in Severe Clostridium difficile Infections. *Clin. Infect. Dis.* **2018**, *66*, 645–650. [CrossRef] [PubMed]
4. Map of Clinical Trials Involving Fecal Microbiota Transplantation. Available online: https://www.clinicaltrials.gov/ct2/results/map?term=fecal+microbiota+transplantation&map (accessed on 9 January 2020).
5. Mukhopadhya, I.; Segal, J.P.; Carding, S.R.; Hart, A.L.; Hold, G.L. The gut virome: The missing link between gut bacteria and host immunity? *Therap. Adv. Gastroenterol.* **2019**, *12*. [CrossRef] [PubMed]
6. Ianiro, G.; Bruno, G.; Lopetuso, L.; Beghella, F.; Laterza, L.; D'Aversa, F.; Gigante, G.; Cammarota, G.; Gasbarrini, A. Role of Yeasts in Healthy and Impaired Gut Microbiota: The Gut Mycome. *Curr. Pharm. Des.* **2014**, *20*, 4565–4569. [CrossRef]
7. Human Microbiome Project Consortium. Structure, function and diversity of the healthy human microbiome. *Nature* **2012**, *486*, 207–214. [CrossRef]
8. Claesson, M.J.; O'Toole, P.W. Evaluating the latest high-throughput molecular techniques for the exploration of microbial gut communities. *Gut Microbes* **2010**, *1*, 277–278. [CrossRef]
9. D'Amore, R.; Ijaz, U.Z.; Schirmer, M.; Kenny, J.G.; Gregory, R.; Darby, A.C.; Shakya, M.; Podar, M.; Quince, C.; Hall, N. A comprehensive benchmarking study of protocols and sequencing platforms for 16S rRNA community profiling. *BMC Genomics* **2016**, *17*, 55. [CrossRef]
10. Lau, J.T.; Whelan, F.J.; Herath, I.; Lee, C.H.; Collins, S.M.; Bercik, P.; Surette, M.G. Capturing the diversity of the human gut microbiota through culture-enriched molecular profiling. *Genome Med.* **2016**, *8*, 72. [CrossRef]
11. Hiergeist, A.; Glasner, J.; Reischl, U.; Gessner, A. Analyses of Intestinal Microbiota: Culture versus Sequencing. *ILAR J.* **2015**, *56*, 228–240. [CrossRef]
12. Fraher, M.H.; O'Toole, P.W.; Quigley, E.M.M. Techniques used to characterize the gut microbiota: A guide for the clinician. *Nat. Rev. Gastroenterol. Hepatol.* **2012**, *9*, 312–322. [CrossRef] [PubMed]
13. Gupta, S.; Mortensen, M.S.; Schjorring, S.; Trivedi, U.; Vestergaard, G.; Stokholm, J.; Bisgaard, H.; Krogfelt, K.A.; Sorensen, S.J. Amplicon sequencing provides more accurate microbiome information in healthy children compared to culturing. *Commun. Biol.* **2019**, *2*, 291. [CrossRef]
14. Wilson, B.C.; Vatanen, T.; Cutfield, W.S.; O'Sullivan, J.M. The Super-Donor Phenomenon in Fecal Microbiota Transplantation. *Front. Cell. Infect. Microbiol.* **2019**, *9*, 2. [CrossRef] [PubMed]
15. Olesen, S.W.; Gerardin, Y. Re-evaluating the evidence for fecal microbiota transplantation "super-donors" in inflammatory bowel disease. *medRxiv* **2020**, 19011635. [CrossRef]
16. Ng, S.C.; Kamm, M.A.; Yeoh, Y.K.; Chan, P.K.S.; Zuo, T.; Tang, W.; Sood, A.; Andoh, A.; Ohmiya, N.; Zhou, Y.; et al. Scientific frontiers in faecal microbiota transplantation: Joint document of Asia-Pacific Association of Gastroenterology (APAGE) and Asia-Pacific Society for Digestive Endoscopy (APSDE). *Gut* **2020**, *69*, 83–91. [CrossRef]
17. El-Salhy, M.; Hatlebakk, J.G.; Gilja, O.H.; Bråthen Kristoffersen, A.; Hausken, T. Efficacy of faecal microbiota transplantation for patients with irritable bowel syndrome in a randomised, double-blind, placebo-controlled study. *Gut* **2020**, *69*, 859–867. [CrossRef]
18. Bilinski, J.; Grzesiowski, P.; Sorensen, N.; Madry, K.; Muszynski, J.; Robak, K.; Wroblewska, M.; Dzieciatkowski, T.; Dulny, G.; Dwilewicz-Trojaczek, J.; et al. Microbiota Transplantation in Patients With Blood Disorders Inhibits Gut Colonization With Antibiotic-Resistant Bacteria: Results of a Prospective, Single-Center Study. *Clin. Infect. Dis.* **2017**, *65*, 364–370. [CrossRef]
19. Cammarota, G.; Ianiro, G.; Kelly, C.R.; Mullish, B.H.; Allegretti, J.R.; Kassam, Z.; Putignani, L.; Fischer, M.; Keller, J.J.; Costello, S.P.; et al. International consensus conference on stool banking for faecal microbiota transplantation in clinical practice. *Gut* **2019**, *68*, 2111–2121. [CrossRef]
20. Molecular Probes LIVE/DEAD BacLight Bacterial Viability and Counting Kit (L34856)—Protocol. Available online: https://assets.thermofisher.com/TFS-Assets/LSG/manuals/mp34856.pdf (accessed on 31 May 2020).
21. Herlemann, D.P.; Labrenz, M.; Jurgens, K.; Bertilsson, S.; Waniek, J.J.; Andersson, A.F. Transitions in bacterial communities along the 2000 km salinity gradient of the Baltic Sea. *ISME J.* **2011**, *5*, 1571–1579. [CrossRef]
22. Klindworth, A.; Pruesse, E.; Schweer, T.; Peplies, J.; Quast, C.; Horn, M.; Glockner, F.O. Evaluation of general 16S ribosomal RNA gene PCR primers for classical and next-generation sequencing-based diversity studies. *Nucleic Acids Res.* **2013**, *41*, e1. [CrossRef]

23. Rodriguez-R, L.M.; Gunturu, S.; Tiedje, J.M.; Cole, J.R.; Konstantinidis, K.T. Nonpareil 3: Fast Estimation of Metagenomic Coverage and Sequence Diversity. *mSystems* **2018**, *3*. [CrossRef]
24. Bolyen, E.; Rideout, J.R.; Dillon, M.R.; Bokulich, N.A.; Abnet, C.C.; Al-Ghalith, G.A.; Alexander, H.; Alm, E.J.; Arumugam, M.; Asnicar, F.; et al. Reproducible, interactive, scalable and extensible microbiome data science usin QIIME 2. *Nat. Biotechnol.* **2019**, *37*, 852–857. [CrossRef]
25. Callahan, B.J.; McMurdie, P.J.; Rosen, M.J.; Han, A.W.; Johnson, A.J.A.; Holmes, S.P. DADA2: High-resolution sample inference from Illumina amplicon data. *Nat. Methods* **2016**, *13*, 581–583. [CrossRef] [PubMed]
26. Quast, C.; Pruesse, E.; Yilmaz, P.; Gerken, J.; Schweer, T.; Yarza, P.; Peplies, J.; Glöckner, F.O. The SILVA ribosomal RNA gene database project: Improved data processing and web-based tools. *Nucleic Acids Res.* **2012**, *41*, D590–D596. [CrossRef] [PubMed]
27. Katoh, K.; Standley, D.M. MAFFT multiple sequence alignment software version 7: Improvements in performance and usability. *Mol. Biol. Evol.* **2013**, *30*, 772–780. [CrossRef]
28. Price, M.N.; Dehal, P.S.; Arkin, A.P. FastTree 2—Approximately Maximum-Likelihood Trees for Large Alignments. *PLoS ONE* **2010**, *5*. [CrossRef] [PubMed]
29. Vazquez-Baeza, Y.; Pirrung, M.; Gonzalez, A.; Knight, R. EMPeror: A tool for visualizing high-throughput microbial community data. *Gigascience* **2013**, *2*, 16. [CrossRef]
30. Mandal, S.; Van Treuren, W.; White, R.A.; Eggesbo, M.; Knight, R.; Peddada, S.D. Analysis of composition of microbiomes: A novel method for studying microbial composition. *Microb. Ecol. Health Dis.* **2015**, *26*, 27663. [CrossRef]
31. Wickham, H. *ggplot2*, 2nd ed.; Use R! Springer International Publishing: Berlin/Heidelberg, Germany, 2016; ISBN 978-3-319-24275-0.
32. Wilke, C. Cowplot—Streamlined Plot Theme and Plot Annotations for Ggplot2. Available online: https://github.com/wilkelab/cowplot (accessed on 7 January 2020).
33. Kassambara, A. Ggpubr: 'Ggplot2' Based Publication Ready Plots. Available online: https://github.com/kassambara/ggpubr (accessed on 7 January 2020).
34. Barb, J.J.; Oler, A.J.; Kim, H.-S.; Chalmers, N.; Wallen, G.R.; Cashion, A.; Munson, P.J.; Ames, N.J. Development of an Analysis Pipeline Characterizing Multiple Hypervariable Regions of 16S rRNA Using Mock Samples. *PLoS ONE* **2016**, *11*, e0148047. [CrossRef]
35. David, L.A.; Maurice, C.F.; Carmody, R.N.; Gootenberg, D.B.; Button, J.E.; Wolfe, B.E.; Ling, A.V.; Devlin, A.S.; Varma, Y.; Fischbach, M.A.; et al. Diet rapidly and reproducibly alters the human gut microbiome. *Nature* **2014**, *505*, 559–563. [CrossRef]
36. Ott, S.J.; Waetzig, G.H.; Rehman, A.; Moltzau-Anderson, J.; Bharti, R.; Grasis, J.A.; Cassidy, L.; Tholey, A.; Fickenscher, H.; Seegert, D.; et al. Efficacy of Sterile Fecal Filtrate Transfer for Treating Patients with Clostridium difficile Infection. *Gastroenterology* **2017**, *152*, 799–811.e7. [CrossRef] [PubMed]
37. Papanicolas, L.E.; Choo, J.M.; Wang, Y.; Leong, L.E.X.; Costello, S.P.; Gordon, D.L.; Wesselingh, S.L.; Rogers, G.B. Bacterial viability in faecal transplants: Which bacteria survive? *EBioMedicine* **2019**, *41*, 509–516. [CrossRef] [PubMed]
38. Rajan, S.K.; Lindqvist, M.; Brummer, R.J.; Schoultz, I.; Repsilber, D. Phylogenetic microbiota profiling in fecal samples depends on combination of sequencing depth and choice of NGS analysis method. *PLoS ONE* **2019**, *14*, e0222171. [CrossRef]
39. Lloyd-Price, J.; Abu-Ali, G.; Huttenhower, C. The healthy human microbiome. *Genome Med.* **2016**, *8*, 51. [CrossRef] [PubMed]
40. Peled, J.U.; Gomes, A.L.C.; Devlin, S.M.; Littmann, E.R.; Taur, Y.; Sung, A.D.; Weber, D.; Hashimoto, D.; Slingerland, A.E.; Slingerland, J.B.; et al. Microbiota as Predictor of Mortality in Allogeneic Hematopoietic-Cell Transplantation. *N. Engl. J. Med.* **2020**, *382*, 822–834. [CrossRef]
41. Shafquat, A.; Joice, R.; Simmons, S.L.; Huttenhower, C. Functional and phylogenetic assembly of microbial communities in the human microbiome. *Trends Microbiol.* **2014**, *22*, 261–266. [CrossRef]
42. Jumas-Bilak, E.; Carlier, J.-P.; Jean-Pierre, H.; Mory, F.; Teyssier, C.; Gay, B.; Campos, J.; Marchandin, H. *Acidaminococcus intestini* sp. nov., isolated from human clinical samples. *Int. J. Syst. Evol. Microbiol.* **2007**, *57*, 2314–2319. [CrossRef]
43. Cook, G.M.; Rainey, F.A.; Chen, G.; Stackebrandt, E.; Russell, J.B. Emendation of the description of *Acidaminococcus fermentans*, a trans-aconitate- and citrate-oxidizing bacterium. *Int. J. Syst. Bacteriol.* **1994**, *44*, 576–578. [CrossRef]

44. Rajilic-Stojanovic, M.; Smidt, H.; de Vos, W.M. Diversity of the human gastrointestinal tract microbiota revisited. *Environ. Microbiol.* **2007**, *9*, 2125–2136. [CrossRef]
45. Stanislawski, M.A.; Lozupone, C.A.; Wagner, B.D.; Eggesbo, M.; Sontag, M.K.; Nusbacher, N.M.; Martinez, M.; Dabelea, D. Gut microbiota in adolescents and the association with fatty liver: The EPOCH study. *Pediatr. Res.* **2018**, *84*, 219–227. [CrossRef]
46. Lun, H.; Yang, W.; Zhao, S.; Jiang, M.; Xu, M.; Liu, F.; Wang, Y. Altered gut microbiota and microbial biomarkers associated with chronic kidney disease. *Microbiologyopen* **2019**, *8*, e00678. [CrossRef] [PubMed]
47. Meehan, C.J.; Beiko, R.G. A phylogenomic view of ecological specialization in the Lachnospiraceae, a family of digestive tract-associated bacteria. *Genome Biol. Evol.* **2014**, *6*, 703–713. [CrossRef] [PubMed]
48. Rocas, I.N.; Siqueira, J.F.J. Characterization of Dialister species in infected root canals. *J. Endod.* **2006**, *32*, 1057–1061. [CrossRef] [PubMed]
49. Hiranmayi, K.V.; Sirisha, K.; Ramoji Rao, M.V.; Sudhakar, P. Novel Pathogens in Periodontal Microbiology. *J. Pharm. Bioallied Sci.* **2017**, *9*, 155–163. [CrossRef]
50. Vermeire, S.; Joossens, M.; Verbeke, K.; Wang, J.; Machiels, K.; Sabino, J.; Ferrante, M.; Van Assche, G.; Rutgeerts, P.; Raes, J. Donor Species Richness Determines Faecal Microbiota Transplantation Success in Inflammatory Bowel Disease. *J. Crohns. Colitis* **2016**, *10*, 387–394. [CrossRef]
51. Kump, P.; Wurm, P.; Grochenig, H.P.; Wenzl, H.; Petritsch, W.; Halwachs, B.; Wagner, M.; Stadlbauer, V.; Eherer, A.; Hoffmann, K.M.; et al. The taxonomic composition of the donor intestinal microbiota is a major factor influencing the efficacy of faecal microbiota transplantation in therapy refractory ulcerative colitis. *Aliment. Pharmacol. Ther.* **2018**, *47*, 67–77. [CrossRef] [PubMed]

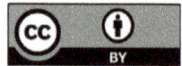

© 2020 by the authors. Licensee MDPI, Basel, Switzerland. This article is an open access article distributed under the terms and conditions of the Creative Commons Attribution (CC BY) license (http://creativecommons.org/licenses/by/4.0/).

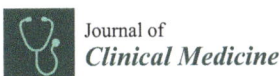

Review

Fecal Microbiota Transplantation: Screening and Selection to Choose the Optimal Donor

Stefano Bibbò [1,2], Carlo Romano Settanni [1,2], Serena Porcari [1,2], Enrico Bocchino [2], Gianluca Ianiro [1,2], Giovanni Cammarota [1,2] and Antonio Gasbarrini [1,2,*]

[1] UOC Medicina Interna e Gastroenterologia, Dipartimento di Scienze Mediche e Chirurgiche, Fondazione Policlinico Universitario "A. Gemelli" IRCCS, 00168 Roma, Italy; stefano.bibbo@policlinicogemelli.it (S.B.); carlosettanni@hotmail.it (C.R.S.); porcariserena89@gmail.com (S.P.); gianluca.ianiro@hotmail.it (G.I.); giovanni.cammarota@unicatt.it (G.C.)
[2] Istituto di Patologia Speciale Medica, Università Cattolica del Sacro Cuore, 00168 Roma, Italy; enrico.bocchino01@gmail.com
* Correspondence: antonio.gasbarrini@unicatt.it

Received: 28 April 2020; Accepted: 2 June 2020; Published: 5 June 2020

Abstract: In the past decade, fecal microbiota transplantation (FMT) has rapidly spread worldwide in clinical practice as a highly effective treatment option against recurrent *Clostridioides difficile* infection. Moreover, new evidence also supports a role for FMT in other conditions, such as inflammatory bowel disease, functional gastrointestinal disorders, or metabolic disorders. Recently, some studies have identified specific microbial characteristics associated with clinical improvement after FMT, in different disorders, paving the way for a microbiota-based precision medicine approach. Moreover, donor screening has become increasingly more complex over years, along with standardization of FMT and the increasing number of stool banks. In this narrative review, we discuss most recent evidence on the screening and selection of the stool donor, with reference to recent studies that have identified specific microbiological features for clinical conditions such as *Clostridioides difficile* infection, irritable bowel syndrome, inflammatory bowel disease, and metabolic disorders.

Keywords: gut microbiota; precision medicine; *Clostridium difficile*; inflammatory bowel disease; ulcerative colitis; irritable bowel disease; metabolic syndrome

---

1. Fecal Microbiota Transplantation: A New Old Therapy

In the last decade, multiple studies have expanded knowledge in the field of gut microbiota, including pathogenesis, diagnosis, and therapeutics [1]. To date, the therapeutic modulation of the intestinal microbiota is performed with traditional approaches such as antibiotics and probiotics, or increasingly through fecal microbiota transplantation (FMT), which is defined as the transfer of fecal material from a healthy donor into the gastrointestinal tract of a recipient [2].

Fecal material has been used in medicine since almost two thousand years. The first description of the use of fecal material for medical purposes dates back to about 1700 years ago; traditional Chinese medicine in particular had perceived the potential role of this biological material and used it for several clinical indications such as gastrointestinal, nervous system, skin, and gynecological diseases [3]. In Western countries, the first description of ancestral FMT dates to the 17th century, when Fabricius Acquapendente reported the transplantation of feces for the cure of animals unable to ruminate [4]. More recently, anecdotal use has been reported during the Second World War. German soldiers residing in North Africa suffered from recurrent episodes of diarrhea that they treated by eating camel stool, being inspired from the local practice of the Bedouins [5]. Western medicine began to study the potential role of FMT only in the second half of the 20th century. Firstly in 1958, Ben Eiseman reported the successfully treatment of four patients with pseudomembranous colitis using fecal enemas [6], and over 20 year later, Schwan et al. reported new evidence supporting the efficacy of FMT in *C. difficile* infection (CDI) [7]. In the following years, several other reports came out, and a growing body of evidence showed the efficacy of FMT in the treatment of recurrent CDI, and, furthermore, the feasibility of FMT was gradually suggested for other clinical indications.

The first randomized controlled trial that investigated the role of FMT for recurrent CDI was published by van Nood et al. in 2013. They reported that a single infusion of fecal material by nasoduodenal route was superior to standard therapy with vancomycin [8]. In further years, other routes of administration were successfully tested in clinical trials, demonstrating the efficacy of FMT by lower route through colonoscopy [9] or upper administration with capsule [10]. Therefore, the growing interest of the scientific community towards FMT has meant that a large amount of data has been published in the last decade; for this reason, a panel of European experts met in Rome in 2017 to release the first evidence-based consensus report for the use of FMT in clinical practice [11].

Over the years, further issues have emerged, which are still not clarified to date. In particular, in view of the growing number of patients who could benefit from FMT, it is necessary to identify innovative ways to storing fecal material to be used if necessary. Indeed, in the early experiences, FMT was performed only with fresh material from occasional healthy donors, but this approach is not feasible for large-scale use of FMT. To solve this problem, the possibility to create structures to bank the feces after manipulation was suggested, and this approach is supported by the evidence of the effectiveness of FMT performed with frozen material [12]. In consideration of the increasing interest of the scientific community on this topic, a panel of international experts met in Rome in 2019 to define the general guidelines for the creation of stool banks [13]. Despite these efforts, many problems remain to be solved. Above all, the identification of the optimal donor is a fundamental clinical issue of rising relevance. Indeed, the increasing number of clinical indications suggests the need to identify the ideal donor for each disease or patient that cannot be treated indiscriminately with the same fecal biomass. The fascinating idea of identifying the "perfect" intestinal microbiota has motivated the scientific community for at least one century—ever since in the early 20 century Elie Metchnikoff suggested the role of intestinal bacteria in the development of many pathological conditions and health in the homeostasis of the microbial species [14], generating the concepts of "eubiosis" and "dysbiosis," which for years were considered only fascinating hypotheses without strong scientific bases. However, in recent years, the molecular techniques of genomic sequencing have allowed to understand the link between gut microbiota and several diseases [15], giving evidence to this old intuition. In particular, we refer to "eubiosis" as considering a status characterized by a preponderance of potentially beneficial species, while "dysbiosis" is a condition characterized by the loss of homeostasis and by the proliferation of microbial species considered potentially pathogenic and, moreover, favor a "milieu" triggering the hyper-inflammatory state [16]. To date, an increasing number of studies confirm these hypotheses, in particular the reduced diversity of gut microbiota, simply defined as the variety and abundance of species in a defined microbial ecosystem [17,18], which is known to characterize several chronic diseases compared to a control group [19,20]. Therefore, in this narrative review, we report the most recent evidences on the screening and selection of the stool donor, with special efforts to describe findings that may lead to the optimal donor in several disease looking for an "optimal microbiota" to be transplanted (CDI, inflammatory bowel disease (IBD), irritable bowel syndrome (IBS), and other emerging pathological conditions).

2. Fecal Microbiota Transplantation in Clinical Practice

To date, the only recommendation for FMT in clinical practice is the treatment of recurrent CDI, although a large number of emerging indications are being experienced in several studies [21].

CDI is a burdensome clinical issue and represent the most relevant cause of antibiotic-associated diarrhea; its incidence has evolved in recent years and the risk of recurrence after standard antibiotic therapy has widely increased [22,23]. The standard treatment for the first occurrence of CDI is still represented by antibiotic therapy, mainly with metronidazole or vancomycin [24]. However, the clinical success rate of antibiotics in the recurrence of CDI is dramatically decreased, consequently, more effective therapies have been proposed, including FMT [25,26]. The clinical success of FMT, in contrast to the loss of efficacy of standard antibiotic therapy, could be explained by understanding the mechanism of action. In fact, FMT is a restorative treatment of gut microbiota alterations, unlike antibiotics, which is a disruptive treatment; accordingly, the administration of FMT results in a prompt and sustained normalization of microbial community structure and then metabolic activity of gut microbiota [27]. Indeed, CDI develops only in subjects with disruption of gut microbiota [28]; supporting this idea, it was demonstrated that the feces of patients with recurrent CDI have a higher relative abundance of several bacterial family as *Enterobacteriaceae*, *Veillonellaceae*, and *Lactobacillaceae*, and lower relative abundance of *Ruminococcaceae*, *Bacteroidaceae*, and *Lachnospiraceae* [29]. Furthermore, FMT recipients have shown changes in microbial profiles and shifts in the gut microbiota composition towards a profile similar to that of the healthy donor; this finding is obtained in a few days and is observed for at least six months [30].

To date, several systematic review and meta-analyses have shown an overall cure rate of FMT of up to 90% in preventing further CDI recurrence [31,32]. Moreover, a recent meta-analysis has shown that both the upper and the lower route are effective, with a slight advantage of colonoscopy over other techniques [32]. Based on these positive evidences, scientific societies have included FMT among the recommended treatment for recurrent CDI. Already in 2014, FMT was strongly recommended in recurrent CDI by the European Society of Clinical Microbiology and Infectious Disease (ESCMID) [33], while the American College of Gastroenterology (ACG) stated that FMT can be considered after the third recurrence [34]; more recently, the Infectious Disease Society of America (IDSA) confirmed the indication in the treatment of recurrent CDI with FMT [24].

Alongside well-established indications such as CDI, several studies have found emerging clinical conditions for which FMT may represent a promising alternative to standard therapies. Most evidence comes from inflammatory bowel disease (IBD) studies. Several alterations of gut microbiota has been proposed as factors contributing to the development of the aberrant immunological response in IBD [35], but it is still unclear if the perturbations of microbiota are the cause or consequence of the mucosal inflammation associated to IBD [36]. In particular, ulcerative colitis (UC) is the most suitable IBD model for the study of FMT, considering the characteristics of inflammation of the mucosa and the established role of the microbiota in pathogenesis [37]. To date, a little number of clinical trials have reported promising results, but several concerns suggest to better investigate this potential clinical application [38]. According to a Cochrane systematic review of four clinical trials, the overall remission rate at week 8 was 37% (52/140 UC patients) in patients receiving FMT, compared with 18% (24/137 patients) in those receiving placebo; additionally, clinical response and endoscopic remission improved in patients treated with FMT [39]. However, several factors appear to influence the clinical response in UC patients, as the condition during the manipulation of the feces or the donor selection. For instance, anaerobic conditions during the manipulation of stool were associated with better performance considering clinical remission or steroid free response [40]. Donor selection might be a relevant factor considering that a study reported higher success rates with one particular donor compared with other donors [41]. Furthermore, an emerging relevant indication for FMT was represented by the flare of UC associated with concurrent *C. difficile* over infection. A recent clinical trial, including patients affected by UC or Crohn disease with recurrent CDI, reported that FMT has a curative effect on the recurrence of CDI, but has no apparent beneficial effect on the IBD course [42].

Gut microbiota disturbance was also involved in other gastrointestinal diseases such as irritable bowel syndrome (IBS). A systematic reviews with meta-analysis showed that FMT may be beneficial in IBS [43], but this finding is limited by the small number of patients included and by the relevant differences in the design of the studies. In particular, IBS is triggered by multiple factors, and furthermore, is a heterogeneous condition that may require a selection of the donor in each case. For instance, El-Salhy et al. have recently reported that FMT administered through gastroscope was highly effective in IBS if a well-defined donor was chosen with a normal disbyosis index and favorable specific microbial signature [44].

Furthermore, metabolic and hepatic diseases are also considered emerging indications for FMT. There is great interest towards the modulation of the gut microbiota in metabolic syndrome, as two studies reported promising results in improving peripheral insulin sensitivity [45,46]. Unfortunately, the improvement of metabolic profile was not maintained in the long term, and a recent systematic review including three studies reported the absence of significant benefits from FMT in metabolic syndrome [47]. Thus, further studies to clarify the feasibility of this approach in metabolic disorders are needed. Furthermore, FMT was able to reverse encephalopathy derived from disturbed gut-brain axis in patients with liver chronic disease, two clinical studies shown promising results in this field of application [48,49].

FMT was also proposed in the treatment of several other clinical conditions, but evidence is limited and results were reported by small studies; thus, the application is limited to clinical studies and selected cases. For instance, FMT was reported as effective in the decolonization of patients carrier of multi-drug resistant organism [50], in reducing symptoms in autism spectrum disorders [51], or in reliving symptoms and increasing progression free survival in graft versus host disease after hematopoietic stem cell transplant [52].

3. Selection and Screening of Stool Donors

Donor selection represents a fundamental challenge in view of the implementation of FMT programs worldwide. To date, there is a broad debate regarding the preference of donor selection, whether the stool donor should be known to the patient or whether it is preferable to use feces from unrelated donor. Moreover, in the case of non-related donor, fecal material could be banked at dedicated structures that provide support to the hospital that will perform FMT [53].

In particular, the ideal stool donor should be a healthy volunteer, without risk factors for infectious or other chronic diseases, and who is willing to "donate" frequently if needed. Unfortunately, although the conditions do not seem too selective, it is not always easy to identify an adequate number of donors to meet the needs of the FMT program. Indeed, data from large stool bank suggest high rates of donor drop out due to high commitment required [54]; furthermore, physicians often give up FMT because of the complexity and costs of screening [55]. Consequently, to solve these problems, it would be appropriate to implement the undirected donor selection program. Hence, the related donors should be only limited in cases of patient preference. Indeed, undirected donors reduced the likelihood of confidentiality concerns, and then, they are essential for the implementation of stool banking in consideration of easy availability, traceability, and reduction of screening expenses [56].

The screening of potential donors consist in two key landmarks, the preliminary interview and the laboratory testing [13]. A preliminary interview is usually performed by a structured questionnaire that investigated several risk factors to minimize the risk of transferring infections or adverse gut microbiota profile. In particular, the medical interview screen potential donors inquiring about the use of drugs that can alter gut microbiota, known history or risk behaviors for infectious disease, and for disorders potentially associated with the disruption of gut microbiota. The schedule of questions reported in this review (Table 1) includes the most frequently investigated features in leading FMT centers. Obviously, this draft of interview is not mandatory, but can be adapted to the socio-cultural context of potential donors. For example, it would be advisable to carefully investigate the eating habits of potential donors from country where the consumption of raw meat and fish is widespread, thereby increasing the risk of transmission of enteric pathogens, or who eat exotic animals that are potential carriers of unknown pathogens; or seasonal habits that increase the risk to get infected with intestinal pathogens (e.g., summer holidays and risk of sea food of poor quality). These examples allow to understand how the aim of the interview is to early intercept potential risks of pathogen transmission; thus, each center should adapt the medical interview to its socio-cultural context to make it more efficient.

Table 1. Preliminary interview to select donors.

Preliminary Interview – Medical History
Drugs that can alter gut microbiota
Use in the last three months of: ■ Antimicrobial drugs   ■ Immunosuppressant agents   ■ Chemotherapy   Daily use for over three months: ■ Proton pump inhibitors
Disorders potentially associated with the disruption of gut microbiota:
■ Personal history of chronic gastrointestinal disease, including functional gastrointestinal disorders; inflammatory bowel disease; celiac disease; other chronic gastroenterological diseases or recent abnormal gastrointestinal symptoms (e.g., diarrhea, hematochezia, etc.)   ■ Personal history of cancer, including gastrointestinal cancers or polyposis syndrome, and first-degree family history of premature colon cancer   ■ Personal history of systemic autoimmune disorders   ■ Obesity (body mass index > 30) and/or metabolic syndrome/diabetes   ■ Personal history of neurological/neurodegenerative disorders   ■ Personal history of psychiatric/neurodevelopmental conditions
Know history or risk behaviors for infectious disease
■ History of HIV, hepatitis B or C viruses, syphilis, human T-lymphotropic virus I and II   ■ Current systemic infection   ■ Use of illegal drugs   ■ High-risk sexual behavior   ■ Previous tissue/organ transplant   ■ Recent hospitalization or discharge from long-term care facilities   ■ High-risk travel   ■ Needle stick accident in the last six months   ■ Body tattoo, piercing, earring, acupuncture in the last six months   ■ Enteric pathogen infection in the last two months   ■ Acute gastroenteritis with or without confirmatory test in the last two months   ■ History of vaccination with a live attenuated virus in the last two months

The optimal donor correspond at young individual (preferably < 50 years, as suggested by a panel of experts [13] taking into account that increasing age has been associated with altered gut microbiota composition [57]; moreover, aged microbiota could have a negative effect contributing to the inflammatory state of the recipient [58]), although is important to exclude candidates with personal history of malignancies or autoimmune disease [13]. Moreover, there are concerns regarding the exclusion of healthcare workers considering the supposed increased risk of colonization by antibiotic-resistant bacteria; however, available data suggest a low prevalence in this population [59].

Potential donors who have a permissive medical history must undergo to blood and fecal examination to exclude infective disease transmittable trough fecal transfer [13]. The tests may change between the various protocols, but there are some mandatory examinations (Table 2).

Table 2. Donor blood and stool testing.

Blood testing
- Complete blood cell count
- Liver enzyme (Aminotransferases)
- Bilirubin
- Creatinine
- C-reactive protein
- Serology for Hepatitis virus (HAV, HBV, HCV, HEV) and Human immunodeficiency virus (HIV)
Stool testing
- *Clostridium difficile*
- *Giardia lamblia, Cryptosporidium* spp, Isospora and Microsporidia
- Protozoa and helminths and parasites (including *Blastocystis hominis* and *Dientamoeba fragilis*)
- Antibiotic-resistant bacteria
- Common enteric pathogens, including *Salmonella, Shigella, Campylobacter*, shiga toxin-producing *Escherichia coli*, Yersinia, and *Vibrio cholerae*
- Norovirus, rotavirus, adenovirus
- *Helicobacter pylori* fecal antigen

In fact, blood testing should include complete blood cell count, liver enzyme, creatinine, and C-reactive protein to check overall clinical condition, serology for Hepatitis virus, and Human immunodeficiency virus (HIV). Furthermore, blood tests can be considered in case of anomalies of the first round of laboratory tests, endemic spread of some pathogens, emergence of new pathogens or selected cases of recipients (e.g., immunosuppressed). In particular, there is debate about the usefulness of serology for EBV and CMV, as the high prevalence of prior exposure among adult individuals weakens the diagnostic power of this approach, limiting the clinical utility to IgM CMV in donors dedicated to immunosuppressed recipients. Of course, it is not appropriate to exclude subjects with prior exposure to EBV or CMV from the donation because of the unlikely risk of transmission, unless clinical or laboratory suspicion of reactivation. Finally, the candidates could be considered for testing the serology for nematodes, based on social and geographical features and tests availability [13].

Stool testing should include common enteric pathogens, *Clostridium difficile*, fecal parasites, and *Helicobacter pylori* antigen (this last exam only for upper route of FMT delivery). Enteric pathogens, which must also be investigated in asymptomatic subjects, should be detected with conventional methods (culture, microscopy, or antigen test) and/or with molecular diagnosis (PCR-based panels) that have shown a high specificity and sensitivity compared to conventional methods in rapid detection of pathogens [60]. Furthermore, it is mandatory to test all fecal samples for antibiotic-resistant bacteria (including meticillin-resistant *Staphylococcus aureus* (MRSA), vancomycin-resistant Enterococci (VRE), extended-spectrum β-lactamase-producing Enterobacteriaceae, and carbapenem-resistant Enterobacteriaceae/carbapenemase-producing Enterobacteriaceae), considering the burden of the gastrointestinal carriage in asymptomatic subjects [61,62] and the reporting of some serious adverse events associated to sepsis after FMT [13]. Nowadays, due to the emerging Covid-19 pandemic, a panel of international experts has suggested to include in the tests for Sars-CoV-2 a thorough nasopharyngeal swab and/or RNA detection in stool [63].

Finally, if all blood and fecal tests are negative, the candidate is accepted to become a stool donor. Especially in the fecal bank program, the donor should be available to donate on many occasions over time. For this reason, it is advisable to repeat the screening tests every 8–12 weeks and administer a short questionnaire on the same day of the donation to check for any recent-onset harmful events.

In this paragraph we have reported the general rules to select and to screen potential donor for FMT, mainly to treat CDI that is cured by the restorative effect of fecal transfer on gut microbiota. However, for other clinical indications, which find their rationale in the modification of metabolic and inflammatory pathways mediated by gut microbiota, it would be appropriate to identify a specific donor for each case. This issue will be discussed later.

4. Selection of the Optimal Donor for FMT to Treat Specific Disorders

The correct recruitment of healthy donors is essential for a standardized and safe FMT procedure [11,13]. FMT is considered a safe procedure; however, mild adverse effects attributable to FMT are reported in about one third of the recipients, such as self-limiting abdominal discomfort or changes of bowel habits, and unfortunately, about 2–6% of patients experienced serious adverse events, such as infection, relapse of pre-existing disease, or death [64]. Moreover, the difficulty of selecting the appropriate candidates is increasing due to emerging concerns, as the possibility of transmission of putative procarcinogenic bacteria [65] or the potential risk of serious life threatening infections with multi-drug resistant organisms after FMT [66]. Moreover, recent evidences showed that the efficacy of FMT in recurrent CDI treatment, in clinical trials and in other healthcare settings seems to be linked to different variables, such as the delivery methods of fecal infusate, the bowel preparation, the number of infusion, the disease severity, and in particular to the microbial diversity and composition of the transplanted stools [32,44,67]. Since the idea that the success rate of FMT could be related to the gut microbiota or other features of the donor, the term "super-donors" has been introduced to indicate the ideal individuals whose stools could ensure a better outcome for recipients compared to others fecal donations [68]. Therefore, assuming that dysbiosis-related disorders have been associated to different imbalanced microbial signatures [15], in order to restore the eubiosis, it is reasonable to assume that reaching the correct donor-recipient match with targeted FMT based on specific microbial disturbances might be the key to improve FMT response. Accumulating evidence strengthens this hypothesis, leading to discard the concept of "one stool fits all" and to search an optimal donor [68], as in other organ transplantation procedures [69].

4.1. Clostridium Difficile Infection

The research of the ideal donor in recurrent CDI is obviously a widely debated topic of study. For example, one study identified the optimal donor among nine healthy vegetarian or vegan candidates, selecting the candidate who had a balanced Bacteroidetes/Firmicutes ratio, the highest alpha diversity among screened individuals, and high butyrate concentration. After 10 weeks from a single or multiple FMT, none of the 10 patients experienced CDI recurrence [70]. Of interest, the gut virome may also play a role in CDI treatment [71]. Indeed, enteric virome alterations marked by an increase in the abundance of *Caudovirales*, together with a decreased *Caudovirales* diversity, richness, and evenness, have been reported in patients with CDI. Moreover, CD eradication was associated with the colonization of a higher abundance of donor-derived *Caudovirales* contigs detected during follow up. These findings could possibly explain why bacterial fecal filtrate infusion resulted in effective treatment of CDI [72], and shifted the attention on the importance of the bacteriophages and on the potential role of selecting donors on the basis of their gut virome. Finally, some authors reported that selecting specific enteric bacterial strains with bacterial cultures from healthy donors to prepare a stool substitute blend might be a winning strategy to cure recurrent and antibiotic-resistant *C. difficile* colitis [73,74]. However, it is likely that the relevant impact on FMT success in CDI depends on the transfer of a complete fecal microbiome rather than specific bacterial strains; moreover, the promising results reported by the study that transfer the fecal filtrate alone suggest a predominant role for bacteriophages rather than for the specific relative abundance pattern of the gut microbiota of donor, shifting the central role from bacteria to viruses in the therapeutic challenge of FMT in CDI; however, these data are still preliminary and need to be confirmed by further studies.

4.2. Inflammatory Bowel Disease

Many studies analyzed the microbial profile of donors and tried to relate it with clinical and laboratory outcomes in patients with IBD. Clinical outcomes and immunological changes after FMT in patients with IBD were significantly related to the variations of several specific strains in recipients of fecal microbiota [75]. For instance, intensive FMT in UC patients were associated with negative outcomes in case of abundance of *Fusobacterium spp* and *Sutterella spp* in recipients' fecal microbiota after the FMT [76]. Furthermore, a study that involved refractory UC patients reported that pre-treatment with antibiotic plus repeated FMTs using fecal material from donor with a high bacterial richness and high relative abundance of *Akkermansia muciniphila*, unclassified Ruminococcaceae, and *Ruminococcus spp.* was more likely to induce remission compared to antibiotics alone [67]. As also described in other studies [41,77,78], it is plausible that choosing donors based on their taxonomic composition, in particular low or high abundance of specific strains, might reflect the possibility for future trials in IBD. For this purpose, methods aimed at preventing an inflammatory response of the recipient's intestinal immune system by selecting compatible donors on their microbial profiles are under study [79]. Furthermore, the gut virome could represent a potential marker for FMT response in UC patients. In particular, results from a small case series reported that FMT responders already presented, before undergoing to FMT, a significantly lower eukaryotic viral richness than non-responders. Moreover, the richness of donor virome was not associated with the FMT outcome, as instead proposed for bacteria [80].

4.3. Other Emerging Indications

Several preclinical and clinical studies supported the rationale for donor selection based on gut microbial profile in other disorders associated to gut dysbiosis. Indeed, in the field of anti-cancer treatment, it has been reported that microbiota can influence chemotherapy response [81]. Preclinical studies found a clinical improvement in mouse models of melanoma on anti-PD-1 therapy that received FMT from donors with a melanoma "responder-like" microbial signature (with high alpha diversity and abundance of Ruminococcaceae, *Faecalibacterium*, *Bifidobacterium longum*, *Collinsella aerofaciens*, and *Enterococcus faecium*) when compared to mice that received "non responder-like" microbiome (characterized by low microbial diversity and high relative abundance of Bacteroidales) [82,83]. Nevertheless, trials on humans, testing the effect of FMT in increasing the response to cancer therapies, are still in progress [84].

Recently, a randomized placebo-controlled trial of FMT in IBS reported that the abundance of *Streptococcus, Dorea, Lactobacillus,* and *Ruminococcaceae* spp in the donor microbiota was associated with efficacy in relieving IBS symptoms [44]. Interestingly, a small open-label clinical trial evaluated the impact of prolonged FMT with antibiotic pre-treatment in children with autism; authors reported a decrease of gastrointestinal symptoms and an improvement of behavior, together with specific genera increase in recipients (*Bifidobacterium, Prevotella,* and *Desulfovibrio*). Conversely, *Prevotella,* and *Desulfovibrio* were more represented in recipients after FMT than in the donor samples, suggesting that unknown factors changed the intestinal ecosystem, making it more hospitable to these strains [85].

Within the context of metabolic diseases, the effect of allogenic FMT post-Roux-en-Y gastric bypass donors was compared with metabolic syndrome donors on glucose metabolism and other parameters in treatment-naïve patients with metabolic syndrome. The authors assessed a decrease of insulin sensitivity in recipients who received FMT from donors with metabolic syndrome compared with using post-surgical donors. Moreover, they identified several microbial OTUs possibly predictive of metabolic response, suggesting a microbiota-related transmissible mechanism of insulin resistance [86]. Similarly, another study reported a significant increase in insulin sensitivity, together with altered microbiota composition, in patients with metabolic syndrome who received allogenic FMT from lean donors compared to those who underwent autologous FMT [46].

To date, these results appear promising but partially controversial; thus, findings need to be confirmed with stronger evidence and by standardized clinical trial. Further research is needed to identify the favorable microbial signature of donor or other ideal features in disease-specific settings.

5. Conclusions and Future Perspectives

In this review, the stool donor screening process has been described, and recent evidence has been reported that try to identify the optimal donor for each clinical condition (Figure S1).

To date, the clinical characteristics of the donor are well defined; in particular, they are recommended to be a healthy volunteer with a balanced lifestyle, without chronic diseases or family history of metabolic diseases or cancer, and defined laboratory exams must certify the current absence of disease. However, identification of the ideal donor through the microbiological typing of the stool is currently not suitable. First of all, understanding the role of the intestinal microbiota in each chronic disease is an indispensable condition before hypothesizing a personalized approach through FMT. In fact, while the restorative mechanism of FMT in recurrent CDI is now understood, many aspects still need to be understood regarding the treatment of other chronic conditions. Interesting evidence has been reported regarding dysbiosis in IBD or in other chronic conditions, but the contrasting results reported in clinical trials of FMT could be justified by the choice of unsuitable donors. The identification of the microbiological characteristics of the ideal donor for each disease appears to be an achievable goal but still far from being accomplished due to the lack of clinical studies. The current evidence is still limited and insufficient for explaining and resolving the complexity of the interaction between the intestinal barrier and its role in gut-related chronic diseases. However, further studies need to be designed to confirm the encouraging results that have been reported in recent years. In particular, it will be necessary to type the fecal microbiota of the donor and the recipient, and to understand how environmental factors, such as diet, or individual features may benefit (or not) the clinical response to FMT. Understanding the microbial characteristics of the optimal donor, in particular if they are modifiable through lifestyle changes or pharmacological measures, could increase the therapeutic potential of FMT.

Supplementary Materials: The following are available online at http://www.mdpi.com/2077-0383/9/6/1757/s1, Figure S1: Optimal Stool Donor to Treat Specific Disorders.

Author Contributions: Conceptualization, S.B. and A.G.; data curation, S.B., C.R.S. and S.P.; writing—original draft preparation, S.B. and C.R.S.; writing—review and editing, S.B., C.R.S., S.P., E.B., G.I., G.C. and A.G. All authors have read and agreed to the published version of the manuscript.

Funding: This research received no external funding.

Conflicts of Interest: The authors declare no conflict of interest.

References

1. Marchesi, J.R.; Adams, D.H.; Fava, F.; Hermes, G.D.; Hirschfield, G.M.; Hold, G.; Quraishi, M.N.; Kinross, J.; Smidt, H.; Tuohy, K.M.; et al. The gut microbiota and host health: A new clinical frontier. *Gut* **2016**, *65*, 330–339. [CrossRef] [PubMed]
2. Bibbo, S.; Ianiro, G.; Gasbarrini, A.; Cammarota, G. Fecal microbiota transplantation: Past, present and future perspectives. *Minerva Gastroenterol. Dietol.* **2017**, *63*, 420–430. [PubMed]
3. Du, H.; Kuang, T.T.; Qiu, S.; Xu, T.; Gang Huan, C.L.; Fan, G.; Zhang, Y. Fecal medicines used in traditional medical system of China: A systematic review of their names, original species, traditional uses, and modern investigations. *Chin. Med.* **2019**, *14*, 31. [CrossRef] [PubMed]
4. Borody, T.J.; Warren, E.F.; Leis, S.M.; Surace, R.; Ashman, O.; Siarakas, S. Bacteriotherapy using fecal flora: Toying with human motions. *J. Clin. Gastroenterol.* **2004**, *38*, 475–483. [CrossRef] [PubMed]
5. Gasbarrini, G.; Bonvicini, F.; Gramenzi, A. Probiotics History. *J. Clin. Gastroenterol.* **2016**, *50*, S116–S119. [CrossRef]
6. Eiseman, B.; Silen, W.; Bascom, G.S.; Kauvar, A.J. Fecal enema as an adjunct in the treatment of pseudomembranous enterocolitis. *Surgery* **1958**, *44*, 854–859.
7. Schwan, A.; Sjolin, S.; Trottestam, U.; Aronsson, B. Relapsing clostridium difficile enterocolitis cured by rectal infusion of homologous faeces. *Lancet* **1983**, *2*, 845. [CrossRef]

8. Van Nood, E.; Vrieze, A.; Nieuwdorp, M.; Fuentes, S.; Zoetendal, E.G.; de Vos, W.M.; Visser, C.E.; Kuijper, E.J.; Bartelsman, J.F.; Tijssen, J.G.; et al. Duodenal infusion of donor feces for recurrent Clostridium difficile. *N. Engl. J. Med.* **2013**, *368*, 407–415. [CrossRef]
9. Cammarota, G.; Masucci, L.; Ianiro, G.; Bibbo, S.; Dinoi, G.; Costamagna, G.; Sanguinetti, M.; Gasbarrini, A. Randomised clinical trial: Faecal microbiota transplantation by colonoscopy vs. vancomycin for the treatment of recurrent Clostridium difficile infection. *Aliment. Pharmacol. Ther.* **2015**, *41*, 835–843. [CrossRef]
10. Youngster, I.; Russell, G.H.; Pindar, C.; Ziv-Baran, T.; Sauk, J.; Hohmann, E.L. Oral, capsulized, frozen fecal microbiota transplantation for relapsing Clostridium difficile infection. *JAMA* **2014**, *312*, 1772–1778. [CrossRef]
11. Cammarota, G.; Ianiro, G.; Tilg, H.; Rajilic-Stojanovic, M.; Kump, P.; Satokari, R.; Sokol, H.; Arkkila, P.; Pintus, C.; Hart, A.; et al. European consensus conference on faecal microbiota transplantation in clinical practice. *Gut* **2017**, *66*, 569–580. [CrossRef] [PubMed]
12. Lee, C.H.; Steiner, T.; Petrof, E.O.; Smieja, M.; Roscoe, D.; Nematallah, A.; Weese, J.S.; Collins, S.; Moayyedi, P.; Crowther, M.; et al. Frozen vs Fresh Fecal Microbiota Transplantation and Clinical Resolution of Diarrhea in Patients With Recurrent Clostridium difficile Infection: A Randomized Clinical Trial. *JAMA* **2016**, *315*, 142–149. [CrossRef] [PubMed]
13. Cammarota, G.; Ianiro, G.; Kelly, C.R.; Mullish, B.H.; Allegretti, J.R.; Kassam, Z.; Putignani, L.; Fischer, M.; Keller, J.J.; Costello, S.P.; et al. International consensus conference on stool banking for faecal microbiota transplantation in clinical practice. *Gut* **2019**, *68*, 2111–2121. [CrossRef] [PubMed]
14. Cavaillon, J.M.; Legout, S. Centenary of the death of Elie Metchnikoff: A visionary and an outstanding team leader. *Microbes Infect.* **2016**, *18*, 577–594. [CrossRef] [PubMed]
15. Vandana, U.K.; Barlaskar, N.H.; Gulzar, A.B.M.; Laskar, I.H.; Kumar, D.; Paul, P.; Pandey, P.; Mazumder, P.B. Linking gut microbiota with the human diseases. *Bioinformation* **2020**, *16*, 196–208. [CrossRef] [PubMed]
16. Iebba, V.; Totino, V.; Gagliardi, A.; Santangelo, F.; Cacciotti, F.; Trancassini, M.; Mancini, C.; Cicerone, C.; Corazziari, E.; Pantanella, F.; et al. Eubiosis and dysbiosis: The two sides of the microbiota. *New Microbiol.* **2016**, *39*, 1–12.
17. Lozupone, C.A.; Stombaugh, J.I.; Gordon, J.I.; Jansson, J.K.; Knight, R. Diversity, stability and resilience of the human gut microbiota. *Nature* **2012**, *489*, 220–230. [CrossRef]
18. Young, V.B.; Schmidt, T.M. Overview of the gastrointestinal microbiota. *Adv. Exp. Med. Biol.* **2008**, *635*, 29–40.
19. Lin, L.; Zhang, J. Role of intestinal microbiota and metabolites on gut homeostasis and human diseases. *BMC Immunol.* **2017**, *18*, 2. [CrossRef]
20. Forbes, J.D.; Chen, C.Y.; Knox, N.C.; Marrie, R.A.; El-Gabalawy, H.; de Kievit, T.; Alfa, M.; Bernstein, C.N.; Van Domselaar, G. A comparative study of the gut microbiota in immune-mediated inflammatory diseases-does a common dysbiosis exist? *Microbiome* **2018**, *6*, 221. [CrossRef]
21. Allegretti, J.R.; Mullish, B.H.; Kelly, C.; Fischer, M. The evolution of the use of faecal microbiota transplantation and emerging therapeutic indications. *Lancet* **2019**, *394*, 420–431. [CrossRef]
22. Leffler, D.A.; Lamont, J.T. Clostridium difficile Infection. *N. Engl. J. Med.* **2015**, *373*, 287–288. [CrossRef]
23. Desai, K.; Gupta, S.B.; Dubberke, E.R.; Prabhu, V.S.; Browne, C.; Mast, T.C. Epidemiological and economic burden of Clostridium difficile in the United States: Estimates from a modeling approach. *BMC Infect. Dis.* **2016**, *16*, 303. [CrossRef]
24. McDonald, L.C.; Gerding, D.N.; Johnson, S.; Bakken, J.S.; Carroll, K.C.; Coffin, S.E.; Dubberke, E.R.; Garey, K.W.; Gould, C.V.; Kelly, C.; et al. Clinical Practice Guidelines for Clostridium difficile Infection in Adults and Children: 2017 Update by the Infectious Diseases Society of America (IDSA) and Society for Healthcare Epidemiology of America (SHEA). *Clin. Infect. Dis. Off. Publ. Infect. Dis. Soc. Am.* **2018**, *66*, 987–994. [CrossRef]
25. Kumar, V.; Fischer, M. Expert opinion on fecal microbiota transplantation for the treatment of Clostridioides difficile infection and beyond. *Expert Opin. Biol. Ther.* **2020**, *20*, 73–81. [CrossRef]
26. Cammarota, G.; Ianiro, G.; Magalini, S.; Gasbarrini, A.; Gui, D. Decrease in Surgery for Clostridium difficile Infection After Starting a Program to Transplant Fecal Microbiota. *Ann. Intern. Med.* **2015**, *163*, 487–488. [CrossRef]
27. Britton, R.A.; Young, V.B. Interaction between the intestinal microbiota and host in Clostridium difficile colonization resistance. *Trends Microbiol.* **2012**, *20*, 313–319. [CrossRef]

28. Bibbo, S.; Lopetuso, L.R.; Ianiro, G.; Di Rienzo, T.; Gasbarrini, A.; Cammarota, G. Role of microbiota and innate immunity in recurrent Clostridium difficile infection. *J. Immunol. Res.* **2014**, *2014*, 462740. [CrossRef] [PubMed]
29. Weingarden, A.R.; Chen, C.; Bobr, A.; Yao, D.; Lu, Y.; Nelson, V.M.; Sadowsky, M.J.; Khoruts, A. Microbiota transplantation restores normal fecal bile acid composition in recurrent Clostridium difficile infection. *Am. J. Physiol. Gastrointest. Liver Physiol.* **2014**, *306*, G310–G319. [CrossRef] [PubMed]
30. Weingarden, A.; Gonzalez, A.; Vazquez-Baeza, Y.; Weiss, S.; Humphry, G.; Berg-Lyons, D.; Knights, D.; Unno, T.; Bobr, A.; Kang, J.; et al. Dynamic changes in short- and long-term bacterial composition following fecal microbiota transplantation for recurrent Clostridium difficile infection. *Microbiome* **2015**, *3*, 10. [CrossRef] [PubMed]
31. Quraishi, M.N.; Widlak, M.; Bhala, N.; Moore, D.; Price, M.; Sharma, N.; Iqbal, T.H. Systematic review with meta-analysis: The efficacy of faecal microbiota transplantation for the treatment of recurrent and refractory Clostridium difficile infection. *Aliment. Pharmacol. Ther.* **2017**, *46*, 479–493. [CrossRef] [PubMed]
32. Ianiro, G.; Maida, M.; Burisch, J.; Simonelli, C.; Hold, G.; Ventimiglia, M.; Gasbarrini, A.; Cammarota, G. Efficacy of different faecal microbiota transplantation protocols for Clostridium difficile infection: A systematic review and meta-analysis. *United Eur. Gastroenterol. J.* **2018**, *6*, 1232–1244. [CrossRef] [PubMed]
33. Debast, S.B.; Bauer, M.P.; Kuijper, E.J. European Society of Clinical M Infectious D. European Society of Clinical Microbiology and Infectious Diseases: Update of the treatment guidance document for Clostridium difficile infection. *Clin. Microbiol. Infect.* **2014**, *20*, 1–26. [CrossRef] [PubMed]
34. Surawicz, C.M.; Brandt, L.J.; Binion, D.G.; Ananthakrishnan, A.N.; Curry, S.R.; Gilligan, P.H.; McFarland, L.V.; Mellow, M.; Zuckerbraun, B.S. Guidelines for diagnosis, treatment, and prevention of Clostridium difficile infections. *Am. J. Gastroenterol.* **2013**, *108*, 478–498. [CrossRef]
35. Cammarota, G.; Ianiro, G.; Cianci, R.; Bibbo, S.; Gasbarrini, A.; Curro, D. The involvement of gut microbiota in inflammatory bowel disease pathogenesis: Potential for therapy. *Pharmacol. Ther.* **2015**, *149*, 191–212. [CrossRef]
36. Khan, I.; Ullah, N.; Zha, L.; Bai, Y.; Khan, A.; Zhao, T.; Che, T.; Zhang, C. Alteration of Gut Microbiota in Inflammatory Bowel Disease (IBD): Cause or Consequence? IBD Treatment Targeting the Gut Microbiome. *Pathogens* **2019**, *8*, 126. [CrossRef]
37. Lopetuso, L.R.; Ianiro, G.; Allegretti, J.R.; Bibbo, S.; Gasbarrini, A.; Scaldaferri, F.; Cammarota, G. Fecal transplantation for ulcerative colitis: Current evidence and future applications. *Expert Opin. Biol. Ther.* **2020**, *20*, 343–351. [CrossRef]
38. Cammarota, G.; Ianiro, G. FMT for ulcerative colitis: Closer to the turning point. *Nat. Rev. Gastroenterol. Hepatol.* **2019**, *16*, 266–268. [CrossRef]
39. Imdad, A.; Nicholson, M.R.; Tanner-Smith, E.E.; Zackular, J.P.; Gomez-Duarte, O.G.; Beaulieu, D.B.; Acra, S. Fecal transplantation for treatment of inflammatory bowel disease. *Cochrane Database Syst. Rev.* **2018**, *11*, CD012774. [CrossRef]
40. Costello, S.P.; Conlon, M.A.; Andrews, J.M. Fecal Microbiota Transplantation for Ulcerative Colitis-Reply. *JAMA* **2019**, *321*, 2240–2241. [CrossRef]
41. Moayyedi, P.; Surette, M.G.; Kim, P.T.; Libertucci, J.; Wolfe, M.; Onischi, C.; Armstrong, D.; Marshall, J.K.; Kassam, Z.; Reinisch, W.; et al. Fecal Microbiota Transplantation Induces Remission in Patients With Active Ulcerative Colitis in a Randomized Controlled Trial. *Gastroenterology* **2015**, *149*, 102–109. [CrossRef] [PubMed]
42. Tariq, R.; Disbrow, M.B.; Dibaise, J.K.; Orenstein, R.; Saha, S.; Solanky, D.; Loftus, E.V.; Pardi, D.S.; Khanna, S. Efficacy of Fecal Microbiota Transplantation for Recurrent, C. Difficile Infection in Inflammatory Bowel Disease. *Inflamm. Bowel Dis.* **2019**. [CrossRef] [PubMed]
43. Ianiro, G.; Eusebi, L.H.; Black, C.J.; Gasbarrini, A.; Cammarota, G.; Ford, A.C. Systematic review with meta-analysis: Efficacy of faecal microbiota transplantation for the treatment of irritable bowel syndrome. *Aliment. Pharmacol. Ther.* **2019**, *50*, 240–248. [CrossRef] [PubMed]
44. El-Salhy, M.; Hatlebakk, J.G.; Gilja, O.H.; Brathen Kristoffersen, A.; Hausken, T. Efficacy of faecal microbiota transplantation for patients with irritable bowel syndrome in a randomised, double-blind, placebo-controlled study. *Gut* **2020**, *69*, 859–867. [CrossRef]

45. Vrieze, A.; Van Nood, E.; Holleman, F.; Salojarvi, J.; Kootte, R.S.; Bartelsman, J.F.; Dallinga-Thie, G.M.; Ackermans, M.T.; Serlie, M.J.; Oozeer, R.; et al. Transfer of intestinal microbiota from lean donors increases insulin sensitivity in individuals with metabolic syndrome. *Gastroenterology* **2012**, *143*, 913–916. [CrossRef]
46. Kootte, R.S.; Levin, E.; Salojarvi, J.; Smits, L.P.; Hartstra, A.V.; Udayappan, S.D.; Hermes, G.; Bouter, K.E.; Koopen, A.M.; Holst, J.J.; et al. Improvement of Insulin Sensitivity after Lean Donor Feces in Metabolic Syndrome Is Driven by Baseline Intestinal Microbiota Composition. *Cell Metab.* **2017**, *26*, 611–619. [CrossRef]
47. Zhang, Z.; Mocanu, V.; Cai, C.; Dang, J.; Slater, L.; Deehan, E.C.; Walter, J.; Madsen, K.L. Impact of Fecal Microbiota Transplantation on Obesity and Metabolic Syndrome-A Systematic Review. *Nutrients* **2019**, *11*, 2291. [CrossRef]
48. Bajaj, J.S.; Fagan, A.; Gavis, E.A.; Kassam, Z.; Sikaroodi, M.; Gillevet, P.M. Long-term Outcomes of Fecal Microbiota Transplantation in Patients With Cirrhosis. *Gastroenterology* **2019**, *156*, 1921–1923. [CrossRef]
49. Bajaj, J.S.; Salzman, N.H.; Acharya, C.; Sterling, R.K.; White, M.B.; Gavis, E.A.; Fagan, A.; Hayward, M.; Holtz, M.L.; Matherly, S.; et al. Fecal Microbial Transplant Capsules Are Safe in Hepatic Encephalopathy: A Phase 1, Randomized, Placebo-Controlled Trial. *Hepatology* **2019**, *70*, 1690–1703. [CrossRef]
50. Huttner, B.D.; de Lastours, V.; Wassenberg, M.; Maharshak, N.; Mauris, A.; Galperine, T.; Zanichelli, V.; Kapel, N.; Bellanger, A.; Olearo, F.; et al. A 5-day course of oral antibiotics followed by faecal transplantation to eradicate carriage of multidrug-resistant Enterobacteriaceae: A randomized clinical trial. *Clin. Microbiol. Infect.* **2019**, *25*, 830–838. [CrossRef]
51. Kang, D.W.; Adams, J.B.; Coleman, D.M.; Pollard, E.L.; Maldonado, J.; McDonough-Means, S.; Caporaso, J.G.; Krajmalnik-Brown, R. Long-term benefit of Microbiota Transfer Therapy on autism symptoms and gut microbiota. *Sci. Rep.* **2019**, *9*, 5821. [CrossRef] [PubMed]
52. Qi, X.; Li, X.; Zhao, Y.; Wu, X.; Chen, F.; Ma, X.; Zhang, F.; Wu, D. Treating Steroid Refractory Intestinal Acute Graft-vs.-Host Disease With Fecal Microbiota Transplantation: A Pilot Study. *Front. Immunol.* **2018**, *9*, 2195. [CrossRef]
53. Woodworth, M.H.; Carpentieri, C.; Sitchenko, K.L.; Kraft, C.S. Challenges in fecal donor selection and screening for fecal microbiota transplantation: A review. *Gut Microbes* **2017**, *8*, 225–237. [CrossRef]
54. Kassam, Z.; Dubois, N.E.; Ling, K.; Ramakrisnha, B.; Quazi, T.; Allegretti, J.R.; Fischer, M.; Kelly, C.R.; Budree, S.; Panchal, P.; et al. 512—Donor Health Screening for Fecal Microbiota Transplantation: Prospective Evaluation of 15,317 Candidate Donors. *Gastroenterology* **2019**, *156*, S100–S101. [CrossRef]
55. Bakken, J.S.; Polgreen, P.M.; Beekmann, S.E.; Riedo, F.X.; Streit, J.A. Treatment approaches including fecal microbiota transplantation for recurrent Clostridium difficile infection (RCDI) among infectious disease physicians. *Anaerobe* **2013**, *24*, 20–24. [CrossRef] [PubMed]
56. Edelstein, C.; Daw, J.R.; Kassam, Z. Seeking safe stool: Canada needs a universal donor model. *CMAJ Can. Med. Assoc. J. L'Assoc. Med. Can.* **2016**, *188*, E431–E432. [CrossRef] [PubMed]
57. Odamaki, T.; Kato, K.; Sugahara, H.; Hashikura, N.; Takahashi, S.; Xiao, J.Z.; Abe, F.; Osawa, R. Age-related changes in gut microbiota composition from newborn to centenarian: A cross-sectional study. *BMC Microbiol.* **2016**, *16*, 90. [CrossRef] [PubMed]
58. Fransen, F.; van Beek, A.A.; Borghuis, T.; Aidy, S.E.; Hugenholtz, F.; van der Gaast-de Jongh, C.; Savelkoul, H.F.J.; De Jonge, M.I.; Boekschoten, M.V.; Smidt, H.; et al. Aged Gut Microbiota Contributes to Systemical Inflammaging after Transfer to Germ-Free Mice. *Front. Immunol.* **2017**, *8*, 1385. [CrossRef]
59. Decker, B.K.; Lau, A.F.; Dekker, J.P.; Spalding, C.D.; Sinaii, N.; Conlan, S.; Henderson, D.K.; Segre, J.A.; Frank, K.M.; Palmore, T.N. Healthcare personnel intestinal colonization with multidrug-resistant organisms. *Clin. Microbiol. Infect. Off. Publ. Eur. Soc. Clin. Microbiol. Infect. Dis.* **2018**, *24*, 82.e81–82.e84. [CrossRef] [PubMed]
60. Zboromyrska, Y.; Vila, J. Advanced PCR-based molecular diagnosis of gastrointestinal infections: Challenges and opportunities. *Expert Rev. Mol. Diagn.* **2016**, *16*, 631–640. [CrossRef] [PubMed]
61. Vasilakopoulou, A.; Karakosta, P.; Vourli, S.; Tarpatzi, A.; Varda, P.; Kostoula, M.; Antoniadou, A.; Pournaras, S. Gastrointestinal Carriage of Vancomycin-Resistant Enterococci and Carbapenem-Resistant Gram-Negative Bacteria in an Endemic Setting: Prevalence, Risk Factors, and Outcomes. *Front. Public Health* **2020**, *8*, 55. [CrossRef] [PubMed]
62. Shenoy, E.S.; Paras, M.L.; Noubary, F.; Walensky, R.P.; Hooper, D.C. Natural history of colonization with methicillin-resistant Staphylococcus aureus (MRSA) and vancomycin-resistant Enterococcus (VRE): A systematic review. *BMC Infect. Dis.* **2014**, *14*, 177. [CrossRef]

63. Ianiro, G.; Mullish, B.H.; Kelly, C.R.; Sokol, H.; Kassam, Z.; Ng, S.; Fischer, M.; Allegretti, J.R.; Masucci, L.; Zhang, F.; et al. Screening of faecal microbiota transplant donors during the COVID-19 outbreak: Suggestions for urgent updates from an international expert panel. *Lancet Gastroenterol. Hepatol.* **2020**, *5*, 430–432. [CrossRef]
64. Wang, S.; Xu, M.; Wang, W.; Cao, X.; Piao, M.; Khan, S.; Yan, F.; Cao, H.; Wang, B. Systematic Review: Adverse Events of Fecal Microbiota Transplantation. *PLoS ONE* **2016**, *11*, e0161174. [CrossRef]
65. Drewes, J.L.; Corona, A.; Sanchez, U.; Fan, Y.; Hourigan, S.K.; Weidner, M.; Sidhu, S.D.; Simner, P.J.; Wang, H.; Timp, W.; et al. Transmission and clearance of potential procarcinogenic bacteria during fecal microbiota transplantation for recurrent Clostridioides difficile. *JCI Insight* **2019**, *4*. [CrossRef] [PubMed]
66. DeFilipp, Z.; Bloom, P.P.; Torres Soto, M.; Mansour, M.K.; Sater, M.R.A.; Huntley, M.H.; Turbett, S.; Chung, R.T.; Chen, Y.B.; Hohmann, E.L. Drug-Resistant E. coli Bacteremia Transmitted by Fecal Microbiota Transplant. *N. Engl. J. Med.* **2019**, *381*, 2043–2050. [CrossRef] [PubMed]
67. Kump, P.; Wurm, P.; Grochenig, H.P.; Wenzl, H.; Petritsch, W.; Halwachs, B.; Wagner, M.; Stadlbauer, V.; Eherer, A.; Hoffmann, K.M.; et al. The taxonomic composition of the donor intestinal microbiota is a major factor influencing the efficacy of faecal microbiota transplantation in therapy refractory ulcerative colitis. *Aliment. Pharmacol. Ther.* **2018**, *47*, 67–77. [CrossRef]
68. Wilson, B.C.; Vatanen, T.; Cutfield, W.S.; O'Sullivan, J.M. The Super-Donor Phenomenon in Fecal Microbiota Transplantation. *Front. Cell. Infect. Microbiol.* **2019**, *9*, 2. [CrossRef]
69. Black, C.K.; Termanini, K.M.; Aguirre, O.; Hawksworth, J.S.; Sosin, M. Solid organ transplantation in the 21(st) century. *Ann. Transl. Med.* **2018**, *6*, 409. [CrossRef]
70. Barnes, D.; Ng, K.; Smits, S.; Sonnenburg, J.; Kassam, Z.; Park, K.T. Competitively Selected Donor Fecal Microbiota Transplantation: Butyrate Concentration and Diversity as Measures of Donor Quality. *J. Pediatr. Gastroenterol. Nutr.* **2018**, *67*, 185–187. [CrossRef] [PubMed]
71. Zuo, T.; Wong, S.H.; Lam, K.; Lui, R.; Cheung, K.; Tang, W.; Ching, J.Y.L.; Chan, P.K.S.; Chan, M.C.W.; Wu, J.C.Y.; et al. Bacteriophage transfer during faecal microbiota transplantation in Clostridium difficile infection is associated with treatment, outcome. *Gut* **2018**, *67*, 634–643. [PubMed]
72. Ott, S.J.; Waetzig, G.H.; Rehman, A.; Moltzau-Anderson, J.; Bharti, R.; Grasis, J.A.; Cassidy, L.; Tholey, A.; Fickenscher, H.; Seegert, D.; et al. Efficacy of Sterile Fecal Filtrate Transfer for Treating Patients With Clostridium difficile Infection. *Gastroenterology* **2017**, *152*, 799–811. [CrossRef]
73. Emanuelsson, F.; Claesson, B.E.; Ljungstrom, L.; Tvede, M.; Ung, K.A. Faecal microbiota transplantation and bacteriotherapy for recurrent Clostridium difficile infection: A retrospective evaluation of 31 patients. *Scand. J. Infect. Dis.* **2014**, *46*, 89–97. [CrossRef] [PubMed]
74. Petrof, E.O.; Gloor, G.B.; Vanner, S.J.; Weese, S.J.; Carter, D.; Daigneault, M.C.; Brown, E.M.; Schroeter, K.; Allen-Vercoe, E. Stool substitute transplant therapy for the eradication of Clostridium difficile infection: 'RePOOPulating' the gut. *Microbiome* **2013**, *1*, 3. [CrossRef]
75. Zou, M.; Jie, Z.; Cui, B.; Wang, H.; Feng, Q.; Zou, Y.; Zhang, X.; Yang, H.; Wang, J.; Zhang, F.; et al. Fecal microbiota transplantation results in bacterial strain displacement in patients with inflammatory bowel diseases. *FEBS Open Bio* **2020**, *10*, 41–55. [CrossRef]
76. Paramsothy, S.; Kamm, M.A.; Kaakoush, N.O.; Walsh, A.J.; van den Bogaerde, J.; Samuel, D.; Leong, R.W.L.; Connor, S.; Ng, W.; Paramsothy, R.; et al. Multidonor intensive faecal microbiota transplantation for active ulcerative colitis: A randomised placebo-controlled trial. *Lancet* **2017**, *389*, 1218–1228. [CrossRef]
77. Vermeire, S.; Joossens, M.; Verbeke, K.; Wang, J.; Machiels, K.; Sabino, J.; Ferrante, M.; Van Assche, G.; Rutgeerts, P.; Raes, J. Donor Species Richness Determines Faecal Microbiota Transplantation Success in Inflammatory Bowel Disease. *J. Crohn's Colitis* **2016**, *10*, 387–394. [CrossRef]
78. Tian, Y.; Zhou, Y.; Huang, S.; Li, J.; Zhao, K.; Li, X.; Wen, X.; Li, X.A. Fecal microbiota transplantation for ulcerative colitis: A prospective clinical study. *BMC Gastroenterol.* **2019**, *19*, 116. [CrossRef]
79. Ponce-Alonso, M.; Garcia-Fernandez, S.; Aguilera, L.; Rodriguez-de-Santiago, E.; Foruny, J.R.; Roy, G.; DelCampo, R.; Canton, R.; Lopez-Sanroman, A. P782 A new compatibility test for donor selection for faecal microbiota transplantation in ulcerative colitis. *J. Crohn's Colitis* **2017**, *11*, S480–S481. [CrossRef]
80. Conceicao-Neto, N.; Deboutte, W.; Dierckx, T.; Machiels, K.; Wang, J.; Yinda, K.C.; Maes, P.; Van Ranst, M.; Joossens, M.; Raes, J.; et al. Low eukaryotic viral richness is associated with faecal microbiota transplantation success in patients with UC. *Gut* **2018**, *67*, 1558–1559. [CrossRef] [PubMed]

81. Panebianco, C.; Andriulli, A.; Pazienza, V. Pharmacomicrobiomics: Exploiting the drug-microbiota interactions in anticancer therapies. *Microbiome* **2018**, *6*, 92. [CrossRef] [PubMed]
82. Gopalakrishnan, V.; Spencer, C.N.; Nezi, L.; Reuben, A.; Andrews, M.C.; Karpinets, T.V.; Prieto, P.A.; Vicente, D.; Hoffman, K.; Wei, S.C.; et al. Gut microbiome modulates response to anti-PD-1 immunotherapy in melanoma patients. *Science* **2018**, *359*, 97–103. [CrossRef] [PubMed]
83. Matson, V.; Fessler, J.; Bao, R.; Chongsuwat, T.; Zha, Y.; Alegre, M.L.; Luke, J.J.; Gajewski, T.F. The commensal microbiome is associated with anti-PD-1 efficacy in metastatic melanoma patients. *Science* **2018**, *359*, 104–108. [CrossRef]
84. Mullard, A. Oncologists tap the microbiome in bid to improve immunotherapy outcomes. *Nat. Rev. Drug Discov.* **2018**, *17*, 153–155. [CrossRef]
85. Kang, D.W.; Adams, J.B.; Gregory, A.C.; Borody, T.; Chittick, L.; Fasano, A.; Khoruts, A.; Geis, E.; Maldonado, J.; McDonough-Means, S.; et al. Microbiota Transfer Therapy alters gut ecosystem and improves gastrointestinal and autism symptoms: An open-label study. *Microbiome* **2017**, *5*, 10. [CrossRef]
86. De Groot, P.; Scheithauer, T.; Bakker, G.J.; Prodan, A.; Levin, E.; Khan, M.T.; Herrema, H.; Ackermans, M.; Serlie, M.J.M.; de Brauw, M.; et al. Donor metabolic characteristics drive effects of faecal microbiota transplantation on recipient insulin sensitivity, energy expenditure and intestinal transit time. *Gut* **2019**, 502–512. [CrossRef]

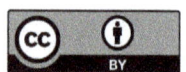

© 2020 by the authors. Licensee MDPI, Basel, Switzerland. This article is an open access article distributed under the terms and conditions of the Creative Commons Attribution (CC BY) license (http://creativecommons.org/licenses/by/4.0/).

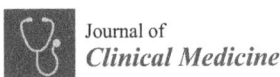

Article

Comparative Study of Salivary, Duodenal, and Fecal Microbiota Composition Across Adult Celiac Disease

Simona Panelli [1,2], Enrica Capelli [2,3], Giuseppe Francesco Damiano Lupo [2,3,4], Annalisa Schiepatti [5], Elena Betti [6], Elisabetta Sauta [7], Simone Marini [3], Riccardo Bellazzi [3,7], Alessandro Vanoli [8], Annamaria Pasi [9], Rosalia Cacciatore [9], Sara Bacchi [2,3], Barbara Balestra [10], Ornella Pastoris [10], Luca Frulloni [11], Gino Roberto Corazza [6], Federico Biagi [5] and Rachele Ciccocioppo [11,*]

[1] Department of Biomedical and Clinical Sciences "L. Sacco", Pediatric Clinical Research Center "Invernizzi", University of Milan, 20122 Milan, Italy; simona.panelli1@unimi.it
[2] Laboratory of Immunology and Genetic Analysis, Department of Earth and Environmental Science, University of Pavia, 27100 Pavia, Italy; enrica.capelli@unipv.it (E.C.); giuseppe.lupo01@universitadipavia.it (G.F.D.L.); sara.bacchi01@universitadipavia.it (S.B.)
[3] Centre for Health Technologies, University of Pavia, 27100 Pavia, Italy; simone.marini@unipv.it (S.M.); riccardo.bellazzi@unipv.it (R.B.)
[4] Department for Sustainable Food Processes, Università Cattolica del Sacro Cuore, 29122 Piacenza, Italy
[5] Gastroenterology Unit, I.R.C.C.S. Pavia, I.C.S. Maugeri, University of Pavia, 27100 Pavia, Italy; salinana@hotmail.it (A.S.); federico.biagi@icsmaugeri.it (F.B.)
[6] Department of Internal Medicine and Therapeutics, Fondazione I.R.C.C.S. Policlinico San Matteo and University of Pavia, 27100 Pavia, Italy; elena.betti19@gmail.com (E.B.); gr.corazza@smatteo.pv.it (G.R.C.)
[7] Laboratory of Bioinformatics, Mathematical Modelling and Synthetic Biology, Department of Electrical, Computer and Biomedical Engineering, University of Pavia, 27100 Pavia, Italy; elisabetta.sauta01@universitadipavia.it
[8] Unit of Anatomic Pathology, Department of Molecular Medicine, University of Pavia and Fondazione I.R.C.C.S. Policlinico San Matteo, 27100 Pavia, Italy; a.vanoli@smatteo.pv.it
[9] Laboratory of Immunogenetics, Department of Transfusion Medicine and Immuno-Hematology, Fondazione I.R.C.C.S. Policlinico S. Matteo, 27100 Pavia, Italy; a.pasi@smatteo.pv.it (A.P.); r.cacciatore@smatteo.pv.it (R.C.)
[10] Laboratory of Pharmacogenetics, Department of Biology and Biotechnology, University of Pavia, 27100 Pavia, Italy; barbara.balestra@unipv.it (B.B.); ornella.pastoris@unipv.it (O.P.)
[11] Gastroenterology Unit, Department of Medicine, A.O.U.I. Borgo Roma and University of Verona, 37134 Verona, Italy; luca.frulloni@univr.it
* Correspondence: rachele.ciccocioppo@univr.it; Tel.: +39-045-8124578; Fax: +39-045-8027495

Received: 29 February 2020; Accepted: 10 April 2020; Published: 13 April 2020

Abstract: Background: Growing evidence suggests that an altered microbiota composition contributes to the pathogenesis and clinical features in celiac disease (CD). We performed a comparative analysis of the gut microbiota in adulthood CD to evaluate whether: (i) dysbiosis anticipates mucosal lesions, (ii) gluten-free diet restores eubiosis, (iii) refractory CD has a peculiar microbial signature, and (iv) salivary and fecal communities overlap the mucosal one. Methods: This is a cross-sectional study where a total of 52 CD patients, including 13 active CD, 29 treated CD, 4 refractory CD, and 6 potential CD, were enrolled in a tertiary center together with 31 controls. A 16S rRNA-based amplicon metagenomics approach was applied to determine the microbiota structure and composition of salivary, duodenal mucosa, and stool samples, followed by appropriate bioinformatic analyses. Results: A reduction of both α- and β-diversity in CD, already evident in the potential form and achieving nadir in refractory CD, was evident. Taxonomically, mucosa displayed a significant abundance of *Proteobacteria* and an expansion of *Neisseria*, especially in active patients, while treated celiacs showed an intermediate profile between active disease and controls. The saliva community mirrored the mucosal one better than stool. Conclusion: Expansion of pathobiontic species anticipates villous atrophy and achieves the maximal divergence from controls in refractory CD. Gluten-free diet results in incomplete recovery. The overlapping results between mucosal and salivary samples indicate the use of saliva as a diagnostic fluid.

Keywords: celiac disease; enteropathy; microbiota; gluten; therapy

1. Introduction

The discovery of the gut microbiota universe and the growing understanding of its role in health and disease have radically changed the current point of view on the pathogenesis of noncommunicable diseases [1]. Among these, celiac disease (CD) represents a privileged situation since both the external (gluten) and internal (tissue transglutaminase) antigens as well as the predisposing human leukocyte antigen haplotypes have been identified [2]. However, although gluten is widely ingested, tissue transglutaminase is a ubiquitous enzyme, and the frequency of at-risk alleles in the general population approaches 40%, only a small proportion of subjects eventually develop enteropathy [3]. Additional factors have therefore been invoked to explain the onset and maintenance of loss of gluten tolerance and mucosal damage. Recently, evidence has been accumulated on the presence of perturbations of the microbiota composition [4] not only in active CD (ACD) [5] but also in a consistent proportion of treated patients (TCD) [6]. Whether dysbiosis represents an epiphenomenon of the enteropathy or, conversely, it contributes to the development of mucosal damage still remains unknown.

On this basis, we firstly aimed to characterize the mucosal microbiota of an adult CD population, including ACD, TCD, refractory CD (RCD), and potential CD (PCD), and compare it to non-CD controls by using the amplicon metagenomics approach. Secondly, since it is unlikely that the most studied bacterial consortium, i.e., fecal microbiota, represents the composition at the level of duodenal mucosa, we also collected and analysed salivary samples to assess whether they mirror the profile at mucosal level better than feces.

2. Patients and Methods

2.1. Study Population

A total of 83 cases were recruited at the Department of Internal Medicine, Fondazione I.R.C.C.S. Policlinico San Matteo (Pavia, Italy) from November 1st, 2015 to June 30th, 2018. They included 52 CD patients, comprehensive of all the possible combinations of diet and villous atrophy (Table 1), i.e., 13 ACD, 29 TCD, 4 RCD, 6 PCD, and 31 patients with functional dyspepsia [7] who served as controls (C). The demographic and clinical features of all recruited cases are shown in Table 2. No significant differences regarding age and comorbidities were found among the groups, albeit the statistical analysis was not performed with the potential and refractory ones due to the small sample size. Diagnoses of PCD, ACD, TCD, and RCD were made on the basis of widely accepted criteria [8] and histological examination of mucosal lesions [9]. The adherence to gluten-free diet (GFD) was evaluated by means of a five-level score, with scores ranging 0 to 2 meaning absence or poor adherence and scores ranging 3 to 4 being indicative of good adherence [10]. Moreover, all enrolled cases followed a Mediterranean diet, and there were no vegan/vegetarian patients.

Table 1. Variables in the celiac population.

Variable	With Villous Atrophy	Without Villous Atrophy
Gluten-containing diet	Active celiac disease	Potential celiac disease
Gluten-free diet	Refractory celiac disease	Treated celiac disease

Table 2. Demographic and clinical features of study cohort.

	Celiac Patients				Controls
	Potential	Active	Treated	Refractory	Functional Dyspepsia
Number of cases	6	13	29	4	31
female:male ratio	3:3	11:2	20:9	4:0	24:7
Mean age at enrolment in years (± standard deviation)	41 ± 14	35 ± 6	37 ± 6	53 ± 15	44 ± 17
Median body mass index as kg/h^2 (25th–75th)	22.4 (19.1–25.6)	21.3 (19.8–22.7)	20.5 (19.9–26.1)	16.9 (15.4–17.0)	22.1 (20.0–24.2)
Median time on a GFD in years (range)	5 cases no GFD 1 case on GFD since one year	No GFD	3.0 (2–7)	17 (11.2–22)	No GFD
Good adherence to GFD (score 3–4)	1	Not applicable	27	4	Not applicable
Poor adherence to GFD (score 0–2)	0	Not applicable	2	0	Not applicable
Autoimmunity	1	4	10	1	8
HLA-DQ2 [+ve]	6	8	17	3	10
HLA-DQ8 [+ve]	0	0	1	1	3
HLA-DQ2/DQ8 [+ve]	0	3	2	0	1
HLA-DQ2/DQ8 [-ve]	0	0	0	0	8
Unknown	0	2	10	0	9

Abbreviations: GFD: gluten-free diet; HLA: Human Leukocyte Antigen; [+ve]: positive; [-ve]: negative.

Patients were excluded if they had recent (within 4 weeks) or current use of medications that could affect bowel function and/or microbiota composition, such as antibiotics, prebiotics, probiotics, opioids, nonsteroidal anti-inflammatory drugs, proton pump inhibitors, laxatives, steroids, or antidiarrheal drugs.

The protocol was approved by the local Ethics Committee (protocol number 20150003822), and each enrolled case gave written informed consent.

2.2. Biological Samples

Saliva

Saliva samples were collected by direct spitting into a sterile plastic tube at least two hours after tooth brushing and before endoscopy. Smoking, and food and drink intake were forbidden since midnight. After collection, salivary samples were kept at −80 °C till analysis.

Mucosa

In all cases, four perendoscopic specimens from duodenal mucosa were formalin-fixed and paraffin-embedded for traditional histology and immunohistochemistry, while two samples were snap-frozen and stored at −80 °C until use. In RCD patients, four additional biopsies were collected for intraepithelial lymphocyte phenotyping.

Stool

Samples were collected at home by patients within 24 h before the endoscopy and kept at −20 °C till delivery in the hospital where they were frozen at −80 °C.

2.3. Extraction and Quantification of DNA

DNA was extracted from each biological sample by using commercial kits (all from Qiagen; Hilden, Germany) and following the manufacturer's instructions according to the suggested procedure for bacteria (DNeasy® Blood & Tissue Handbook). Specifically, the QIAamp DNA Stool Mini kit was used for feces; the QIAamp DNA Blood Mini Kit was used for saliva; and the DNeasy Blood and Tissue Kit was used for duodenal biopsies. More in depth, stool samples were first solubilized in a buffer provided in the kit in order to remove polymerase chain reaction inhibitors contained in feces; then, the DNA extraction was performed applying the same procedures used for the other sample biotypes. The DNA concentration of each sample was assessed fluorometrically.

2.4. Production of 16S rRNA Amplicons (V3–V4 Regions) and Sequencing

For amplicon production, the V3–V4 hypervariable regions of the prokariotic 16S rRNA gene were targeted [11]. Polymerase chain reaction was performed in a 50-µL volume containing template DNA, 1× HiFi HotStart Ready Mix (Kapa Biosystems; Wilmington, MA, USA) and 0.5 µM of each primer. The cycling program, performed on a MJ Mini thermal cycler (Promega corp.; Madison, WI), included an initial denaturation cycle (95 °C for 3 min), followed by a variable number of cycles (25 for saliva; 30 for feces and mucosa) at 94 °C for 30 sec, at 55 °C for 30 sec, at 72 °C for 30 sec, and at a final extension (72 °C for 5 min) [12,13]. Cleanup of amplicons was performed using Agencourt AMPure XP SPRI magnetic beads (ThermoFisher Scientific; Waltham, MA, USA). Illumina sequencing libraries were finally constructed through the link of indices (Nextera XT Index Kit, Illumina; San Diego, CA, USA), quantified using a Qubit 2.0 Fluorometer (ThermoFisher Scientific), normalized, and pooled. Libraries underwent paired-end sequencing on an Illumina MiSeq platform at BMR Genomics (Padua, Italy).

2.5. Power Calculation

In this cross-sectional observational study, a convenience sample of 80 cases will be enrolled, possibly distributed as follows: 10 potential CD patients, 10 complicated CD patients, 20 active CD patients, 20 treated CD patients, and 20 non-CD patients. The effect size (mean difference/standard deviation) that can be elicited, given the sample size and 80% power, was computed based on the primary endpoint, i.e., the comparison of the microbiota composition between CD groups (potential, active, treated, and refractory) and non-CD patients (controls). A conservative alpha of 0.001 was used, given the multiple endpoints and comparisons planned. The effect size that can be discovered on the basis of these hypotheses will be 1.8 when comparing potential and treated patients to controls and 1.4 when comparing active and treated patients to controls.

2.6. Bioinformatics Analysis

An ad hoc bioinformatics pipeline was built up under the R environment [14] Raw sequences were processed using USEARCH (version 10.0.240). Paired reads were merged, and low-quality reads were discarded. Filtered reads were assigned to different taxonomic levels (from phylum to species) and organised into operational taxonomic units (OTUs). Sequences were clustered at 97% nucleotide similarity, and chimeric ones were filtered out; their taxonomy was assessed through the Greengenes 16S rRNA bacterial database (version 13.8) [15]. Data were normalized with the Total Sum Scaling method, and normalized OTUs were used to investigate community diversity in each sample biotype. The observed richness and the Chao1 [16] and Shannon [17] indices were calculated to analyse the within-sample species richness (α-diversity). The β-diversity analysis was conducted to estimate the between-sample diversity, using the generalized UniFrac index as a distance metric [18]. The resulting phylogenetic matrices were represented by multidimensional scaling. Permutational Multivariate Analysis of Variance (PERMANOVA) was performed for β-diversity analysis to statistically assess the grouping of samples by diagnosis. Microbial profiles obtained for each taxonomic level and for each sample biotype were compared among patient groups using the Mann–Whitney U-test, the

Kruskal–Wallis Rank Sum test, and a 20% cutoff for prevalence. For all the statistical analyses, the significance threshold (p-value) was set to 0.05, and all the obtained p values were corrected for multiple testing with the Benjamini–Hochberg method.

3. Results

3.1. Overall Structure of Salivary, Mucosal, and Fecal Bacterial Communities

To investigate the shift in structure and composition of the mucosal, salivary, and fecal bacterial communities across patient groups, 209 out of 249 expected samples (77 mucosal, 76 salivary, and 56 fecal) underwent sequencing and processing, since in some cases (one ACD, two C, and three TCD) the samples displayed degradation of the nucleic acid due to poor conservation. A total of 3.5 million high-quality reads were obtained, of which 5,327,971 were for mucosal, 4,993,425 were for salivary, and 3,208,768 were for fecal samples. All the obtained sequences were classified into 5556 OTUs, representing 26 phyla, 52 classes, 89 orders, 156 familiae, 315 genera, and 186 species (spp.) (see Table S1: Taxonomic assignment across sample biotypes in the study cohort). The relative distribution of the phyla is shown in Figure 1, where a critical decrease of *Firmicutes* and *Actinobacteria* and an expansion of *Proteobacteria* at mucosal and salivary levels appear evident in all CD groups, mostly in ACD and RCD, in comparison with the C group that does not normalize in TCD. By contrast, no clear differences are evident at the stool level probably due to the high variability among samples. As regards the relative distribution of genera, as in Figure 2, an expansion of *Neisseria* and a reduction of *Streptococcus* in CD groups with respect to the C group emerge in both mucosal and salivary communities, whereas *Bacteroides* is the predominant one in the stool consortium.

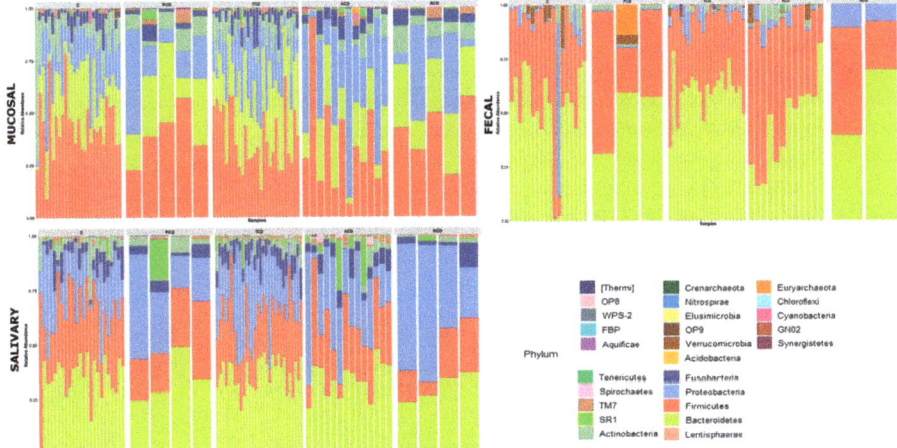

Figure 1. Phylum-level classification of bacteria identified in individual mucosal, salivary, and fecal samples belonging to the five study groups: Each bar represents the relative contribution of phylum-level profiles of each subject enrolled in the study as indicated on the top of each panel (ACD: active celiac disease, C: control subjects, PCD: potential celiac disease, RCD: refractory celiac disease, and TCD: treated celiac disease). Twenty-six different phyla were identified across the three biotypes and are represented by different colors as indicated in the legend. The relative distribution of phyla among study groups indicates a critical decrease of *Firmicutes* and *Actinobacteria* and an expansion of *Proteobacteria* at mucosal and salivary levels in all celiac groups, mostly in ACD and RCD, in comparison with the C group that does not normalize in TCD. By contrast, no clear differences are evident in the stools.

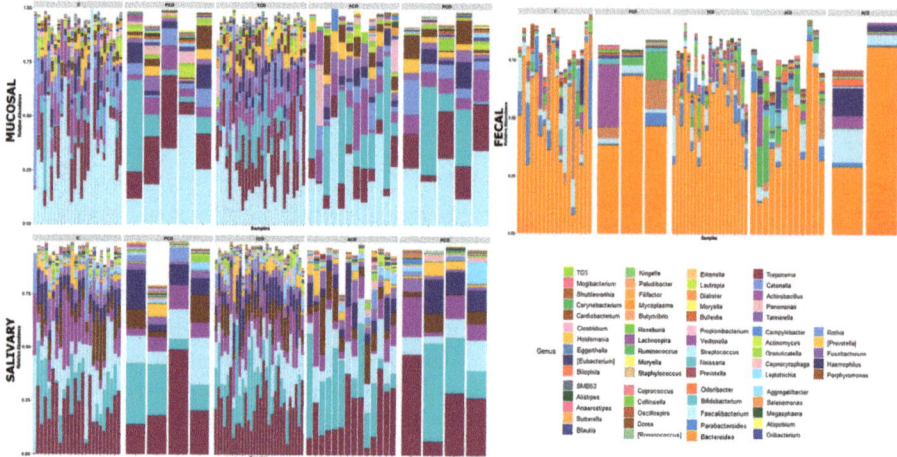

Figure 2. Genus-level classification of bacteria identified in individual mucosal, salivary, and fecal samples belonging to the five study groups: Each bar represents the relative contribution of genus-level profiles with an abundance of at least 1% in each considered sample as indicated on the top of each panel. Sixty-nine different genera were identified across the three biotypes and are represented by different colors as indicated in the legend. An expansion of *Neisseria* and a reduction of *Streptococcus* in celiac groups with respect to controls emerge in both mucosal and salivary communities, whereas *Bacteroides* is the predominant one in the stool consortium.

The within-sample diversity (α-diversity) was evaluated by computing observed richness and the Chao1 and Shannon indices, of which the single values are shown in Table S2: α-diversity indices for each sample. Figure 3 shows a critical reduction of both observed richness and Shannon index in all CD groups in comparison to the C group at the mucosal level, while the Chao1 index yields significant differences when comparing ACD and PCD with C. The group that fails to be significantly discriminated despite the apparent reduction is the RCD one, possibly because of the small sample size. The salivary community shows the highest richness and Chao1 index in ACD and the lowest in RCD, while PCD and TCD display values similar to the C group. At variance with salivary samples at the fecal level, only the Shannon index produces significant differences between groups, with ACD and TCD showing higher values than C.

The comparison of β-diversity reveals significant differences only in mucosal bacterial community distribution, when considering all groups of patients (Figure 4A) and the following pairwise comparisons: TCD versus ACD (Figure 4B), and ACD versus C (Figure 4C).

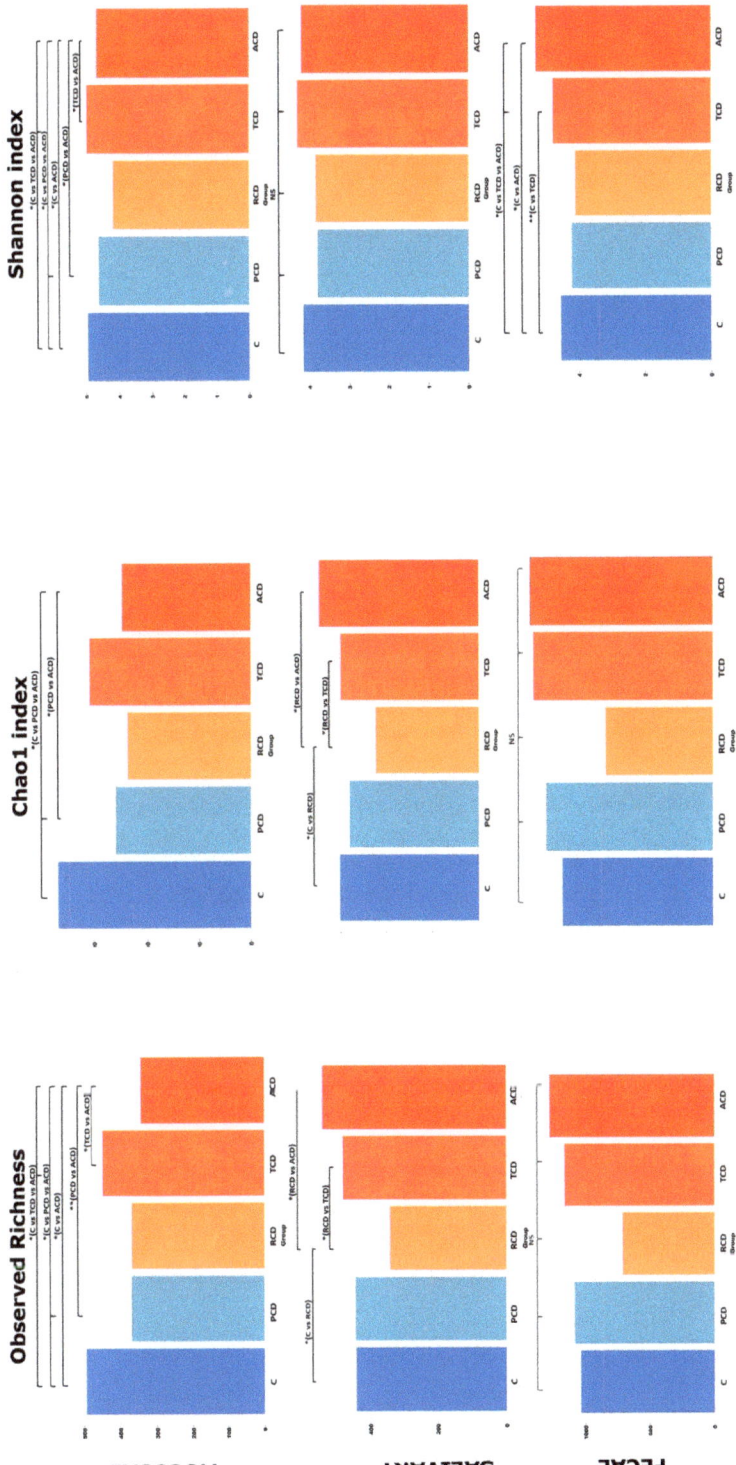

Figure 3. Alpha-diversity: Overall comparison of mucosal, salivary, and fecal microbiota structure. Observed richness and the Chao1 (representing community richness) and Shannon (representing diversity) indices are presented. The bars depict the mean of relative abundances rates. Significant (* $p < 0.05$; ** $p < 0.01$) comparisons between patient categories are indicated over the bars.

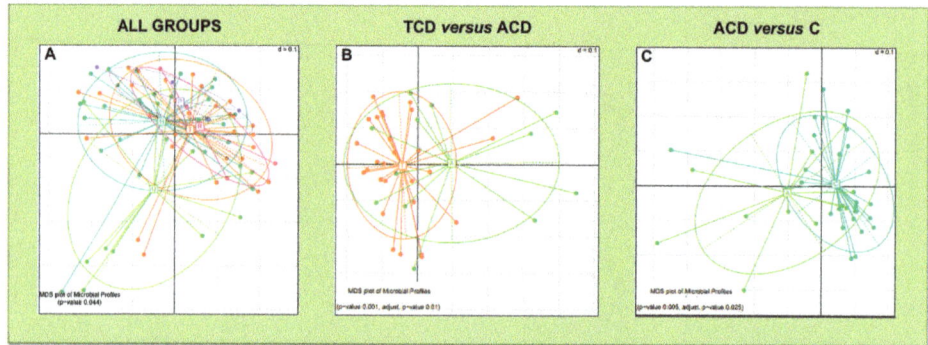

Figure 4. Beta-diversity comparison for the mucosal microbiota: Multidimensional Scaling (MDS) plots of mucosal samples for which the Permutational Multivariate Analysis of Variance test detected a significant separation of study groups in terms of bacterial community composition. The microbiota phylogenetic distances were evaluated through the generalized UniFrac distance. Each point represents the microbiota composition of one sample. Panel (**A**): all patient groups were compared. Panel (**B**): TCD versus ACD comparison. Panel (**C**): ACD versus C comparison. Each point represents the microbiota composition of one sample.

3.2. Taxonomy-Based Analyses of Mucosal Community

As shown in Table 3, the phylum distribution is indicative of a decrease in *Actinobacteria* and an increase in *Proteobacteria* in all celiac groups, with ACD being that with the greatest deviation with respect to C. A different pattern is observed for *Bacteroidetes* that are decreased in ACD and increased in the other CD groups in comparison to C. Although *Firmicutes* are the most abundant phylum, accounting for a portion of bacterial diversity ranging from a maximum of 43.6% in C to a minimum of 34.8% in ACD, with the other CD groups displaying intermediate values (39.5% in PCD, 37.5% in TCD, and 40.16% in RCD), no significant differences are seen. Moving on to bacterial families within the last phylum, the *Streptococcaceae* show the lowest value in TCD, the *Veillonellaceae* are the lowest in ACD, and the *Lachnospiraceace* are the lowest in both ACD and RCD, whereas a critical decrease of *Gemellaceae* in PCD, ACD, and TCD in comparison to C and RCD is clearly evident. Within *Bacteroidetes*, only the *Prevotellaceae* show differences, with ACD displaying a decrease and the other CD groups displaying an increase in comparison to C. Concerning *Actinobacteria*, the *Micrococcaceae* show a critical reduction in CD groups, achieving the nadir in ACD, whilst RCD mirrors C. Finally, within the *Proteobacteria*, *Neisseriaceae* show a robust increase in all CD groups, mostly in ACD, in comparison with C. This situation is perfectly overlapped by the profile observed for the genus *Neisseria*. Among the other genera, *Streptococcus* spp. presents an opposite trend, since it is reduced in CD, especially in ACD and, to a lesser extent, in TCD, while the relative abundance found in PCD and RCD was closer to the profile detected in C. Within the same phylum of *Firmicutes* (*Peptoniphilaceae* family), *Parvimonas* spp. shows a particular profile, with a value in PCD double the level found in C, while it is the half of the C group in the other CD groups. At the species level, it is interesting to note that *Prevotellae* increase in all CD groups with respect to C, except in ACD. By contrast, *Rothia aerea* displays values in CD groups similar to C, except in PCD, where its relative abundance is decreased, and in RCD, where it appears increased.

Table 3. Taxa displaying significantly different relative abundances in mucosal biopsies.

Taxon	Relative Abundance (%)					Comparisons * in Which Statistical Analysis Produced p-Values < 0.05
	C	PCD	TCD	ACD	RCD	
Phyla						
Bacteroidetes	20.76	25.19	28.08	18.20	24.60	C versus TCD (0.021) C versus TCD versus ACD (0.017) TCD versus ACD (0.019)
Actinobacteria	11.1	7.57	7.94	4.15	7.56	C versus TCD versus ACD (0.030) C versus ACD (0.012) C versus PCD versus ACD (0.035) TCD versus ACD (0.038)
Proteobacteria	17.89	20.92	19.21	35.48	20.71	C versus TCD versus ACD (0.045) C versus ACD (0.016) TCD versus ACD (0.036)
Families						
Phylum: Firmicutes						
Streptococcaceae	25.77	23.39	18.34	22.77	23.10	C versus TCD (0.041)
Gemellaceae	2.17	0.91	1.51	0.83	2.30	C versus TCD versus ACD (0.027) C versus ACD (0.011) C versus PCD versus ACD (0.022)
Veillonellaceae	7.37	6.54	8.95	4.50	9.39	C versus TCD versus ACD (0.035) T versus ACD (0.0090) ACD versus RCD (0.035)
Lachnospiraceae	2.71	2.50	3.26	2.00	1.67	TCD versus ACD (0.023)
Phylum: Bacteroidetes						
Prevotellaceae	12.1	17.95	17.80	6.80	15.93	C versus TCD versus ACD (0.0030) PCD versus ACD (0.045) TCD versus ACD (0.00040) ACD versus RCD (0.020)
Phylum: Actinobacteria						
Micrococcaceae	7.51	4.44	4.98	2.27	6.26	C versus ACD (0.029) ACD versus RCD (0.0061)
Phylum: Proteobacteria						
Neisseriaceae	3.95	10.46	7.91	16.14	14.90	C versus ACD (0.034)
Genera						
Phylum: Firmicutes; Family: Streptococcaceae						
Streptococcus spp.	28.17	25.52	19.76	15.60	24.42	C versus TCD (0.023) C versus TCD versus ACD (0.013) C versus PCD versus ACD (0.048) C versus ACD (0.016)
Phylum: Firmicutes; Family: Peptoniphilaceae						
Parvimonas spp.	0.74	1.39	0.45	0.32	0.34	PCD versus ACD (0.020) C versus PCD versus ACD (0.038)
Phylum: Firmicutes; Family: Veillonellaceae						
Veillonella spp.	7.2	5.49	8.57	4.44	8.65	C versus TCD versus ACD (0.038) TCD versus ACD (0.009)
Phylum: Proteobacteria; Family: Neisseriaceae						
Neisseria spp.	4.07	11.16	8.10	17.02	14.74	C versus PCD versus ACD (0.038) C versus ACD (0.034) C versus TCD versus ACD (0.049)

Table 3. Cont.

Taxon	Relative Abundance (%)					Comparisons * in Which Statistical Analysis Produced p-Values < 0.05
	C	PCD	TCD	ACD	RCD	
Phylum: *Bacteroidetes*; Family: *Prevotellaceae*						
Prevotella spp.	13.18	18.90	18.82	7.55	16.92	ACD versus RCD (0.020) PCD versus ACD (0.026) TCD versus ACD (0.0004)
Phylum: *Actinobacteria*; Family: *Actinomycetaceae*						
Actinomyces spp.	1.66	1.71	1.42	0.66	0.82	TCD versus ACD (0.044)
Phylum: *Actinobacteria*; Family: *Micrococcaceae*						
Rothia spp.	8.10	4.60	5.35	2.47	6.72	ACD versus RCD (0.0061) C versus ACD (0.027)
Species						
Phylum: *Bacteroidetes*; Family: *Prevotellaceae*						
Prevotella melaninogenica	23.1	35.71	32.5	14.36	29.67	C versus TCD (0.035) C versus TCD versus ACD (0.0052) PCD versus ACD (0.015) TCD versus ACD (0.0019)
Prevotella copri	0.73	1.32	1.07	1.59	2.58	TCD versus ACD (0.027)
Prevotella pallens	3.24	2.84	4.85	1.40	1.58	TCD versus ACD (0.034)
Prevotella nigrescens	0.26	2.45	0.46	0.38	1.42	C versus PCD versus ACD (0.003) PCD versus ACD (0.003) C versus PCD (0.002)
Phylum: *Actinobacteria*; Family: *Micrococcaceae*						
Rothia aerea	0.45	0.080	0.47	0.040	1.13	RCD versus TCD (0.026) TCD versus ACD (0.025) C versus ACD (0.034) ACD versus RCD (0.0009)
Rothia mucilaginosa	19.17	12.47	13.13	10.00	17.74	ACD versus RCD (0.045)

Abbreviations: C = controls; PCD = potential celiac disease, ACD = active celiac disease; TCD = treated celiac disease; RCD = refractory celiac disease. * The following comparisons were performed: C versus PCD; C versus TCD; C versus ACD; C versus TCD versus ACD; C versus ACD; PCD versus ACD; PCD versus ACD versus C; TCD versus RCD; ACD versus TCD; and ACD versus RCD.

3.3. Taxonomy-Based Analyses of Salivary Community

Also, in this ecosystem, *Firmicutes* is the most represented phylum, accounting for 33% of the bacterial diversity in C and falling to around 25% in TCD, ACD, and PCD and to 17% in RCD. *Bacteroidetes*, on the other hand, show more homogeneous values, ranging from 30.04% in RCD to 36.6% in TCD, with the other groups being around 33%. Interestingly, the *SR1* phylum displays a relative abundance <1% in both C (0.96%) and RCD (0.78%), whilst it rises to almost 5% in the other CD groups (4.68% in PCD and TCD and 4.23% in ACD). The comparisons between the relative abundances of taxa that yielded statistically significant differences are presented in Table 4. Within the phyla, *Proteobacteria* are increased in CD, especially in RCD, with respect to C. At the family level, again, the RCD condition differs from the other CD groups since it displays a marked reduction of *Fusobacteriaceae* and *Lachnospiraceace*. Noteworthily, within genera, *Neisseria* spp. presents a trend overlapping what was observed at the mucosal level, being critically increased in PCD, ACD, and RCD and close to C in TCD.

Table 4. Taxa displaying significantly different relative abundances in saliva samples.

Taxon	Relative Abundance (%)					Comparisons * in Which Statistical Analysis Produced p-Values < 0.05
	C	PCD	TCD	ACD	RCD	
Phyla						
Proteobacteria	20.51	27.71	24.03	26.35	45.11	TCD versus RCD (0.024)
Families						
Phylum: *Fusobacteria*						
Fusobacteriaceae	4.50	2.95	5.43	4.16	1.66	ACD versus RCD (0.025) TCD versus RCD (0.0088)
Phylum: *Firmicutes*						
Lachnospiraceae	1.11	0.66	0.97	0.82	0.22	TCD versus RCD (0.0038) ACD versus RCD (0.033)
Genera						
Phylum: *Proteobacteria*; Family: *Neisseriaceae*						
Neisseria spp.	10.08	18.66	15.10	20.44	21.69	C versus ACD (0.049)
Phylum: *Proteobacteria*; Family: *Moraxellaceae*						
Acinetobacter spp	2.08	0.0099	0.068	0.016	0.069	C versus ACD (0.032)
Phylum: *Fusobacteria*; Family: *Fusobacteriaceae*						
Fusobacterium spp.	4.62	2.99	5.54	4.27	2.44	TCD versus RCD (0.032)
Phylum: *Firmicutes*; Family: *Lachnospiraceae*						
Oribacterium spp.	0.40	0.21	0.38	0.26	0.09	TCD versus ACD (0.038) TCD versus RCD (0.037)
Species						
Phylum: *Bacteroidetes*; Family: *Porphyromonadaceae*						
Porphyromonas endodontalis	1.35	0.65	0.76	4.07	1.66	C versus T versus A (0.039)

3.4. Taxonomy-Based Analyses of Fecal Community

From Table 5, it emerges that TCD and RCD display values of relative abundances of phyla similar to C whereas ACD invariably shows a profile significantly different from TCD, except for *Proteobacteria*. At the family level, all CD groups are characterised by an increase of *Ruminococcaceae*, while *Veillonellaceae* appear decreased in ACD. Moreover, PCD displays an increased abundance in *Erysipelitrichaceae*, while RCD has an increase in *Pasteurellaceae*, which are suppressed in the other CD groups in comparison to C. Within genera, *Blautia*, *Coprococcus*, and *Roseburia* spp. show a strong increase in ACD in comparison to all the other groups, together with *Ruminococcus* spp. that appears increased even in PCD. Interestingly, *Veillonella* spp. and *Haemophilus* spp strongly increase in RCD while *Bifidobacterium* spp. and *Parabacteriodes* spp. abundance is negligible with respect to all the other groups. Finally, at the species level, the great increase of *Faecalibacterium prausnitzii* and *Veillonella dispar* emerges in RCD, whilst *Bifodobacterium longum*, that is increased in both PCD and ACD, appears suppressed. Also, *Roseburia faecis* appeares increased in ACD in comparison with other groups, at variance with *Bacteroides eggerthii* that displays negligible levels in both ACD and RCD, whilst it is increased in TCD.

Table 5. Taxa displaying significantly different relative abundances in stool samples.

Taxon	Relative Abundance (%)					Comparisons * in Which Statistical Analysis Produced p Values < 0.05
	C	PCD	TCD	ACD	RCD	
Phyla						
Bacteroidetes	51.97	49.23	59.99	44.27	54.5	TCD versus ACD (0.0027) C versus TCD versus ACD (0.025)
Firmicutes	36.39	42.3	34.21	47.83	36.10	TCD versus ACD (0.020)
Actinobacteria	1.96	4.6	0.82	2.93	0.098	TCD versus ACD (0.029)
Proteobacteria	6.90	0.78	3.96	3.12	9.27	ACD versus RCD (0.044)
Coriobacteriaceae	0.14	0.67	0.12	1.39	0.0093	C versus TCD versus ACD (0.0066) C versus PCD versus ACD (0.015) TCD versus ACD (0.0063) ACD versus RCD (0.044)
Families						
Philum: *Firmicutes*						
Clostridiaceae	0.18	0.23	0.57	0.63	0.11	C versus TCD versus ACD (0.020) C versus PCD versus ACD (0.029) C versus TCD (0.037)
Veillonellaceae	6.35	4.66	6.35	2.40	8.85	C versus ACD (0.046)
Erysipelitrichaceae	0.30	2.21	0.44	1.14	0.12	C versus TCD versus ACD (0.0090) C versus PCD versus ACD (0.012) TCD versus ACD (0.0070) C versus ACD (0.0050)
Ruminococcaceae	23.52	23.81	13.94	23.52	18.47	TCD versus ACD (0.016)
Philum: *Actinobacteria*						
Coriobacteriaceae	0.14	0.67	0.12	1.39	0.009	C versus PCD versus ACD (0.015)
Philum: *Proteobacteria*						
Enterobacteriaceae	0.46	0.27	2.13	1.84	0.01	TCD versus RCD (0.038) ACD versus RCD (0.028)
Pasteurellaceae	2.32	0.17	0.41	0.56	5.86	TCD versus RCD (0.028) ACD versus RCD (0.044)
Genera						
Philum: *Firmicutes*; Family: *Lachnospiraceae*						
Blautia spp.	0.53	0.94	0.88	3.12	0.46	C versus TCD versus ACD (0.016) C versus ACD (0.0059) C versus PCD versus ACD (0.022)
Coprococcus spp.	0.31	0.57	0.47	1.10	0.094	C versus TCD versus ACD (0.008) C versus ACD (0.0030) C versus PCD versus ACD (0.011) TCD versus ACD (0.017)
Roseburia spp.	0.81	0.17	1.50	1.72	0.39	PCD versus ACD (0.043)
Philum: *Firmicutes*; Family: *Ruminococcaceae*						
Ruminococcus spp.	3.62	14.22	2.22	8.75	0.12	ACD versus RCD (0.044) TCD versus ACD (0.047) PCD versus ACD versus C (0.037) TCD versus RCD (0.030)

Table 5. Cont.

Taxon	Relative Abundance (%)					Comparisons * in Which Statistical Analysis Produced p Values < 0.05
	C	PCD	TCD	ACD	RCD	
Philum: *Firmicutes*; Family: *Clostridiaceae*						
Dorea spp.	0.88	0.36	0.3	1.03	0.19	C versus TCD versus ACD (0.008) C versus ACD (0.012) C versus PCD versus ACD (0.027) TCD versus ACD (0.0031)
Philum: *Firmicutes*; Family: *Veillonellaceae*						
Veillonella spp.	0.095	0.021	0.32	0.16	8.67	RCD versus TCD (0.029) ACD versus RCD (0.028)
Philum: *Firmicutes*; Family: *Acidaminococcaceae*						
Megasphaera spp.	0.079	0.0037	1.20	0.02	0.08	RCD versus TCD (0.044)
Philum: *Proteobacteria*; Family: *Pasteurellaceae*						
Haemophilus spp.	0.96	0.19	0.50	0.80	7.69	TCD versus RCD (0.038) ACD versus RCD (0.043)
Philum: *Actinobacteria*; Family: *Bifidobacteriaceae*						
Bifidobacterium spp.	1.65	1.15	0.89	2.62	0.11	TCD versus ACD (0.045)
Philum: *Bacteroidetes*; Family: *Porphyromonadaceae*						
Parabacteriodes spp.	6.89	2.77	4.23	3.11	1.41	TCD versus ACD (0.029)
Species						
Philum: *Firmicutes*; Family: *Lachnospiraceae*						
Roseburia fecis	0.99	0.19	0.93	2.76	0.74	C versus TCD versus ACD (0.049) C versus PCD versus ACD (0.044) C versus ACD (0.022)
Philum: *Firmicutes*; Family: *Ruminococcaceae*						
Faecalibacterium prausnitzii	13.90	11.05	9.49	15.42	27.48	TCD versus RCD (0.049)
Philum: *Firmicutes*; Family: *Veillonellaceae*						
Veillonella dispar	0.45	0.15	1.77	0.80	22.44	TCD versus RCD (0.029) ACD versus RCD (0.027)
Philum: *Actinobacteria*; Family: *Bifidobacteriaceae*						
Bifodobacterium longum	1.40	2.07	0.80	4.99	0.008	C versus TCD versus ACD (0.011) C versus ACD (0.016) TCD versus ACD (0.004) C versus PCD versus ACD (0.045)
Philum: *Bacteroidetes*; Family: *Bacteroidaceae*						
Bacteroides eggerthii	2.49	11.07	6.68	0.46	0	TCD versus ACD (0.046)

In summary, the relative distribution of the most abundant phyla and genera in the study cohort is represented in Figures 5 and 6, respectively. It becomes evident that the salivary profiles mirror the condition at the mucosal level better than the fecal ones. The distribution of the five most abundant families is shown in Figure S1: Plot of relative abundances of the five most abundant families retrieved in each sample biotype, where, again, *Neisseriaceae* represents the most abundant one in both ACD and RCD mucosal and salivary samples.

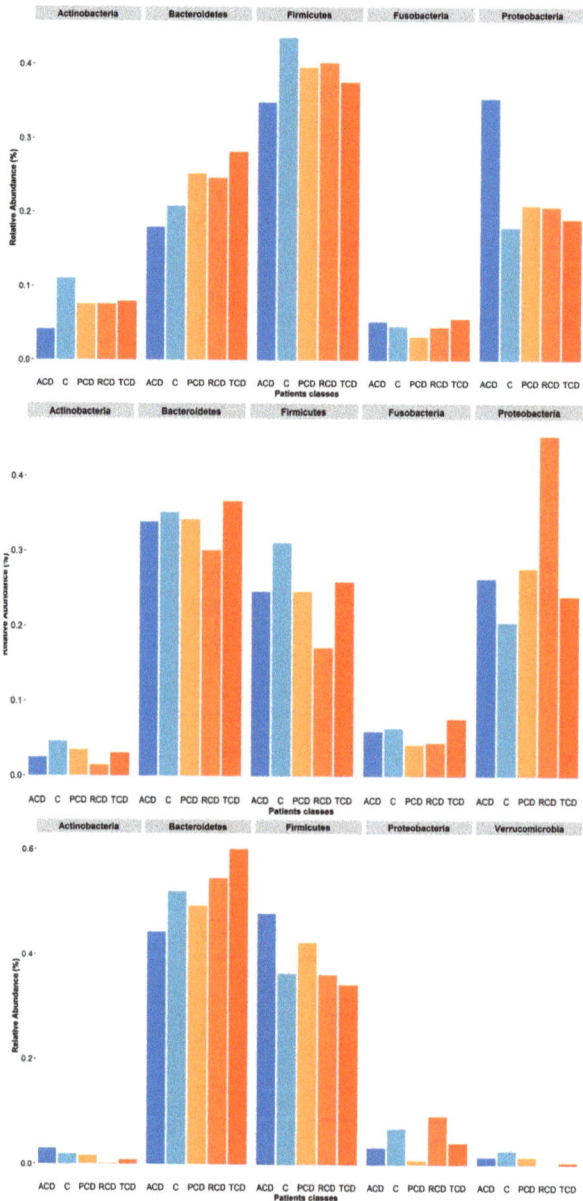

Figure 5. Plot of relative abundances of the five most abundant phyla retrieved in each sample biotype: At mucosal level (upper panel), although *Firmicutes* is the most abundant phylum, it is reduced in the ACD group as *Actinobacteria*. A parallel increase of the *Proteobacteria* is found in this group, while an expansion of *Bacteroidetes* in the RCD group and a reduction of *Fusobacteria* in the PCD one are evident. In the salivary samples (central panel), the most abundant phylum is *Bacteroidetes*. Again, *Firmicutes* is reduced in the ACD group as *Actinobacteria* in comparison to the C group. Interestingly, the RCD group shows a decrease of all phyla but *Proteobacteria*. In the stool samples (lower panel), the two most abundant phyla are *Bacteroidetes* and *Firmicutes*, with the other phyla showing negligible values. Noteworthily, the former is decreased in the ACD group and increased in the TCD group in comparison to C, while the latter is increased in the ACD and PCD groups.

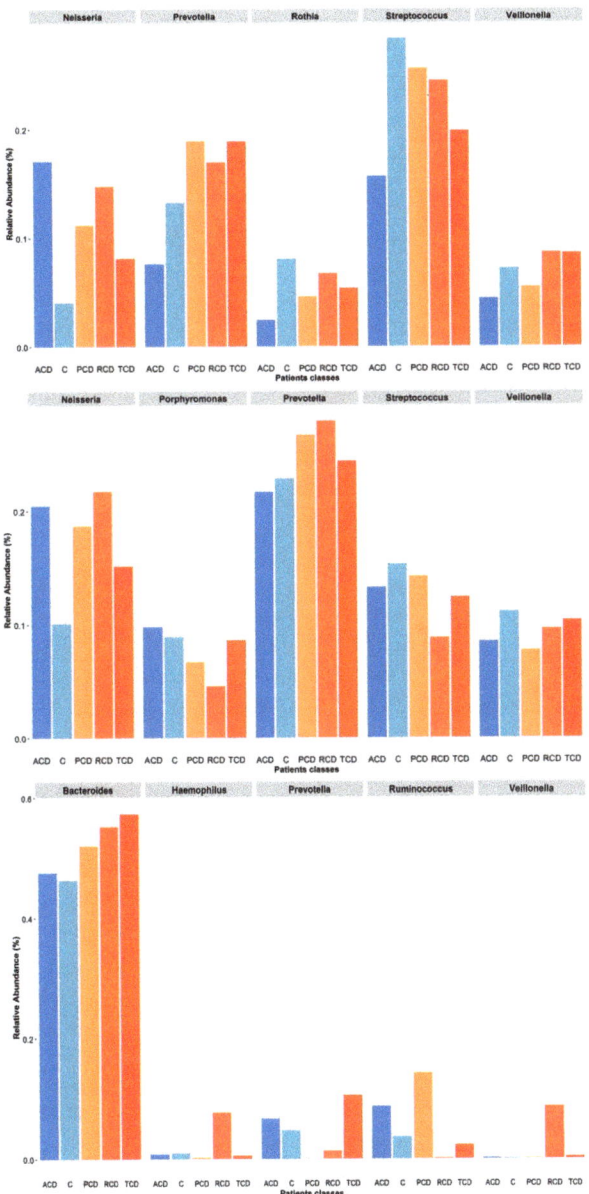

Figure 6. Plot of relative abundances of the five most abundant genera retrieved in each sample biotype: At the mucosal level (upper panel), all the most abundant genera are decreased in the ACD group but *Neisseria* as in all the other celiac groups with respect to the C one. Interestingly, *Prevotella* abundance is increased in the PCD, RCD, and TCD groups. In the salivary samples (central panel), again, *Neisseria* abundance is critically increased in all celiac groups with respect to the C one while *Prevotella* is increased only in the PCD, RCD, and TCD groups. Finally, in the stool samples (lower panel), the most abundant genus is *Bacteroides* that is increased in all celiac groups, with the other genera showing negligible values. Notably, the *Haemophilus* and *Veillonella* genera are critically increased only in the RCD group while the *Prevotella* is absent in the PCD group that displays a robust increase of the *Ruminococcus* as in the ACD group.

4. Discussion

In spite of the considerable understanding of the mechanisms leading to mucosal injury [19], the role of environmental factors in CD pathogenesis remains elusive and, consequently, the treatment is far from optimal. Perturbations of the gut microbiota (dysbiosis) and viral infections have been suggested to trigger the first hit of mucosal inflammation [20,21]. In this regard, a series of elegant experiments has provided some mechanistic insights showing that both gluten- and amylase-trypsin inhibitor-derived peptides generated by pathobiont species, such as *Pseudomonas aeriginosa*, are able to disrupt the epithelial barrier, to activate protease-activated receptors-2 signalling, and to recruit intraepithelial lymphocytes in sensitized mice with a susceptible genetic background [22,23]. Nonetheless, gut mucosa may also harbour gluten-degrading bacteria, such as *Rothia* spp. [24] and *Lactobacillus* spp. [25], with the potential to dampen the harmful effects of gluten peptides. When considering studies carried out in adulthood CD, the few performed on duodenal mucosa invariably found a decrease in the relative abundance of *Firmicutes* and an increase of *Proteobacteria*, together with changes of microbiota structure and composition [6,26,27]. However, the small sample size and the lack of a control group do not allow any firm conclusions to be drawn. On the other side, in the vast majority of studies carried out in paediatric CD, the analyses were carried out on stool samples [28]. Since this analysis may miss changes associated with duodenal inflammation or may find others not causally related to the disease process, we sought to investigate the structure and composition of gut microbiota directly at the duodenal level, the main site of tissue injury. We found marked alterations of the ecological indices in CD in terms of reduction of bacterial richness and diversity with respect to dyspeptic patients used as controls. Worthy of note, those suffering from PCD displayed mucosal indices similar to those with active enteropathy (ACD and RCD). This evidence reinforces the hypothesis that a significant shift of the microbiota composition anticipates the development of mucosal lesions [20]. When considering the data obtained in the groups with active enteropathy, we found the lowest values of α-diversity indices in the three bacterial communities of the RCD group. ACD also showed a reduced microbial richness that, together with a *Proteobacteria*-rich microbiota, has been repeatedly associated with chronic inflammatory conditions [29], including CD [6,26,27]. The TCD group shows intermediate values of both α- and β-diversity comprised between those of ACD and C ones, thus confirming that the GFD does not completely restore a healthy microbiota [6,27].

Moving on to the taxonomic analysis, our results definitely confirm the decrease of *Firmicutes* and increase of *Proteobacteria* in the duodenal mucosa of ACD patients, whereas *Bacteroidetes* displayed a mixed pattern, being decreased in ACD and increased in all the other CD groups, mostly in RCD. Remarkably, Wacklin and coworkers identified *Proteobacteria* as the most abundant phylum in biopsies of TCD patients who suffered from persistent abdominal symptoms [6,27]. It is known that a balanced gut microbiota is capable of inhibiting uncontrolled expansion of *Proteobacteria*, while a bloom of this phylum has been proposed as reflecting an unstable structure [28,29]. Noteworthily, the profiles of the phyla distribution in salivary samples almost completely mirror those found at the mucosal level, except for *Proteobacteria* that were found predominantly increased in RCD, whilst no substantial correspondence with the other consortia was found in fecal samples.

A further interesting point is the enrichment of the genus *Neisseria* (phylum *Proteobacteria*) and the corresponding family *Neisseriaceae* in duodenal biopsies of ACD patients, in agreement with previous evidence [26]. Our study enlarges the picture since an increased abundance of *Neisseria* spp. is already evident in PCD, reaches its maximum in ACD and RCD, and then lowers in TCD, although without reaching control levels. This evidence reinforces the hypothesis that it represents a disease-triggering factor instead of a pure consequence of intestinal damage. Moreover, the behaviour of the gluten-degradator species *Rothia* [30] in RCD mucosa should be pointed out since its abundance was similar to controls and significantly higher than in the other CD groups. The reason remains elusive, although it is conceivable that a long-lasting presence of undigested gluten peptides in the gut lumen may select those species with a high capability of degrading them. On the other hand, the depletion of this species in PCD might contribute to loss of gluten tolerance since an incomplete digestion generates oligopeptides with high immunogenicity [2].

Finally, in the salivary ecosystem, it emerges that the SR1 phylum rises from a rate of less than 1% in controls and refractory patients to about 5% in PCD, ACD, and TCD. This is a relatively recently described phylum [31], of which the abundance increases in the oral cavity of subjects with periodontal disease [32]. Another particular trend observed was the critical decrease of both *Lechnospiraceae* and *Fusobacteriaceae* in RCD, whereas they were increased in mucosal samples of noncomplicated CD patients. The taxonomic composition of the fecal community also suggests the existence of a pattern specific for RCD if considering the strong increase of *Pasteurellaceae* and, within this family, of the genus *Haemophilus* spp., in accordance with Cheng et al. [33]. Other taxa generally thought to be protective against inflammation, such as *Faecalibacterium prausnitzii* [34], display a boom in RCD. Therefore, despite the obvious limited number of RCD cases, the presence of particular changes to the microbiota composition in both saliva and fecal samples offers important opportunities for screening those cases transitioning to RCD. In addition, the recent finding of full recovery of duodenal architecture and clinical picture in a patient suffering from RCD following fecal microbiota transplantation for *Clostridium difficile* infection strengthens the relevance of our data [35].

Certainly, our work has some limitations, including the limited sample size. However, it should be pointed out that only those patients who agreed to collect all biological samples were enrolled and that PCD and RCD are rare conditions. Furthermore, despite the oral cavity hardly representing the environment at the duodenal level, we found that saliva displays a microbiota structure and composition more similar to mucosal ones than feces. We also acknowledge that dyspepsia does not represent a real control condition; nonetheless a peculiar dysbiosis, largely dominated by the phylum *Proteobacteria*, genus *Neisseria*, clearly emerged in CD, even before the development of enteropathy. Moreover, the presence of an altered community structure not only in ACD but also in TCD clearly points to the need for additional non-dietary therapies. Since these findings are largely retrievable in the oral cavity, salivary analysis seems a useful tool to capture CD specific signatures. Taken together, our data pave the way for larger studies and support the utility of gut microbiota manipulation for preventive and therapeutic purposes in adulthood CD.

Supplementary Materials: The following are available online at http://www.mdpi.com/2077-0383/9/4/1109/s1, Figure S1: Plot of relative abundances of the five most abundant families retrieved in each sample biotype; Table S1: Taxonomic assignment across sample biotypes (mucosal, salivary and fecal) in the study cohort; Table S2: α-diversity indices for each sample.

Author Contributions: R.C., E.C. and F.B. designed the study. G.F.D.L., S.B. and E.C. were responsible for sample handling and for amplicon production and sequencing. S.M., E.S. and R.B. conceived, designed and implemented the metagenomic pipelines. The operational taxonomic unit abundances were calculated by S.P. and B.B. Phylogenetic analysis was done by S.P., G.F.D.L., S.B. and E.C. Bioinformatic analysis was conceived and implemented by E.S., S.M. and R.B., A.S., E.B. and F.B. were responsible for patient selection and for sample collection and storage. A.V. was responsible for histopathology examination. A.P. and R.C. conducted the human leukocyte antigen genotyping. O.P. was responsible for project and resource administration. R.C. and S.P. wrote the manuscript with contributions from E.C., A.S., E.S. and F.B. L.F. and G.R.C. critically revised the article for important intellectual content. All authors agreed to be personally accountable for the author's own contributions and for ensuring that questions related to the accuracy or integrity of any part of the work, even ones in which the author was not personally involved, are appropriately investigated, resolved, and documented in the literature. All authors have read and agreed to the published version of the manuscript.

Funding: This study was funded by a grant from the Fondazione Celiachia (Italy), project number: N. 016_FC_2015. This source of funding did not influence the study design; collection, analysis, and interpretation of data; writing of the manuscript; or decision to submit the article for publication.

Acknowledgments: The authors wish to thank Susan West for her thorough revision of the English text and doctor Laura Vanelli for performing the flow cytometric analysis of intraepithelial lymphocytes.

Conflicts of Interest: The authors declare no conflict of interest

Abbreviations

ACD	active celiac disease
C	control
CD	celiac disease
GFD	gluten-free diet
OTU	operational taxonomic unit
PCD	potential celiac disease
RCD	refractory celiac disease
spp	species
TCD	treated celiac disease

References

1. Young, V.B. The role of the microbiome in human health and disease: An introduction for clinicians. *BMJ* **2017**, *356*, j831. [CrossRef]
2. Stamnaes, J.; Sollid, L.M. Celiac Disease: Autoimmunity in response to food antigen. *Semin. Immunol.* **2015**, *27*, 343–352. [CrossRef]
3. Abadie Sollid, L.M.; Barreiro, L.B.; Jabri, B. Integration of genetic and immunological insights into a model of celiac disease pathogenesis. *Annu. Rev. Immunol.* **2011**, *29*, 493–525. [CrossRef]
4. Verdu, E.F.; Galipeau, H.J.; Jabri, B. Novel players in coeliac disease pathogenesis: Role of the gut microbiota. *Nat. Rev. Gastroenterol. Hepatol.* **2015**, *12*, 497–506. [CrossRef] [PubMed]
5. Nistal, E.; Caminero, A.; Herrán, A.R.; Perez-Andres, J.; Vivas, S.; Ruiz de Morales, J.M.; Saenz de Miera, L.E.; Casqueiro, J. Study of duodenal bacterial communities by 16S rRNA gene analysis in adults with active celiac disease vs non-celiac disease controls. *J. Appl. Microbiol.* **2016**, *120*, 1691–1700. [CrossRef] [PubMed]
6. Wacklin, P.; Laurikka, P.; Lindfors, K.; Collin, P.; Salmi, T.; Lähdeaho, M.-L.; Saavalainen, P.; Mäki, M.; Mättö, J.; Kurppa, K.; et al. Altered duodenal microbiota composition in celiac disease patients suffering from persistent symptoms on a long-term gluten-free diet. *Am. J. Gastroenterol.* **2014**, *109*, 1933–1941. [CrossRef] [PubMed]
7. Drossman, D.A. The functional gastrointestinal disorders and the Rome III process. *Gastroenterology* **2006**, *130*, 1377–1390. [CrossRef]
8. Ludvigsson, J.F.; Leffler, D.A.; Bai, J.C.; Biagi, F.; Fasano, A.; Green, P.H.R.; Hadjivassiliou, M.; Kaukinen, K.; Kelly, C.P.; Leonard, J.N.; et al. The Oslo definitions for coeliac disease and related terms. *Gut* **2013**, *62*, 43–52. [CrossRef]
9. Corazza, G.R.; Villanacci, V.; Zambelli, C.; Milione, M.; Luinetti, O.; Vindigni, C.; Chioda, C.; Albarello, L.; Bartolini, D.; Donato, F. Comparison of the interobserver reproducibility with different histologic criteria used in celiac disease. *Clin. Gastroenterol. Hepatol.* **2007**, *5*, 838–843. [CrossRef]
10. Biagi, F.; Andrealli, A.; Bianchi, P.I.; Marchese, A. A gluten-free diet score to evaluate dietary compliance in patients with coeliac disease. *Br. J. Nutr.* **2009**, *102*, 882–887. [CrossRef]
11. Takahashi, S.; Tomita, J.; Nishioka, K.; Hisada, T.; Nishijima, M. Development of a prokaryotic universal primer for simultaneous analysis of bacteria and archaea using Next-Generation Sequencing. *PLoS ONE* **2014**, *9*, e105592. [CrossRef] [PubMed]
12. Sinha, R.; Chen, J.; Amir, A.; Vogtmann, E.; Shi, J.; Inman, K.S.; Flores, R.; Sampson, J.; Knight, R.; Chia, N. Collecting fecal samples for microbiome analyses in epidemiology studies. *Cancer Epidemiol. Biomark.* **2016**, *25*, 407–416. [CrossRef] [PubMed]
13. Huse, S.M.; Young, V.B.; Morrison, H.G.; Antonopoulos, D.A.; Kwon, J.; Dalal, S.; Arrieta, R.; Hubert, N.A.; Shen, L.; Vineis, J.H.; et al. Comparison of brush and biopsy sampling methods of the ileal pouch for assessment of mucosa-associated microbiota of human subjects. *Microbiome* **2014**, *2*, 5. [CrossRef] [PubMed]
14. R Development Core Team. *R: A Language and Environment for Statistical Computing*; R Foundation for Statistical Computing: Vienna, Austria, 2008; ISBN 3-900051-07-0. Available online: http://www.R-project.org (accessed on 31 March 2019).
15. DeSantis, T.Z.; Hugenholtz, P.; Larsen, N.; Rojas, M.; Brodie, E.L.; Keller, K.; Huber, T.; Dalevi, D.; Hu, P.; Andersen, G.L. Greengenes, a chimera-checked 16S rRNA gene database and workbench compatible with ARB. *Appl. Environ. Microb.* **2006**, *72*, 5069–5072. [CrossRef] [PubMed]

16. Chao, A.; Chazdon, R.L.; Colwell, R.K.; Shen, T.-J. Abundance-based similarity indices and their estimation when there are unseen species in samples. *Biometrics* **2006**, *62*, 361–371. [CrossRef] [PubMed]
17. Hughes, J.B.; Hellmann, J.J.; Ricketts, T.H.; Bohannan, B.J.M. Counting the uncountable: Statistical approaches to estimating microbial diversity. *Appl. Environ. Microbiol.* **2001**, *67*, 4399–4406. [CrossRef] [PubMed]
18. Chen, J.; Bittinger, K.; Charlson, S.E.; Hoffmann, C.; Lewis, J.; Wu, G.D.; Collman, R.G.; Bushman, F.D.; Li, H. Associating microbiome composition with environmental covariates using generalized UniFrac distances. *Bioinformatics* **2012**, *28*, 2106–2113. [CrossRef]
19. Meresse, B.; Malamut, G.; Cerf-Bensussan, N. Celiac disease: An immunological jigsaw. *Immunity* **2012**, *36*, 907–919. [CrossRef]
20. Caminero, A.; Verdu, E.F. Celiac disease: Should we care about microbes? *Am. J. Physiol. Gastrointest. Liver Physiol.* **2019**, *317*, G161–G170. [CrossRef]
21. Kemppainen, K.M.; Lynch, K.F.; Liu, E.; Lonnrot, M.; Simell, V.; Briese, T.; Koletzko, S.; Hagopian, W.; Rewers, M.; She, J.-X.; et al. Factors that increase risk of celiac disease autoimmunity after a gastrointestinal infection in early life. *Clin. Gastroenterol. Hepatol.* **2017**, *15*, 694–702. [CrossRef]
22. Caminero, A.; McCarville, J.L.; Galipeau, H.J.; Deraison, C.; Bernier, S.P.; Constante, M.; Rolland, C.; Meisel, M.; Murray, J.A.; Yu, X.B.; et al. Duodenal bacterial proteolytic activity determines sensitivity to dietary antigen through protease-activated receptor-2. *Nat. Commun.* **2019**, *10*, 1198. [CrossRef] [PubMed]
23. Caminero, A.; McCarville, J.L.; Zevallos, V.F.; Pigrau, M.; Yu, X.B.; Jury, J.; Galipeau, H.J.; Clarizio, A.V.; Casqueiro, J.; Murray, J.A.; et al. Lactobacilli degrade wheat amylase trypsin inhibitors to reduce intestinal dysfunction induced by immunogenic wheat prteins. *Gastroenterology* **2019**, *156*, 2266–2280. [CrossRef] [PubMed]
24. Zamakhchari, M.; Wei, G.; Dewhirst, F.; Lee, J.; Schuppan, D.; Oppenheim, F.G.; Helmerhoest, E.J. Identification of Rothia bacteria as gluten-degrading natural colonizers of the upper gastro-intestinal tract. *PLoS ONE* **2011**, *6*, e24455. [CrossRef] [PubMed]
25. Caminero, A.; Galipeau, H.J.; McCarville, J.L.; Johnston, C.W.; Bernier, S.P.; Russell, A.K.; Jury, J.; Herran, A.R.; Casqueiro, J.; Tye-Din, J.A.; et al. Duodenal bacteria from patients with celiac disease and healthy subjects distinctly affect gluten breakdown and immunogenicity. *Gastroenterology* **2016**, *151*, 670–683. [CrossRef] [PubMed]
26. D'Argenio, V.; Casaburi, G.; Precone, V.; Pagliuca, C.; Colicchio, R.; Sarnataro, D.; Discepolo, V.; Kim, S.M.; Russo, I.; Del Vecchio Blanco, G.; et al. Metagenomics reveals dysbiosis and a potentially pathogenic N. flavescens strain in duodenum of adult celiac patients. *Am. J. Gastroenterol.* **2016**, *111*, 879–890. [CrossRef]
27. Wacklin, P.; Kaukinen, K.; Tuovinen, E.; Collin, P.; Lindfors, K.; Partanen, J.; Maki, M.; Matto, J. The duodenal microbiota composition of adult celiac disease is associated with the clinical manifestations of the disease. *Inflamm. Bowel. Dis.* **2013**, *19*, 934–941. [CrossRef]
28. Sanz, Y. Microbiome and gluten. *Ann. Nutr. Metab.* **2015**, *67*, 28–41. [CrossRef]
29. Shin, N.-R.; Whon, T.W.; Bae, J.-W. Proteobacteria: Microbial signature of dysbiosis in gut microbiota. *Trends Biotechnol.* **2015**, *33*, 496–503. [CrossRef]
30. Tian, N.; Wei, G.; Schuppan, D.; Helmerhorst, E. Effect of Rothia mucilaginosa enzymes on gliadin (gluten) structure, deamidation, and immunogenic epitopes relevant to celiac disease. *Am. J. Physiol. Gastrointest. Liver Physiol.* **2014**, *307*, G769–G776. [CrossRef]
31. Dewhirst, F.E.; Chen, T.; Izard, J.; Paster, B.J.; Tanner, A.C.R.; Yu, W.-H.; Lakshmanan, A.; Wade, W.G. The human oral microbiome. *J. Bacteriol.* **2010**, *192*, 5002–5017. [CrossRef]
32. Griffen, A.L.; Beall, C.J.; Campbell, J.H.; Firestone, N.D.; Kumar, P.S.; Yang, Z.K.; Podar, M.; Leys, E.J. Distinct and complex bacterial profiles in human periodontitis and health revealed by 16S pyrosequencing. *ISME J.* **2012**, *6*, 1176–1185. [CrossRef] [PubMed]
33. Cheng, J.; Kalliomaki, M.; Heilig, H.G.H.; Palva, A.; Lahteenoja, H.; de Vos, W.M.; Salojarvi, J.; Satokari, R. Duodenal microbiota composition and mucosal homeostasis in pediatric celiac disease. *BMC Gastroenterol.* **2013**, *13*, 113. [CrossRef] [PubMed]

34. Hakansson, A.; Molin, A. Gut microbiota and inflammation. *Nutrients* **2011**, *3*, 637–682. [CrossRef] [PubMed]
35. van Beurden, Y.H.; van Gils, T.; van Gils, N.A.; Kassam, Z.; Mulder, C.J.J.; Aparicio-Pages, N. Serendipity in refractory celiac disease: Full recovery of duodenal villi and clinical symptoms after fecal microbiota transfer. *J. Gastroenterol. Liver Dis.* **2016**, *25*, 385–388. [CrossRef]

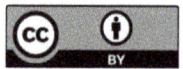

© 2020 by the authors. Licensee MDPI, Basel, Switzerland. This article is an open access article distributed under the terms and conditions of the Creative Commons Attribution (CC BY) license (http://creativecommons.org/licenses/by/4.0/).

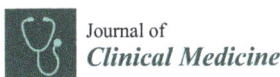

Article

Transient and Persistent Gastric Microbiome: Adherence of Bacteria in Gastric Cancer and Dyspeptic Patient Biopsies after Washing

Malene R. Spiegelhauer [1,*], Juozas Kupcinskas [2,3], Thor B. Johannesen [4], Mindaugas Urba [2,3], Jurgita Skieceviciene [3], Laimas Jonaitis [2], Tove H. Frandsen [1], Limas Kupcinskas [2,3], Kurt Fuursted [4] and Leif P. Andersen [1]

1. Department of Clinical Microbiology, Rigshospitalet, Henrik Harpestrengs Vej 4A, 2100 Copenhagen, Denmark; Tove.Havnhoj.Frandsen@rsyd.dk (T.H.F.); leif.percival.andersen@regionh.dk (L.P.A.)
2. Department of Gastroenterology, Lithuanian University of Health Sciences, Eiveniu str. 2, LT-50009 Kaunas, Lithuania; juozas.kupcinskas@lsmuni.lt (J.K.); mindaugas.urba@lsmuni.lt (M.U.); laimas.jonaitis@lsmuni.lt (L.J.); limas.kupcinskas@lsmuni.lt (L.K.)
3. Institute for Digestive Research, Lithuanian University of Health Sciences, Eiveniu str. 2, LT-50009 Kaunas, Lithuania; jurgita.skieceviciene@lsmuni.lt
4. Department of Clinical Microbiology and Infection Control, Statens Serum Institute, Artillerivej 5, 2300 Copenhagen, Denmark; THEJ@ssi.dk (T.B.J.); kfu@ssi.dk (K.F.)
* Correspondence: malene.spiegelhauer@outlook.com; Tel.: +45-2585-2011

Received: 21 April 2020; Accepted: 13 June 2020; Published: 16 June 2020

Abstract: *Helicobacter pylori* is a common colonizer of the human stomach, and long-term colonization has been related to development of atrophic gastritis, peptic ulcers and gastric cancer. The increased gastric pH caused by *H. pylori* colonization, treatment with antibiotics or proton pump inhibitors (PPI) may allow growth of other bacteria. Previous studies have detected non-*Helicobacter* bacteria in stomach biopsies, but no conclusion has been made of whether these represent a transient contamination or a persistent microbiota. The aim of this study was to evaluate the transient and persistent bacterial communities of gastric biopsies. The washed or unwashed gastric biopsies were investigated by cultivation and microbiota analysis (16S rRNA gene-targeted amplicon sequencing) for the distribution of *H. pylori* and other non-*Helicobacter* bacteria. The number of cultured non-*Helicobacter* bacteria decreased in the washed biopsies, suggesting that they might be a transient contamination. No significant differences in the bacterial diversity were observed in the microbiome analysis between unwashed and washed biopsies. However, the bacterial diversity in biopsies shown *H. pylori*-positive and *H. pylori*-negative were significantly different, implying that *H. pylori* is the major modulator of the gastric microbiome. Further large-scale studies are required to investigate the transient and persistent gastric microbiota.

Keywords: gastric microbiota; transient; persistent; culture; microbiome; sequencing; *Helicobacter pylori*

---

1. Introduction

1.1. Helicobacter Pylori *Colonization of the Stomach*

Helicobacter is a group of Gram-negative, curved or spiral-shaped bacteria, of which *Helicobacter pylori* is the most commonly known species [1]. *H. pylori* is able to colonize the human stomach by moving through the gastric mucin layer, and long-term colonization may increase the risk for development of atrophic gastritis, peptic ulcers and ultimately gastric cancer [2–5].

Approximately 30% of adults in developed countries and 80% of adults in developing countries are colonized with *H. pylori*, and of these, 1–3% further develop gastric cancer [6,7].

H. pylori has only been shown as a natural colonizer in humans, but another *Helicobacter* species capable of gastric colonization in humans is *Helicobacter heilmanii* [8,9]. The prevalence of infection with *H. heilmanii* is much lower than of *H. pylori* and it has been described less than 0.5% of patients undergoing upper gastric endoscopy [10].

Due to gastric peristalsis, mucus thickness, low pH and secretion of bile and acid, it was initially believed that no bacteria could survive in the inhospitable stomach environment [2,3,11]. Later, studies detected *H. pylori* as the only bacterium in stomachs with a healthy low pH, while more bacteria were detected at higher pH [12]. The mucus thickness and viscosity are pH-dependent, and a decreased acidity caused by *H. pylori* colonization, atrophic gastritis, treatment with antibiotics or proton pump inhibitors (PPI) may reduce the acidic protection of the stomach, leading to bacterial overgrowth and a higher diversity [13–16]. An alteration of the gastric bacterial composition has also been reported in cases of gastric cancer, with an increase of both oral and intestinal bacterial groups [16]. Recent studies have described the presence of a non-*Helicobacter* gastric microbiota, suggesting that other bacteria are able to live in the strict environment of the stomach [13].

1.2. Previous Studies of the Gastric Microbiota

Initial studies on gastric bacterial communities were reported in the 1980s [17]. Since then, several studies have investigated the presence of *H. pylori* and non-*Helicobacter* bacteria by cultivation methods and DNA-based methods [16,17]. Zilberstein et al. cultured gastric biopsies in aerobic and anaerobic conditions and found *Veillonella*, *Lactobacillus* and *Clostridium* to be the predominant bacterial groups [18]. They concluded that species of these bacterial groups may be transiently present [18]. Li et al. performed 16S rRNA gene amplicon sequencing on gastric biopsies from healthy people and patients with gastritis and observed a community dominated by species of *Prevotella*, *Streptococcus*, *Veillonella*, *Rothia* and *Haemophilus* [14]. Similar results were obtained by Bik et al. by 16S rRNA gene amplicon sequencing, where the dominating genera were found to be *Streptococcus*, *Prevotella*, *Rothia*, *Fusobacterium* and *Veillonella* [2]. A study by Delgado et al. on healthy patients identified *Lactobacillus* as one of the most abundant genera in the stomach as well as *Streptococcus* and *Propionibacterium* by 16S rRNA gene amplicon pyrosequencing [19]. A study by Dicksved et al. detected a bacterial community of *Streptococcus*, *Lactobacillus*, *Veillonella* and *Prevotella*, with a low abundance of *Helicobacter* [20]. The study found no significant differences in the gastric bacterial communities of patients with gastric cancer or dyspepsia [8]. Maldonado-Contreras et al. investigated the microbial composition by 16S rRNA gene amplicon hybridization and found non-*Helicobacter* bacteria such as *Proteobacteria*, *Firmicutes*, *Actinobacteria* and *Bacteroidetes* to be dominating [21]. Yu et al. identified similar phyla in the gastric stomach area and other body sites [22]. The authors performed a functional profiling of the stomach microbiota and concluded that though similar phyla were present in these areas, the microbiota of the different areas presented different functions [22]. A systematic review by Rajilic-Stojanovic et al. compared the results of papers investigating the gastric microbiota by next-generation sequencing (NGS) [16]. Approximately 2/3 of the described papers detected species of *Prevotella*, *Streptococcus*, *Veillonella*, *Neisseria*, *Fusobacterium* and *Haemophilus* and have described that the microbiota is subject-specific and differ between individuals [16]. More than 65% of the bacterial groups found in the stomach have also been identified in the human oral cavity, and many bacteria identified in the stomach may originate from the oral cavity or as reflux from the intestine [3]. Previous studies have not been conclusive about whether the detected non-*Helicobacter* bacteria represent a transient contamination of the stomach or if they belong to the persistent gastric microbiota.

1.3. H. pylori *and the Non-Helicobacter Microbial Community*

The human stomach has been described to contain a core microbiome mainly consisting of *Prevotella, Streptococcus, Veillonella, Rothia* and *Haemophilus* spp., influenced by diet, inflammation and medication [3]. However, the effect of *H. pylori* colonization on the bacterial diversity has not been established yet. Andersson et al. investigated the bacterial composition with 16S rRNA gene amplicon pyrosequencing and found complex microbial communities with a great diversity in the absence of *H. pylori* [23]. When present, *H. pylori* accounted for 90% of the bacteria, and diversity was decreased [23]. This agrees with other findings of a large variation in the bacterial community depending on the presence or absence of *H. pylori* [4,12,16,21]. The study by Maldonado-Contreras associated *H. pylori* colonization with an increase of *Proteobacteria*, *Spirochetes* and *Acidobacteria* and decrease of *Actinobacteria*, *Bacteroidetes* and *Firmicutes* [21]. Other studies have opposed the suggestion that the diversity of bacteria in the stomach is negatively affected by the presence of *H. pylori* [2,22,24]. As such, the significance of *H. pylori* on the presence of other bacteria in the gastric environment remains unknown. In a study by Sanduleanu et al., the non-*Helicobacter* bacteria in the stomach were found to contaminate both the gastric juices and the mucosa during gastric acid inhibition [15]. A study by Li et al. investigated the effect of washing on the bacterial content of gastric biopsies [14]. The majority of bacteria remained in the biopsies even after several washing steps, and in particular, *Streptococcus* were not removed [14]. Colonization with *H. pylori* has been associated with increased inflammation and development of gastric atrophy, which may cause overgrowth of other bacteria as the environment turns less acidic [25]. The presence of a complex microbial community in an atrophic stomach may further promote inflammation, malignancies and cancer development [25].

1.4. Microbial Effects on the Development of Gastric Cancer

H. pylori is classified as a class I carcinogen, and colonization with this species is associated with an increased risk for gastric cancer [26]. The precise mechanism for this development is not known in detail, but it may be affected by diet and interactions with the gastric microbiota [27]. It has been hypothesized that the presence of a specific microbiota promotes inflammation and that other bacteria in addition to *H. pylori* may further promote cancer development [26]. The pH is usually increased in the stomachs of gastric cancer patients, resulting in atrophic gastritis and subsequent loss of *H. pylori*, as the environment becomes less acidic [28]. Several studies of the gastric microbiota in the settings of gastric cancer have been performed. A study by Dicksved et al. compared the microbiota of biopsies from patients with gastric cancer and dyspepsia by terminal restriction fragment length polymorphism [20]. They identified complex compositions of bacteria in gastric cancer biopsies but with no significant differences in the microbial compositions compared to dyspepsia patient biopsies [20]. A low abundance of *H. pylori* and a dominance of species from *Streptococcus*, *Lactobacillus*, *Veillonella* and *Prevotella* were observed in biopsies from gastric cancer patients [20]. Another study by Ferreira et al. investigated the bacterial composition in biopsies from patients with atrophic gastritis and gastric cancer [29]. They detected a reduced microbial diversity in gastric cancer patients and found an abundance of less than 5% *H. pylori* in most gastric cancer patients [29]. Based on calculations of a microbial dysbiosis index, the presence of a dysbiotic microbiota in the gastric cancer patients was suggested, compared to the microbiota of individuals with atrophic gastritis [29]. In particular, the microbiota of gastric cancer biopsies showed increased abundances of the groups *Actinobacteria* and *Firmicutes*, while the presence of the groups *Bacteroidetes* and *Fusobacteria* were decreased [29]. Yu et al. analyzed the microbiota of gastric cancer biopsies and identified *H. pylori* as the most abundant bacterial species present, followed by bacteria associated with the oral environment [22]. A decrease in *Proteobacteria* and increase in *Bacteroidetes*, *Firmicutes* and *Spirochetes* were observed in gastric cancer tissue, but comparisons of microbiota in the corpus and antrum areas of the stomach showed no differences [22]. An altered bacterial composition has also been reported in cases of gastric cancer, with an increase of both oral and intestinal bacterial groups [16].

1.5. Definition of Persistent and Transient Microbiota and Microbiome

In this study, the gastric microbiota is defined as the persistent bacteria that adhere to the gastric mucosa. The gastric microbiome is defined as the collection of microbial genes in the stomach, which also include the community of non-adherent, transient bacteria [30]. Previous studies have not been able to agree on whether the bacteria identified in the stomach represent a true microbiota or are contamination from the oral cavity. It is therefore not clear which bacteria belong to the true gastric microbiota.

The main aim of this study was to investigate the presence of persistent and transient bacterial communities by comparing the changes in bacterial composition of washed and unwashed gastric biopsies. It is the first comprehensive attempt to distinguish between the transient and resident bacteria of the stomach using 16S rRNA gene sequencing.

The second aim of this study was to investigate and compare the gastric microbiota of gastric cancer patients and dyspepsia patients. The results will contribute to the ongoing debate about whether the process of gastric carcinogenesis is mediated through a microbial shift caused by *H. pylori*. Biopsies from both cancerous and non-cancerous tissue were included, and dyspepsia patients were involved as controls of a healthy microbiota.

The hypothesis of our experimental setup is that *H. pylori* is the only true gastric microbiota of the stomach and will be the predominant bacterium that is able to remain in the washed biopsies. Although other studies have shown the presence of non-*Helicobacter* bacteria in the stomach, these will be expected to be present at least in the unwashed biopsies, as transient contamination from other niches [3].

2. Experimental Section/Materials and Methods

2.1. Sampling of Gastric Biopsies

Twenty-two patients with dyspepsia and twelve patients with gastric cancer were included in the study. The distribution was 68% female ($n = 23$ patients), 32% male ($n = 11$ patients) and an age range of 22–91 years (median 53 years). Clinical information about the patients is listed in Table 1. The exclusion criteria for the patients were age below 18 years, a previous history of *H. pylori* eradication, use of PPI within the last 3 months, use of antibiotics within the last 3 months, and previous treatment of gastric cancer. Three antral biopsies were taken about 4 cm from pylorus from patients with dyspepsia ($n = 22$ patients) by gastroscopy. From patients with gastric cancer ($n = 12$ patients), three antrum biopsies were taken about 4 cm from pylorus, and three biopsies were taken from the cancer area in the corpus. The biopsies were obtained between November 2017 and June 2019. The first biopsy was immediately used for histology to examine the presence of *H. pylori*. Histological slides were stained with haematoxylin/eosin, and a Giemsa stain was used to confirm the presence or absence of *H. pylori*. Figure 1 shows a histological sample positive for *H. pylori* infection.

Table 1. Clinical data of patients included in the study.

Diagnosis	Mean Age (years)	Gender	*H. pylori* Status (Histology)	Lauren Classification	G Stage	Proximal/Distal Part
Gastric adenocarcinoma ($n = 12$)	62.2	Female ($n = 5$)	Negative ($n = 9$)	Diffuse ($n = 6$)	2 ($n = 5$)	Proximal ($n = 3$)
		Male ($n = 7$)	Positive ($n = 3$)	Intestinal ($n = 4$)	3 ($n = 7$)	Distal ($n = 9$)
				Mixed ($n = 2$)		
Dyspepsia ($n = 22$)	48.1	Female ($n = 18$)	Negative ($n = 11$)	NA	NA	NA
		Male ($n = 4$)	Positive ($n = 11$)			

NA: Not applicable.

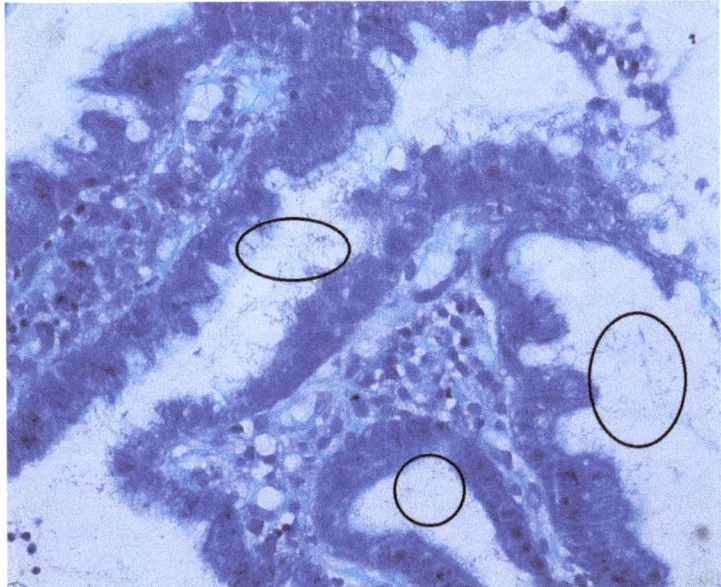

Figure 1. The positive results of *Helicobacter pylori* infection by Giemsa stain. Black circles indicate stained *H. pylori* (blue) that are attached to the gastric epithelial cells.

All patients participating in the study have signed an informed consent form. The study protocol has been approved by Kaunas Regional Bioethics Committee (Protocol No: BE-2-10; P1-BE-2-31).

The second biopsy was immediately transferred to the transport medium Portagerm pylori (bioMérieux, Marcy L'Etoile, France) and stored at −80 °C. The third biopsy was placed in a tube with sterile 4 °C PBS, collected by sterile forceps and washed for 15 s in 4 °C PBS and transferred to a new sterile tube containing 4 °C PBS. This step was repeated twice, after which the biopsy was placed in the transport medium Portagerm pylori (bioMérieux, Marcy L'Etoile, France) and stored at −80 °C. These biopsies were then transported to the Copenhagen University Hospital (Rigshospitalet) for culture.

2.2. Culture of Gastric Biopsies and Identification of Single Colonies

Biopsies were cultured on 7% defibrinated horse blood agar plates (SSI Diagnostica A/S, Hillerød, Denmark), placed in serum bouillon with 10% glycerol (SSI Diagnostica, Hillerød, Denmark), and frozen at −80 °C. The agar plates were incubated 6 days at 37 °C in microaerobic conditions (10% CO_2, 5% O_2); the observed growth was noted, and single colonies of each morphology were isolated on new 5% horse blood agar plates (SSI Diagnostica A/S, Hillerød, Denmark). The plates with the isolated cultures were incubated at 37 °C in microaerobic conditions until visible growth was seen (1–3 days). Each isolate was transferred to a MALDI-TOF target plate, treated with 1μL HCAA matrix (Bruker Daltonics, Billerica, MA, USA), analyzed with MALDI-TOF Mass Spectrometry (Bruker Daltonics, Billerica, MA, USA), and the protein profile was compared to the database Compass (Bruker Daltonics, Billerica, MA, USA) to identify the species. The biopsies were then transported to Statens Serum Institute for microbiome analysis (16S rRNA gene amplicon sequencing).

2.3. Microbiome Analysis (16S rRNA Gene Amplicon Sequencing)

DNA was extracted from the biopsies using a QIAamp DNA mini Kit (Qiagen, Hilden, Germany) according to the manufacturer's instruction for tissues. For each batch of DNA extraction, a negative control without sample material was included for downstream analysis. DNA was amplified using a two-step PCR using a modified version of the published universal prokaryotic primers 341F (ACTCCTAYGGGRBGCASCAG) and 806R (ACTCCTAYGGGRBGCASCAG) targeting the V3-V4 regions of the 16S rRNA gene. Amplicons were sequenced on the Illumina MiSeq desktop sequencer (Illumina Inc., San Diego, CA, USA), using the V2 Reagent Kit.

2.3.1. Library Preparation

Purified genomic DNA from each sample was initially amplified in a 25 µL reaction, using the REDExtract-N-Amp PCR ReadyMix (Sigma-Aldrich, St Louis, MO, USA) with 0.4 µM of each 16S rRNA gene primer and 2 µL template. The 16S PCR conditions were the following: an initial denaturation at 95 °C for 2 min, 20 cycles of 95 °C for 30 s, 60 °C for 1 min and 72 °C for 30 s and final elongation at 72 °C for 7 min. This PCR run is referred to as PCR1. The product from PCR1 was prepared for sequencing by a second PCR (referred to as PCR2), using the same PCR protocol as described above. PCR2 attached an adaptor A, an index i5 and a forward sequencing primer site (FSP) in the 5′ end of the amplicons and an adaptor B, an index i7 and a reverse sequencing primer site (RSP) to the 3′ end of the amplicons. DNA was quantified using the Quant-IT^{TM} dsDNA High Sensitive Assay Kit (Thermo Fisher Scientific, Waltham, MA, USA) and PCR2 products were pooled in equimolar amounts between samples. Agencourt AMPure XP bead (Beckman Coulter, Brea, CA, USA) purification was performed to remove undesirable DNA amplicons from the pooled amplicon library (PAL) in a two-step process. First, DNA fragments below 300 nucleotides length were removed by a PAL AMPure beads 10:24 ratio, following the manufacturer's instructions, and eluted in 40 µL TE buffer (AM1). Secondly, large DNA fragments above 1kbp were removed by AM1 to AMPure beads 10:16 ratio as previously described. The resulting AMPure beads purified PAL (bPAL) was diluted to a final concentration of 11.5 pM DNA in a 0.001 N NaOH and used for sequencing on the Illumina MiSeq desktop sequencer (Illumina Inc., San Diego, CA, USA). The library was sequenced with the 500-cycle MiSeq Reagent Kit V2 in a 2 × 250 nt setup (Illumina Inc., San Diego, CA, USA). The sequencing was performed at Statens Serum Institute (SSI).

2.3.2. Bioinformatics

BION-META (http://box.com/bion), a newly developed analytical semi-commercial open-source package for 16S rRNA gene and other reference gene analysis classifying mostly species was used, and the data were processed following the previously described automated steps [31,32]. After BION-META analysis, taxonomy tables were made with the identified phylum, class, order, family, genus, species and number of reads. The data from the sequencing were submitted to European Nucleotide Archive with the accession number PRJEB38558.

2.3.3. Statistics of Microbiome Analysis Results

The ten most abundant genera across all samples are shown in staggered bar plots in which samples are ordered according to a hierarchical clustering based on Bray Curtis dissimilarities and ward-linkage. The difference in the distribution of bacterial groups between biopsies was analyzed with an unpaired t-test using the graphing and statistics program GraphPad Prism version 5.01 (San Diego, CA, USA).

Analysis of the microbiome diversity was performed in the statistical computing program R, version 3.5.0 (R Foundation for Statistical Computing, Vienna, Austria) using the packages phyloseq v.1.24.3 and vegan v. 2.5-2. Figures were created using the packages ggplot2 v.3.2.0 and plotly v. 4.8.0. Alpha-diversity of samples as well as relative abundance of individual genera were compared pairwise between groups with Mann–Whitney rank sum tests and adjusted for multiple testing using Bonferroni correction. Principal coordinate analysis (PCoA) of samples was performed based BIONs species-level classification on Bray Curtis dissimilarity. Within-group similarities were compared to between-group similarities with analysis of similarities (ANOSIM test) using 1000 random permutations to estimate p-value.

3. Results

3.1. Comparison of Bacterial Composition in Unwashed Biopsies and Washed Biopsies

3.1.1. A Decrease in Cultured Bacteria was Observed for the Washed Biopsies

The overall number of cultured non-*Helicobacter* species decreased in the washed biopsies compared to the unwashed biopsies, suggesting that many bacteria do not adhere to the tissue. A total of 27 biopsy pairs showed reduced or no growth in the washed biopsy compared to the growth observed in the unwashed biopsy (Table 2). Only 5 biopsy pairs showed unchanged growth, while 3 showed increased growth.

Table 2. Change in growth of bacterial species cultured from the biopsy pairs.

Growth Result	Dyspepsia Patients	Gastric Cancer Patients
No bacterial growth in either biopsy	8 biopsy pairs	3 biopsy pairs
Growth in unwashed but not in washed biopsy	4 biopsy pairs	5 biopsy pairs
Reduced growth in the washed biopsy	9 biopsy pairs	9 biopsy pairs
Unchanged growth	1 biopsy pairs	4 biopsy pairs
Increased growth in the washed biopsy	0 biopsy pairs	3 biopsy pairs

The total number of colonies of cultured *Streptococcus* spp. decreased, but its relative abundance was higher in the washed biopsies compared to the unwashed biopsies (Figure 2, Table 3). The cultured bacteria in the biopsies were dominated by *Streptococcus* spp., followed by *Rothia* spp. and *Actinomyces* spp. (Table 3).

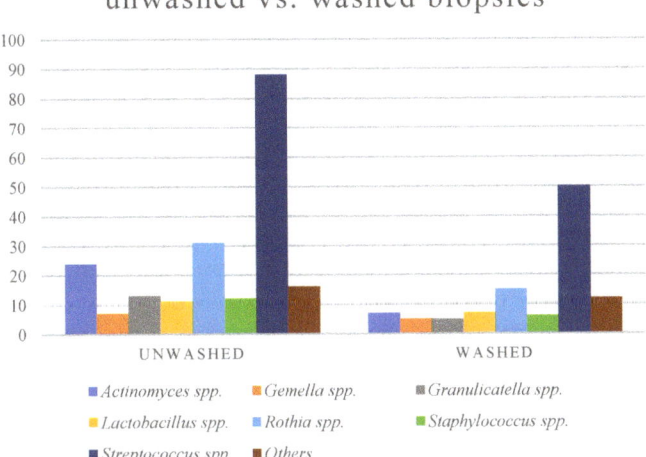

Figure 2. The number of bacterial species isolated from culture of gastric cancer and dyspepsia patient biopsies. "Others" include *Bacillus* spp., *Corynebacterium* spp., *Enterobacter* spp., *Enterococcus* spp., *Haemophilus* spp, *Micrococcus* spp., *Neisseria* spp., and *Stenotrophomonas* spp.

Table 3. Distribution of total cultured bacterial groups.

	Dyspepsia		Gastric Cancer	
	Unwashed	Washed	Unwashed	Washed
Streptococcus spp.	40%	43%	47%	49%
Rothia spp.	16%	14%	15%	14%
Actinomyces spp.	16%	9%	9%	6%
Staphylococcus spp.	8%	6%	4%	6%
Granulicatella spp.	7%	6%	6%	4%
Lactobacillus spp.	4%	3%	7%	8%
Gemella spp.	2%	9%	5%	3%
Enterococcus spp.	1%	3%	6%	8%
Micrococcus spp.	2%	3%	2%	0%
Corynebacterium spp.	2%	3%	-	-
Stenotrophomonas spp.	1%	0%	-	-
Neisseria spp.	1%	0%	-	-
Enterobacter spp.	0%	3%	-	-
Bacillus spp.	-	-	1%	0%
Haemophilus spp.	-	-	0%	3%

3.1.2. Microbiome Analysis

Bacterial DNA was detected in all biopsies, even in those were no growth was observed. The ten most prevalent groups in the microbiome analysis were *Helicobacter* spp., *Streptococcus* spp., *Prevotella* spp., *Escherichia* spp., *Veillonella* spp., *Fusobacterium* spp., *Haemophilus* spp., *Rothia* spp., *Neisseria* spp., and *Alloprevotella* spp. (Figure 3). The average relative abundance of *H. pylori* increased in some of the washed biopsies compared to the unwashed, but this was not always observed in the individual samples (Table 4). The increase in *H. pylori* was therefore not significant. The "other bacteria" belong to over 100 different bacterial groups, of which some species were only present in few biopsies. The bacterial groups that were found in several of the biopsies are among the genera: *Abiotrophia, Aggregatibacter, Atopobium, Campylobacter, Capnocytophaga, Catonella, Corynebaccterium, Dialister, Eubacterium, Filifacter, Flavobacterium, Gemella, Granulicatella, Lachnoanaerobaculum, Lactobacillus, Leptotrichia, Megasphaera, Oribacterium, Parvimonas, Peptostreptococcus, Porphyromonas, Propionibacterium, Selenomonas, Solobacterium, Staphylococcus, Stenotrophomonas, Stomatobaculum* and *Treponema* (Table 5). The relative abundance of other non-*H. pylori* bacteria was similar between unwashed and washed samples, and none of the listed groups showed a significant change in relative abundance in either dyspepsia patients (Figure 3a) or gastric cancer patients (Figure 3b). No significant differences were observed in the bacterial distribution between the patient groups. Comparison of the bacterial diversity within the samples showed no significant differences between the unwashed and washed biopsies (Figure 3c), and similar bacterial species were clustered in both groups (Figure 3d).

Table 4. Mean and standard error of the 10 most common bacterial groups as percentage of total bacterial reads in the microbiome analysis.

	Dyspepsia Biopsiy Pairs (n = 22)		Gastric Cancer Biopsy Pairs (n = 24)	
	Unwashed (% ± SEM)	Washed (% ± SEM)	Unwashed (% ± SEM)	Washed (% ± SEM)
Helicobacter spp.	28.3 ± 7.9	31.2 ± 8.4	11.8 ± 4.4	12.7 ± 5.0
Streptococcus spp.	12.6 ± 1.8	9.6 ± 1.8	21.3 ± 4.3	20.1 ± 4.3
Prevotella spp.	13.9 ± 2.7	11.0 ± 2.5	6.4 ± 1.1	6.1 ± 1.3
Escherichia spp.	7.0 ± 2.9	10.4 ± 3.8	9.5 ± 3.6	11.9 ± 3.6
Veillonella spp.	5.3 ± 0.9	3.4 ± 0.9	3.5 ± 1.0	3.7 ± 0.7
Fusobacterium spp.	4.8 ± 1.0	4.3 ± 1.5	4.2 ± 1.4	3.7 ± 1.2
Haemophilus spp.	4.6 ± 1.3	3.2 ± 0.9	2.4 ± 0.5	2.0 ± 0.5
Rothia spp.	3.5 ± 0.8	1.9 ± 0.6	2.2 ± 0.4	2.0 ± 0.7
Neisseria spp.	2.2 ± 0.7	1.5 ± 0.6	6.5 ± 2.7	6.8 ± 2.5
Alloprevotella spp.	1.5 ± 0.5	1.4 ± 0.4	1.7 ± 0.7	1.8 ± 0.7
Other bacteria	17.4 ± 2.7	17.0 ± 3.1	30.57 ± 5.8	29.3 ± 5.2

Table 5. Mean and standard error of the most common bacterial groups belonging to "other bacteria" as percentage of total bacterial reads in the microbiome analysis.

	Dyspepsia Biopsy Pairs (n = 22)		Gastric Cancer Biopsy Pairs (n = 24)	
	Unwashed (% ± SEM)	Washed (% ± SEM)	Unwashed (% ± SEM)	Washed (% ± SEM)
Abiotrophia spp.	0.013 ± 0.007	0.007 ± 0.009	0.104 ± 0.055	0.128 ± 0.047
Aggregatibacter spp.	0.139 ± 0.043	0.134 ± 0.044	0.103 ± 0.038	0.187 ± 0.086
Atopobium spp.	0.359 ± 0.113	0.31 ± 0.128	0.328 ± 0.064	0.335 ± 0.086
Campylobacter spp.	0.507 ± 0.141	0.452 ± 0.104	0.423 ± 0.121	0.314 ± 0.116
Capnocytophaga spp.	0.455 ± 0.19	0.308 ± 0.123	0.329 ± 0.087	0.274 ± 0.079
Catonella spp.	0.311 ± 0.098	0.212 ± 0.056	0.093 ± 0.027	0.119 ± 0.061
Corynebacterium spp.	0.214 ± 0.112	0.257 ± 0.175	0.047 ± 0.017	0.08 ± 0.033
Dialister spp.	0.304 ± 0.089	0.199 ± 0.083	0.31 ± 0.132	0.242 ± 0.101
Eubacterium spp.	0.123 ± 0.03	0.181 ± 0.059	0.186 ± 0.07	0.277 ± 0.147
Filifactor spp.	0.172 ± 0.076	0.262 ± 0.139	0.043 ± 0.012	0.08 ± 0.044
Flavobcaterium spp.	1.235 ± 0.975	1.27 ± 0.927	0.164 ± 0.063	0.575 ± 0.375
Gemella spp.	0.827 ± 0.228	0.82 ± 0.313	0.861 ± 0.211	1.446 ± 0.433
Granulicatella spp.	1.046 ± 0.219	1.093 ± 0.206	1.333 ± 0.405	1.603 ± 0.431
Lachnoanaerobaculum spp.	0.296 ± 0.066	0.271 ± 0.106	0.457 ± 0.156	0.435 ± 0.137
Lactobacillus spp.	0.013 ± 0.007	0.012 ± 0.006	1.925 ± 1.245	10.5 ± 8.878
Leptotrichia spp.	0.459 ± 0.196	0.967 ± 0.516	0.728 ± 0.362	0.42 ± 0.177
Megasphaera spp	0.554 ± 0.188	0.448 ± 0.143	0.219 ± 0.062	0.196 ± 0.059
Oribacterium spp.	0.432 ± 0.09	0.336 ± 0.11	0.329 ± 0.113	0.632 ± 0.327
Parvimonas spp.	0.229 ± 0.076	0.31 ± 0.188	1.478 ± 0.833	2.508 ± 1.555
Peptostreptococcus spp.	0.135 ± 0.045	0.13 ± 0.066	2.517 ± 1.448	3.319 ± 1.892
Porphyromonas spp.	1.765 ± 0.52	1.607 ± 0.653	0.666 ± 0.198	1.241 ± 0.566
Propionibacterium spp.	0.058 ± 0.031	0.082 ± 0.026	0.141 ± 0.056	0.256 ± 0.107
Selenomonas spp.	0.167 ± 0.059	0.231 ± 0.082	0.087 ± 0.022	0.088 ± 0.031
Solobacterium spp.	0.281 ± 0.062	0.282 ± 0.103	0.674 ± 0.29	0.603 ± 0.217
Staphylococcus spp.	0.403 ± 0.168	0.627 ± 0.153	0.292 ± 0.077	0.728 ± 0.351
Stenotrophomonas spp.	0.679 ± 0.54	1.128 ± 0.769	0.156 ± 0.052	0.495 ± 0.325
Stomatobaculum spp.	0.328 ± 0.12	0.365 ± 0.115	0.561 ± 0.332	0.775 ± 0.483
Treponema spp.	0.211 ± 0.076	0.391 ± 0.218	0.067 ± 0.031	0.056 ± 0.019

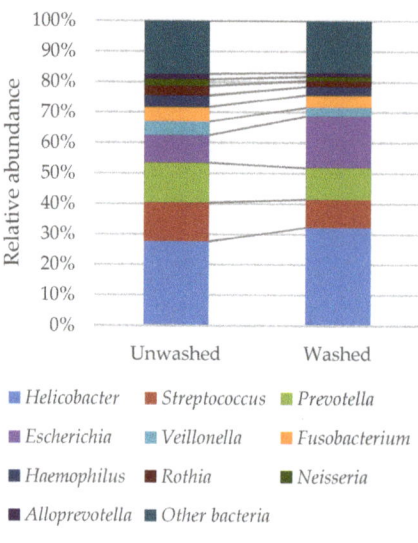

(a)

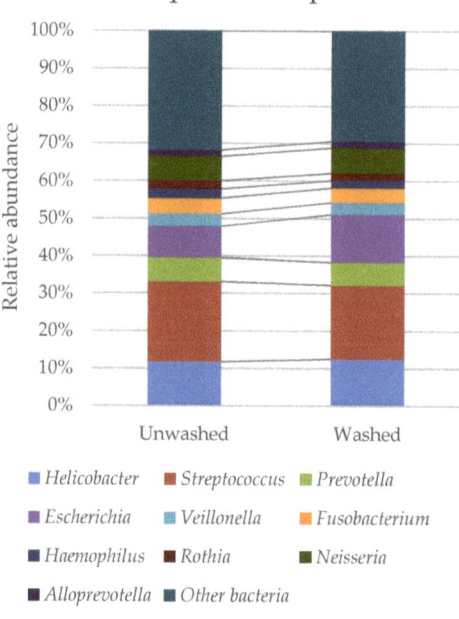

(b)

Figure 3. *Cont.*

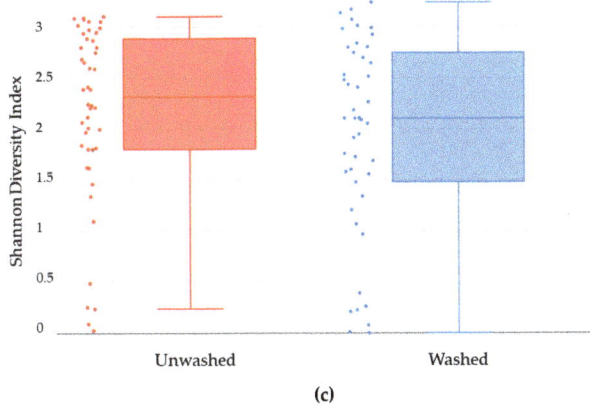

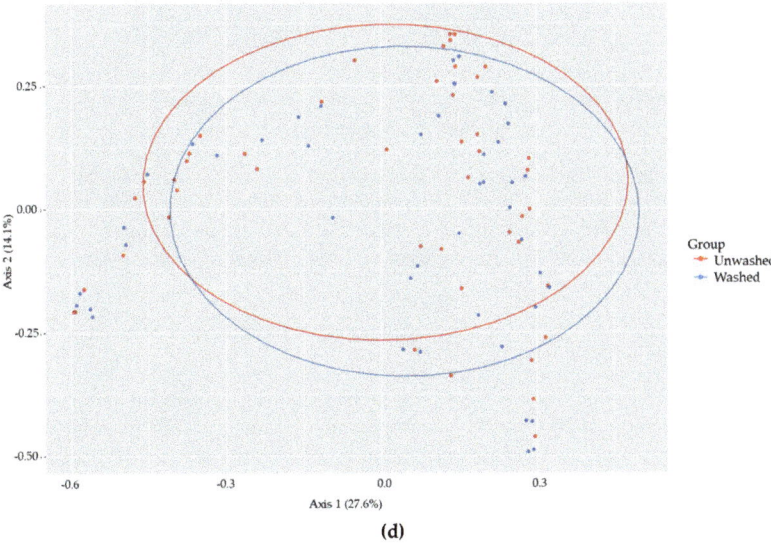

Figure 3. Comparison of the bacterial reads from microbiome analysis of unwashed and washed biopsies from (**a**) dyspepsia patients and (**b**) gastric cancer patients (percentages are listed in Table 4). Comparison of (**c**) the alpha-diversity shown by a Shannon Index, $p = 0.22581$ and (**d**) the beta-diversity between the two groups shown by PCoA plot, $p = 0.801199$, in unwashed biopsies (red) and washed biopsies (blue).

3.2. Comparison of Biopsies from Gastric Cancer Patients and Dyspepsia Patients

3.2.1. Cultured Bacteria were Dominated by *Streptococcus* spp.

The biopsies from dyspepsia patients and gastric cancer patients were dominated by similar cultured bacteria (Figure 4). Species of *Lactobacillus* were cultured from several cancer patient biopsies but only from one dyspepsia patient biopsy (Table 2). The distribution of cultured bacteria in biopsies from gastric cancer patients and dyspepsia patients showed an increase in the relative abundance of *Streptococcus* and a decrease in *Actinomyces* spp. (Table 3, Figure 4).

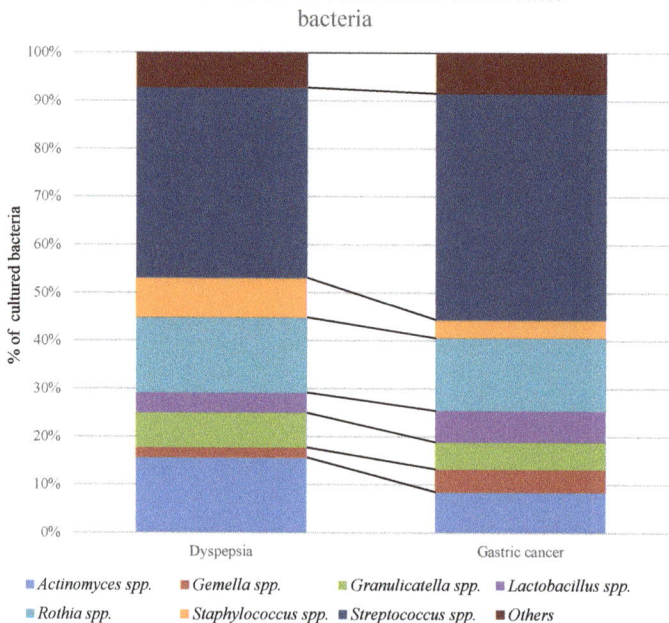

Figure 4. The relative distribution of non-*Helicobacter* bacteria cultured from the unwashed biopsies showed that *Streptococcus* spp. were predominant in both dyspepsia patients and gastric cancer patients. The percentages can be found in Table 3. "Others" include *Bacillus* spp., *Corynebacterium* spp., *Enterobacter* spp., *Enterococcus* spp., *Haemophilus* spp, *Micrococcus* spp., *Neisseria* spp., and *Stenotrophomonas* spp.

3.2.2. Microbiome Analysis Revealed Similar Distributions of Bacteria in Dyspepsia Patients and Gastric Cancer Patients

The average relative abundance of *H. pylori* was not significantly different in untreated biopsies untreated dyspepsia patients and gastric cancer patients (Figure 5a). For most bacterial groups, no significant difference was observed in the distribution of bacteria between dyspepsia patient and gastric cancer patient biopsies. However, a significant increase in the presence of *Prevotella* spp. was observed in dyspepsia patients ($p = 0.0109$) and of "other bacteria" in gastric cancer patients ($p = 0.0349$). This increase in other bacteria may be explained by the dominance of *Enterococcus* spp. in one biopsy pair, where more than 95% of the bacterial reads were identified as this. If this biopsy pair was removed from the data, the difference in "other bacteria" between the patient groups was not significant. The bacterial diversity in biopsies from dyspepsia patients and gastric cancer patients showed no significant differences within the groups (Figure 5b) or between the distribution of species in the groups (Figure 5c).

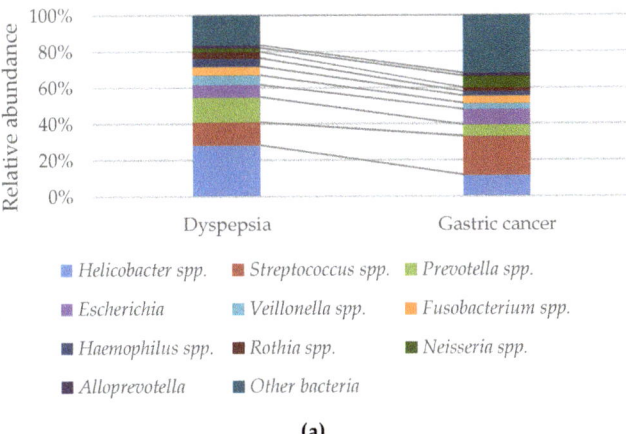

(a)

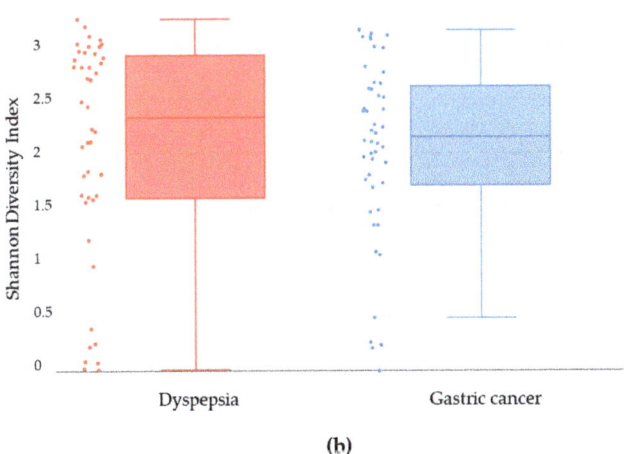

(b)

Figure 5. Cont.

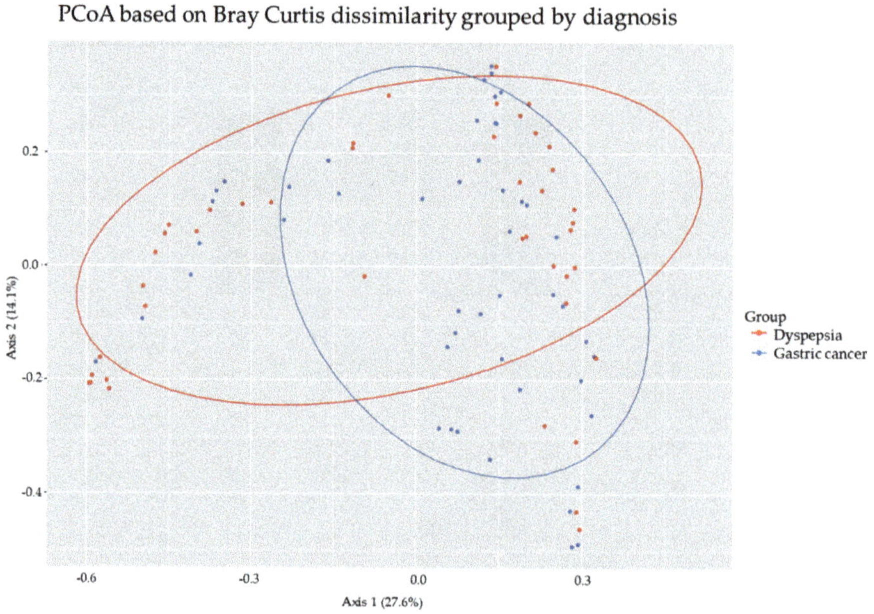

PCoA based on Bray Curtis dissimilarity grouped by diagnosis

(Scatter plot: Axis 1 (27.6%) vs Axis 2 (14.1%); Group: Dyspepsia (red), Gastric cancer (blue))

(c)

Figure 5. (**a**) The average relative abundance of the ten most common bacterial genera of untreated biopsies from dyspepsia patients and gastric cancer patients. Comparison of (**b**) the alpha-diversity shown by a Shannon Index, $p = 0.556831$ and (**c**) the beta-diversity between the two groups shown by PCoA plot, $p = 0.052947$, in biopsies from dyspepsia patients (red) and gastric cancer patients (blue).

A low percentage of the bacterial reads in biopsies from dyspepsia patients were identified as *Lactobacillus* spp. (<0.1% of total bacterial reads). Most biopsy pairs from gastric cancer patients (30 pairs) did not show presence of *Lactobacillus* spp.; 6 biopsy pairs showed a relative abundance of 0–0.5% of total bacterial reads, and 7 biopsy pairs showed a relative abundance of 0.5–2% *Lactobacillus* spp., while three biopsy pairs showed a high relative abundance of *Lactobacillus* spp., which both increased (from 11 to 27%) and decreased (from 23% to 0.4% and from 29% to 5%) between the unwashed and washed biopsies. This difference in *Lactobacillus* spp. abundance was not significant between dyspepsia and gastric cancer patients.

The biopsies from antrum and cancer area of gastric cancer patients showed no significant differences in the distribution of bacterial groups (Figure 6a, Table 6).

The diversity of bacteria in biopsies from antrum and corpus did not show differences in the bacterial diversity within the sample areas (Figure 6b) or between the two sample areas (Figure 6c).

Table 6. Mean and standard error as percentage of the 10 most common bacteria as percentage of total bacterial reads in the microbiome analysis of biopsies from gastric cancer patients (n = 12).

	Antrum Area (% ± SEM)	Cancer Area (% ± SEM)
Helicobacter spp.	14.5 ± 7.3	9.1 ± 4.9
Streptococcus spp.	17.6 ± 5.1	25.1 ± 6.9
Prevotella spp.	7.4 ± 1.6	5.3 ± 1.5
Escherichia spp.	6.1 ± 2.7	12.9 ± 6.6
Veillonella spp.	4.3 ± 1.8	2.7 ± 2.0
Fusobacterium spp.	6.2 ± 2.6	2.1 ± 0.8
Haemophilus spp.	2.2 ± 0.7	2.6 ± 0.9
Rothia spp.	2.8 ± 0.8	1.6 ± 0.5
Neisseria spp.	7.3 ± 4.4	5.6 ± 3.2
Alloprevotella spp.	1.9 ± 1.0	1.5 ± 0.9
Other bacteria	29.6 ± 7.6	34.1 ± 8.8

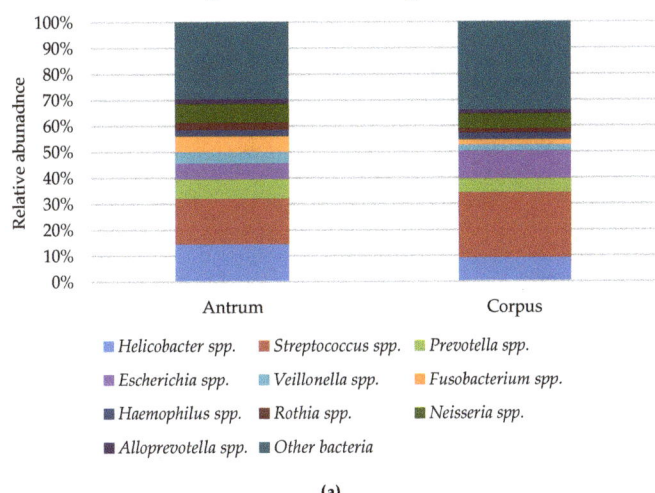

(a)

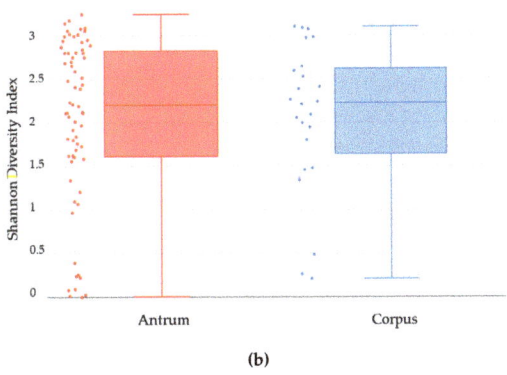

(b)

Figure 6. *Cont.*

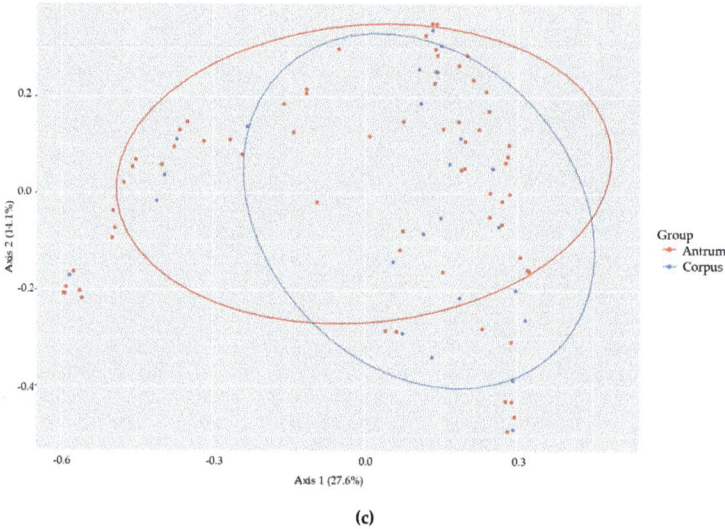

(c)

Figure 6. (a) The relative abundance of bacteria in untreated biopsies from the antrum and corpus area of gastric cancer patients. No significant differences were observed in the distributions of bacteria between the two groups. (Percentages are listed in Table 6). Comparison of (b) the alpha-diversity shown by a Shannon Index, $p = 0.960995$ and (c) the beta-diversity between shown by PCoA plot, $p = 0.111888$, in biopsies from antrum area (red) and corpus area (blue) in the stomach.

3.3. Presence of H. pylori

H. pylori was detected in 14 of 34 patients (41%) by histology. Culture of *H. pylori* was only successful for 4 biopsies from 2 patients, despite incubation for additional days. Microbiome analysis identified DNA from *H. pylori* in 16 of 34 patients (47%), and *H. pylori* was identified as the only species of *Helicobacter* in the biopsies. The difference between culture and 16S rRNA gene amplicon sequencing may be explained by the fastidious nature of *H. pylori*, which may be difficult to culture after storage.

Three different distribution types of *H. pylori* and non-*Helicobacter* were observed; 4 biopsy pairs showed almost complete dominance of *H. pylori* (>90% of total bacterial reads in at least one of the biopsies) (Figure 7a), 16 biopsy pairs showed a mixed relative abundance of *H. pylori* and other bacteria (Figure 7b), and 26 biopsy pairs showed none or less than 1% of total bacterial reads identified as *H. pylori* (Figure 7c).

The biopsies determined positive or negative for *H. pylori* by histology showed significant differences in the bacterial diversity. The *H. pylori*-negative biopsies showed a significantly higher diversity than *H. pylori*-positive biopsies (p-value = 0.004353) (Figure 8a). In addition, a significant difference in the bacterial diversity was observed between biopsies determined positive or negative for *H. pylori* (p-value = 0.0009999), indicating that the presence of *H. pylori* may change the bacterial community to allow for a unique composition (Figure 8b).

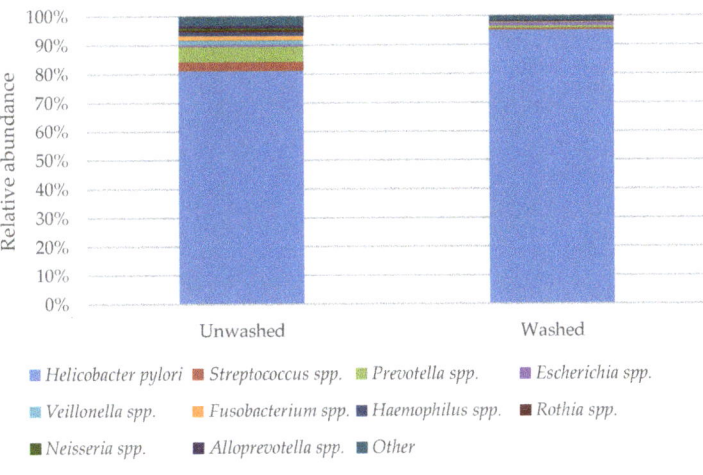

(a)

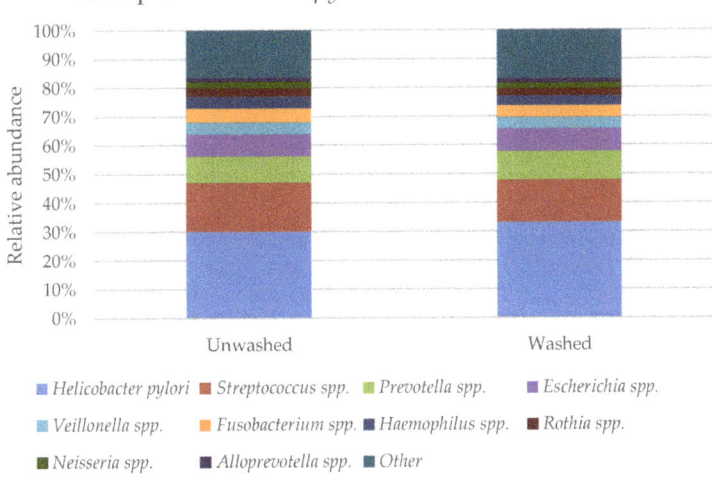

(b)

Figure 7. *Cont.*

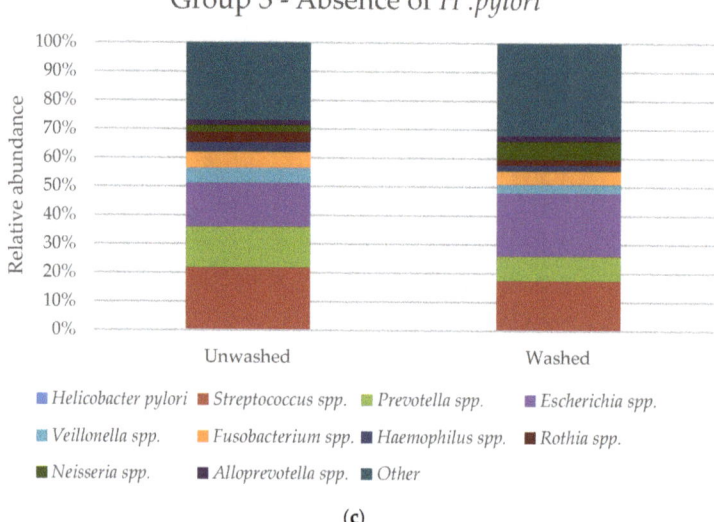

(c)

Figure 7. The average relative abundance divided into three groups based on their distribution of H. pylori and other bacteria by (**a**) dominance of H. pylori, (**b**) mixed presence of non-Helicobacter and H. pylori, and (**c**) absence of H. pylori.

4. Discussion

4.1. Washed Biopsies vs. Unwashed Biopsies

We observed a decreased bacterial growth from the washed biopsies compared to the unwashed biopsies in this study (Figure 2, Table 2). Based on our hypothesis, this might suggest that the bacteria removed by washing were not adhering to the biopsy and should not be considered a part of the gastric microbiota. *Streptococcus* spp. was the most dominant non-*Helicobacter* bacterial group in the biopsies, which may either be attributed to a higher starting concentration in the unwashed biopsy or an increased ability to adhere to the tissue, compared to the other bacteria in the biopsies.

The non-*Helicobacter* species identified in this study have previously been described as commensals of the oral cavity, upper airways and intestinal tract, including species of the dominant groups *Streptococcus*, *Rothia* and *Actinomyces* [11,16,20,21,25]. Intestinal bacteria such as *Enterococcus* spp. and *Escherichia* spp. were also identified with both culture and microbiome analysis and may be a sign of overgrowth from the intestines. Species of *Staphylococcus* were cultured from several biopsies, but the group was not among the 10 most common in the microbiome analysis, where between 0% and 4% of the reads were identified as *Staphylococcus* spp. The high detection in culture compared to microbiome analysis may be explained by selection of growth of *Staphylococcus*, as species of this group are facultative aerobic with a fast growth rate.

Our expectation was that only *H. pylori* would remain in the washed biopsies. This was not the case, as we observed the presence of many bacteria, of which the average relative abundance and diversity within the biopsies did not significantly change in the washed biopsies (Figure 3). This may suggest that some bacterial groups may remain in the biopsies and should be further investigated.

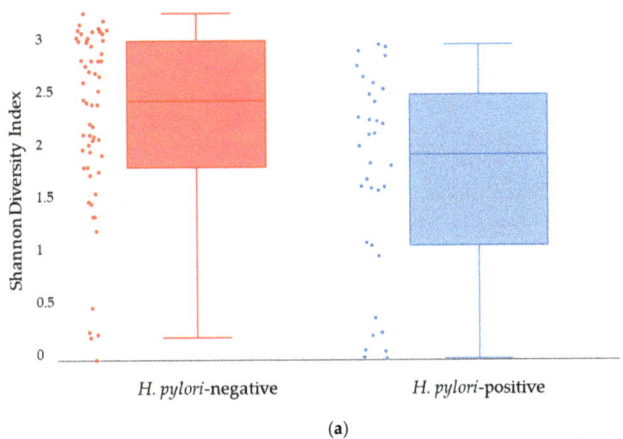

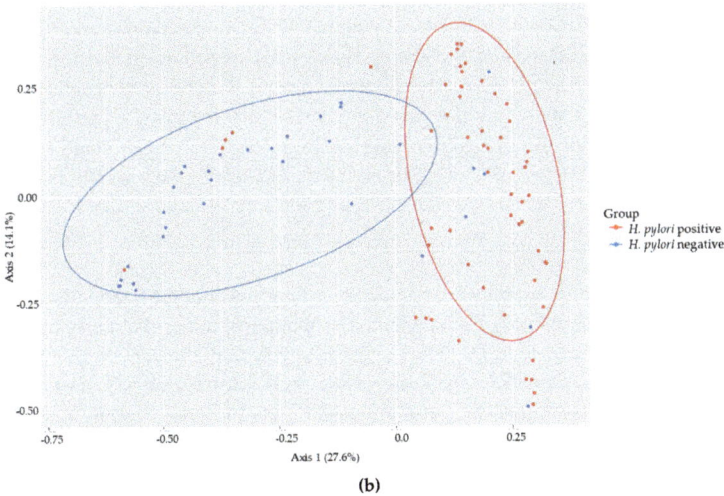

Figure 8. Comparison of the bacterial diversity from biopsies of patients shown negative for *H. pylori* (red) or positive for *H. pylori* (blue). (a) The alpha-diversity shown by a Shannon Index, $p = 0.004353$. (b) The beta-diversity between the two groups shown by PCoA plot, $p = 0.000999.4$.

4.2. Gastric Cancer Patients vs. Dyspepsia Patients

Comparison of the bacterial composition did not reveal significant differences in the bacterial diversity between biopsies from dyspepsia patients or gastric cancer patients. *Lactobacillus* was cultured, and DNA was detected in a higher abundance in biopsies from gastric cancer patients than in biopsies from dyspepsia patients, although not significantly. Development of gastric cancer has been described as a result of dysbiosis, and it is believed that a change in the gastric bacteria towards oral and intestinal bacteria may contribute to this process [19]. However, previous studies have not detected specific bacterial genera in only one of the patient groups [8,19]. It may be discussed if the presence of cancer cells causes alterations in the environment, which leads to changed microbial growth, or if the development is inversed. The increased presence of cultured *Lactobacillus* spp. in gastric cancer patient biopsies may also be an important difference between these patient groups, although the exact function is unknown.

The expected result from this comparison was that a different bacterial composition would be observed in the cancer tissue compared to non-cancer patients, which was not confirmed by our results (Figure 6). To date, no studies have shown a connection between non-*Helicobacter* bacteria and development of pathologies such as gastric cancer in humans [11]. We observed an increased presence of *Lactobacillus* spp. in gastric cancer patient biopsies compared to dyspepsia patient biopsies in both the culture and microbiome analysis but cannot with certainty conclude that this bacterial group is involved in the development of gastric cancer. Four biopsies were positive for culture of *Lactobacillus* spp., where no reads were found in the microbiome analysis. However, 16 biopsies were negative for growth of *Lactobacillus* spp. but positive in the microbiome analysis. 16S rRNA-based analysis is more sensitive, and it is possible to detect the presence of bacteria in small quantities. An explanation for the difference in culture and microbiome results may be that 16S rRNA gene amplicon sequencing is not genus-specific, and as such, the 16S rRNA genes from several bacteria are amplified simultaneously. If *Lactobacillus* spp. are present in small quantities, the presence of a high amount of other DNA may drown it out, and it will not be detected. Combined with a selection in the culture for microaerobic-growing bacteria, the abundance of *Lactobacillus* spp. may appear higher in this experiment setting. This discrepancy between methods should also be considered in future culture- and sequencing-based studies.

A study by Blaser and Atherton discussed whether *H. pylori* is a main driver of gastric cancer development, or if its presence is enough to change the stomach environment and allow for growth of other bacteria, which in turn increase the risk of gastric cancer [28]. The authors agree that long-term colonization causes inflammation and damage to the host tissues but that the mechanism leading to development of gastric cancer is not well defined [28]. In order to fully understand the pathological changes of other non-*Helicobacter* species in the stomach, infection assays should be performed on human cell cultures or model organisms with gastrointestinal tracts more similar to humans.

4.3. Presence of H. pylor in the Biopsies

H. pylori was only cultured from the biopsies of two patients after extended culture, even though its presence in other patients was confirmed by histology and microbiome analysis. Further, microbiome analysis identified *H. pylori* in two biopsies, where the histology result was negative for *H. pylori*. This comparison of methods demonstrates that culture, histology and 16S rRNA gene sequencing are not always in accordance, and investigation of bacterial communities using several methods is preferred. During colonization or prolonged incubation, *H. pylori* take a coccoid form which may be difficult or impossible to culture in vitro [25]. Based on its slow growth and fastidious nature, culture of this species from clinical specimens is expected to be challenging. The culture results are still considered to be valid, as other species were cultivated, and thus, the medium and growth conditions must have been sufficient for bacterial growth. However, in order to culture all the present bacteria in the biopsies, several other medium types and atmospheres might have been considered. The relative distribution of *H. pylori* was expected to increase after wash, along with the removal of contaminating bacteria. This was not always observed (Figure 3). Studies have shown that it is possible to detect *H. pylori* with sensitive DNA-based methods in individuals previously shown negative for *H. pylori* with conventional methods [19]. This may also be the reason why a higher prevalence of *H. pylori* was observed with microbiome analysis compared to histology. The results from microbiome sequencing showed a variable distribution of *H. pylori* and non-*H. pylori* bacteria in the gastric environment. Three overall types of bacterial distribution were observed, suggesting that the stomach is more complex than previously thought (Figure 7). Natural variations in the microbiota caused by the geographical origin of the patients may also be of importance for this. The results from this study contribute to the agreement of a dynamic relationship between *H. pylori* and non-*Helicobacter* bacteria in the stomach, and previous discrepancies between studies may be caused by natural differences between patients. The ten most prevalent groups with microbiome analysis fits with the groups detected in other reported NGS-studies [19].

The biopsies showing positive or negative for *H. pylori* by histology analysis displayed significant differences in the bacterial diversity within and between the groups (Figure 8), suggesting that *H. pylori* may cause changes in the environment to allow for survival of other bacteria as suggested by Blaser and Atherton [28]. Our findings are also in agreement with the study by Maldonado-Contreras, which discovered a difference in the bacterial diversity based on *H. pylori*-status [21]. Patients negative for *H. pylori* presented a higher relative abundance of *Actinobacteria* and *Firmicutes*, whereas *H. pylori*-positive patients presented a higher abundance of *Proteobacteria* and *Acidobacteria*.

The most common bacterial groups identified in the culture and microbiome analysis shows few similarities, and only two genera in the 10 most abundant groups from the microbiome analysis were cultured. However, both *Gemella* and *Granulicatella* were detected in several biopsies but not in high enough reads to be included in the top 10. The difference between the methods may be caused by selection of certain bacteria in the microaerobic incubation. Four of the 10 most common groups have been described as anaerobes or strict anaerobes (*Prevotella*, *Veillonella*, *Fusobacterium*, *Neisseria*), preventing them from growing in the microaerobic environment used in this study. *H. pylori* was detected in 47% of the biopsies by microbiome analysis but only cultured from two biopsy pairs. The biopsies were stored in the transport medium at −80 °C, which might have decreased the viability of *H. pylori*. It may be suggested that other bacteria identified by microbiome analysis were also present in the biopsies but were inhibited by the storage/freezing, and therefore unable to be cultured.

4.4. Limitations

It has been described that 80% of the bacteria that are identified with molecular methods in the human gut cannot successfully be cultured in vitro [16]. As we only cultured the biopsies in microaerobic environment, growth was selected for the microaerobically growing bacteria. The presence of these appeared higher than with microbiome sequencing. Several types of growth conditions and culture media would be required to select growth for all bacteria present in the biopsy.

Culture-independent methods such as 16S rRNA gene amplicon sequencing or microbiome analysis may provide detailed information about the bacterial composition. One disadvantage may be that it does not differentiate between live and dead bacteria and between residents and contamination [2,10,19]. Other methods with the ability to distinguish between active and inactive bacteria, such as immunostaining or analysis of the metabolic activity, may also be considered for future investigations [22].

The results of this study are new as both culturing and sequencing are included as methods of detection, and the effect of washing or presence of *H. pylori* on the bacterial composition and diversity are investigated. Our results showed a decrease in the growth of some bacterial groups from washed biopsies, which are also known oral commensal bacteria. The species that remain in the tissue after wash must thus contain mechanisms for adhesion to avoid being removed.

We present the first comprehensive paper attempting to distinguish between transient and resident bacteria in the stomach using a 16S rRNA gene amplicon sequencing approach and washing of biopsies. One other study has investigated the bacterial content of biopsies with a similar approach [14]. However, the study included only a small number of samples and used a taxon-specific quantitative PCR to define the taxa [14]. Future investigations in gastric microbiota should consider the presence of other bacteria in the stomach that may only be a transient contamination.

5. Conclusions

In conclusion, the number of cultured non-*Helicobacter* bacteria decreased in the washed biopsies, suggesting that they might be a transient contamination from oral cavity; however, in the microbiome analysis, no significant differences in the bacterial diversity were observed between unwashed and washed biopsies. The bacterial diversity in biopsies that were *H. pylori*-positive and *H. pylori*-negative was significantly different, implying that *H. pylori* is the major modulator of gastric microbiome. Further large-scale studies are required to investigate the transient and persistent gastric microbiota. This may include an increased number of samples, investigation of dysbiosis, a wider range of culture conditions and growth media, metatranscriptomic analysis, immunological assays or additional treatment of biopsies.

Author Contributions: Conceptualization, J.K., L.K. and L.P.A.; methodology, J.K., L.K. and L.P.A.; validation, M.R.S., T.B.J., T.H.F., K.F. and L.P.A.; formal analysis, M.R.S., T.B.J. and K.F.; investigation, M.R.S., M.U., J.S. and L.J.; resources, J.K., J.S., K.F. and L.P.A.; data curation, M.R.S., T.B.J. and M.U.; writing—original draft preparation, M.R.S.; writing—review and editing, M.R.S., J.K. and L.P.A.; visualization, M.R.S., T.B.J. and K.F.; supervision, J.K., K.F., L.K. and L.P.A.; project administration, J.K.; funding acquisition, J.K. and L.K. All authors have read and agreed to the published version of the manuscript.

Funding: The collection and processing of samples in Lithuania was funded by Lithuanian Research Council under the grant No. APP-2/2016.

Acknowledgments: The authors would like to acknowledge Justina Arstikyte for excellent work in the lab.

Conflicts of Interest: The authors declare no conflict of interest. The funders had no role in the design of the study; in the collection, analyses or interpretation of data; in the writing of the manuscript or in the decision to publish the results.

References

1. Dewhirst, F.E.; Fox, J.G.; On, S.L.W. Recommended minimal standards for Helicobacter. *Int. J. Syst. Evol. Microbiol.* **2000**, *50*, 2231–2237. [CrossRef]
2. Bik, E.M.; Eckburg, P.B.; Gill, S.R.; Nelson, K.E.; Purdom, E.A.; Francois, F.; Peres-Perez, G.; Blaser, M.J.; Relman, D.A. Molecular analysis of the bacterial microbiota in the human stomach. *Proc. Natl. Acad. Sci. USA* **2006**, *103*, 732–737. [CrossRef]
3. Nardone, G.; Compare, D. The human gastric microbiota: Is it time to rethink the pathogenesis of stomach diseases? *United Eur. Gastroenterol. J.* **2015**, *3*, 255–260. [CrossRef] [PubMed]
4. Llorca, L.; Perez-Perez, G.; Urruzuno, P.; Martinez, M.J.; Iizumi, T.; Gao, Z.; Sohn, J.; Chung, J.; Cox, L.; Simón-Soro, A.; et al. Characterization of the Gastric Microbiota in a Pediatric Population According to Helicobacter Pylori Status. *Pediatri. Infect. Dis. J.* **2017**, *36*, 173–178. [CrossRef] [PubMed]
5. Jonaitis, L.; Pellicano, R.; Kupcinskas, L. *Helicobacter pylori* and nonmalignant upper gastrointestinal diseases. *Helicobacter* **2018**, *23* (Suppl. 1), e12522. [CrossRef]
6. Pérez-Pérez, G.I.; Sack, R.B.; Reid, R.; Reid, R.; Santosham, M.; Croll, J.; Blaser, M.J. Transient and Persistent *Helicobacter pylori* Colonization in Native American Children. *J. Clin. Microbiol.* **2003**, *41*, 2401–2407. [CrossRef] [PubMed]
7. Li, J.; Perez, G.I.P. Is There a Role for the Non-*Helicobacter pylori* Bacteria in the Risk of Developing Gastric Cancer? *Int. J. Mol. Sci.* **2018**, *19*, 1353. [CrossRef]
8. Cover, T.L.; Blaser, M.J. *Helicobacter pylori* in health and disease. *Gastroenterology* **2009**, *136*, 1863–1873. [CrossRef]
9. Smet, A.; Flahou, B.; Mukhopadhya, I.; Ducatelle, R.; Pasmans, F.; Haseobrouck, F.; Hold, G.L. The Other Helicobacters. *Helicobacter* **2011**, *16*, 70–75. [CrossRef]
10. Solnick, J.V.; Schauer, D.B. Emergence of Diverse *Helicobacter* Species in the Pathogenesis of Gastric and Enterohepatic Diseases. *Clin. Microbiol. Rev.* **2001**, *14*, 59–97. [CrossRef]
11. O'Hara, A.M.; Shanahan, F. The gut flora as a forgotten organ. *EMBO Rep.* **2006**, *7*, 688–693. [CrossRef] [PubMed]
12. Ianiro, G.; Molina-Infante, J.; Gasbarrini, A. Gastric Microbiota. *Helicobacter* **2015**, *20*, 68–71. [CrossRef] [PubMed]
13. Engstrand, L.; Lindberg, M. *Helicobacter pylori* and the gastric microbiota. *Best Pract. Res. Clin. Gastroenterol.* **2013**, *27*, 39–45. [CrossRef] [PubMed]
14. Li, X.X.; Wong, G.L.H.; To, K.F.; Wong, V.W.S.; Lai, L.H.; Chow, D.K.; Lau, J.Y.W.; Sung, J.J.Y.; Ding, C. Bacterial microbiota profiling in gastritis without *Helicobacter pylori* infection or non-steroidal anti-inflammatory drug use. *PLoS ONE* **2009**, *4*, e7985. [CrossRef]

15. Sanduleanu, S.; Jonkers, D.; Bruine ADe Hameeteman, W.; Stockbrügger, R.W. Non-*Helicobacter pylori* bacterial flora during acid-suppressive therapy: Differential findings in gastric juice and gastric mucosa. *Aliment. Pharmacol. Ther.* **2001**, *15*, 379–388. [CrossRef]
16. Rajilic-Stojanovic, M.; Figueiredo, C.; Smet, A.; Hansen, R.; Kupcinskas, J.; Rokkas, T.; Andersen, L.; Machado, J.; Ianiro, G.; Gasbarrini, A.; et al. Systematic review: Gastric microbiota in health and disease. *Aliment. Pharmacol. Ther.* **2020**, *51*, 582–602. [CrossRef]
17. Schulz, C.; Schütte, K.; Malfertheiner, P. *Helicobacter pylori* and Other Gastric Microbiota in Gastroduodenal Pathologies. *Dig. Dis.* **2016**, *34*, 210–216. [CrossRef]
18. Zilberstein, B.; Quintanilha, A.G.; Santos, M.A.A.; Pajecki, D.; Moura, E.G.; Alves, P.R.A.; Filho, F.M.; Souza, J.A.U.; Gama-Rodriguez, J. Digestive tract microbiota in healthy volunteers. *Clinics* **2007**, *62*, 47–54. [CrossRef]
19. Delgado, S.; Cabrera-Rubio, R.; Mira, A.; Suarez, A.; Mayo, B. Microbiological Survey of the Human Gastric Ecosystem Using Culturing and Pyrosequencing Methods. *Microb. Ecol.* **2013**, *65*, 763–772. [CrossRef]
20. Dicksved, J.; Lindberg, M.; Rosenquist, M.; Enroth, H.; Jansson, J.K.; Engstrand, L. Molecular characterization of the stomach microbiota in patients with gastric cancer and in controls. *J. Med. Microbiol.* **2009**, *58*, 509–516. [CrossRef]
21. Maldonado-Contreras, A.; Goldfarb, K.C.; Godoy-Vitorino, F.; Karaoz, U.; Contreras, M.; Blaser, M.J.; Brodie, E.L.; Dominguez-Bello, M.G. Structure of the human gastric bacterial community in relation to *Helicobacter pylori* status. *ISME J.* **2011**, *5*, 574–579. [CrossRef]
22. Yu, G.; Torres, J.; Hu, N.; Medrano-Guzman, R.; Herrera-Goepfert, R.; Humphrys, M.S.; Wang, L.; Wang, C.; Ding, T.; Ravel, J.; et al. Molecular Characterization of the Human Stomach Microbiota in Gastric Cancer Patients. *Front. Cell. Infect. Microbiol.* 2017. [CrossRef] [PubMed]
23. Andersson, A.F.; Lindberg, M.; Jakobsson, H.; Bäckhed, F.; Nyrén, P.; Engstrand, L. Comparative analysis of human gut microbiota by barcoded pyrosequencing. *PLoS ONE* **2008**, *3*. [CrossRef]
24. Monstein, È.R.G.; Tiveljung, A.; Kraft, C.H.; Borch, K.Å.; Jonasson, J. Profiling of bacterial flora in gastric biopsies from patients with *Helicobacter pylori*-associated gastritis and histologically normal control individuals by temperature gradient gel electrophoresis and 16S rDNA sequence analysis. *J. Med. Microbiol.* **2000**, *49*, 817–822. [CrossRef]
25. Lofgren, J.L.; Whary, M.T.; Ge, Z.; Muthupalani, S.; Taylor, N.S.; Mobley, M.; Potter, A.; Varro, A.; Eiback, D.; Suerbaum, S.; et al. Lack of Commensal Flora in *Helicobacter pylori*—Infected INS-GAS Mice Reduces Gastritis and Delays Intraepithelial Neoplasia. *Gastroenterology* **2011**, *140*, 210–220. [CrossRef]
26. Abreu, M.T.; Peek, R.M. Gastrointestinal Malignancy and the Microbiome. *Gastroenterology* **2014**, *146*, 1534–1546. [CrossRef]
27. Amieva, M.; Peek, R.M. Pathobiology of *Helicobacter pylori*-induced Gastric Cancer. *Gastroenterology* **2016**, *150*, 64–78. [CrossRef]
28. Blaser, M.J.; Atherton, J.C. *Helicobacter pylori* persistence: Biology and disease. *J. Clin. Investig.* **2004**, *113*, 321–333. [CrossRef]
29. Ferreira, R.M.; Pereira-Marques, J.; Pinto-Ribeiro, I.; Costa, J.L.; Carneiro, F.; Machado, J.C.; Figueiredo, C. Gastric microbial community profiling reveals a dysbiotic cancer-associated microbiota. *Gut* **2018**, *67*, 226–236. [CrossRef]
30. Marchesi, J.R.; Ravel, J. The vocabulary of microbiome research: A proposal. *Microbiome* **2015**, *3*, 31. [CrossRef]
31. Mcdonald, J.E.; Larsen, N.; Pennington, A.; Connoly, J.; Wallis, C.; Rooks, D.J.; Hall, N.; McCarthy, A.J.; Allosin, H.E. Characterising the Canine Oral Microbiome by Direct Sequencing of Reverse-Transcribed rRNA Molecules. *PLoS ONE* **2016**, *11*, e0157046. [CrossRef] [PubMed]
32. Ring, H.C.; Thorsen, J.; Saunte, D.M.; Lilje, B.; Bay, L.; Riis, P.T.; Larsen, N.; Andersen, L.O.; Nielsen, H.V.; Miller, I.M.; et al. The Follicular Skin Microbiome in Patients With Hidradenitis Suppurativa and Healthy Controls. *JAMA Dermatol.* **2017**, *153*, 897–905. [CrossRef] [PubMed]

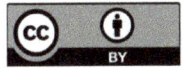

© 2020 by the authors. Licensee MDPI, Basel, Switzerland. This article is an open access article distributed under the terms and conditions of the Creative Commons Attribution (CC BY) license (http://creativecommons.org/licenses/by/4.0/).

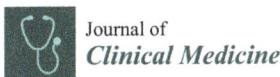
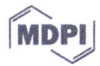

Review

Pancreatic Diseases and Microbiota: A Literature Review and Future Perspectives

Marcantonio Gesualdo, Felice Rizzi *, Silvia Bonetto, Stefano Rizza, Federico Cravero, Giorgio Maria Saracco and Claudio Giovanni De Angelis *

Gastroenterology and Digestive Endoscopy Unit, AOU Città della Salute e della Scienza, University of Turin, 10126 Turin, Italy; marcantonio.gesualdo@gmail.com (M.G.); silvia.bonetto@edu.unito.it (S.B.); stefanorizza@live.it (S.R.); fed.cravero@gmail.com (F.C.); giorgiomaria.saracco@unito.it (G.M.S.)
* Correspondence: rizzifelice91@libero.it (F.R.); eusdeang@hotmail.com (C.G.D.A.)

Received: 13 October 2020; Accepted: 30 October 2020; Published: 1 November 2020

Abstract: Gut microbiota represent an interesting worldwide research area. Several studies confirm that microbiota has a key role in human diseases, both intestinal (such as inflammatory bowel disease, celiac disease, intestinal infectious diseases, irritable bowel syndrome) and extra intestinal disorders (such as autism, multiple sclerosis, rheumatologic diseases). Nowadays, it is possible to manipulate microbiota by administering prebiotics, probiotics or synbiotics, through fecal microbiota transplantation in selected cases. In this scenario, pancreatic disorders might be influenced by gut microbiota and this relationship could be an innovative and inspiring field of research. However, data are still scarce and controversial. Microbiota manipulation could represent an important therapeutic strategy in the pancreatic diseases, in addition to standard therapies. In this review, we analyze current knowledge about correlation between gut microbiota and pancreatic diseases, by discussing on the one hand existing data and on the other hand future possible perspectives.

Keywords: pancreatic diseases; microbiota; microbiome; gut microbiota; acute pancreatitis; chronic pancreatitis; diabetes mellitus; pancreatic ductal adenocarcinoma; pancreatic cystic neoplasms

1. Introduction

The human gastrointestinal (GI) tract is colonized by a rich microbial community consisting of more than 10^{14} microorganisms, defining microbiota, and more than 5,000,000 genes defining microbiome [1,2]. The microbiota is composed of bacteria, viruses and yeasts [3]. In healthy conditions, these microorganisms colonize mucosal surfaces, particularly the large intestine, and talk closely with them; in this way they regulate important physiological functions [4,5]. First, they are involved in metabolism of nutrients and drugs and vitamin production [6]. Then, through food fermentation, bacteria produce some short-chain fatty acids (SCFAs), for example butyrate, which have trophic effects on the GI epithelium [7]. Furthermore, gut microbiota influences the immune system through its antigenic effects. The interaction between gut microbiota, intestinal epithelial cells and the mucosal immune system creates an environment that prevents overgrowth of the host pathogenic microorganisms [8] and limits the colonization of the intestinal tract by foreign pathogens [9–11].

In healthy people gut microbiota is characterized by richness in microorganisms and high diversity of species. This situation is called *eubiosis*. In this microenvironment, bacteria are predominant and represent the main group of microorganisms that are strictly anaerobics and extremophiles. *Firmicutes* and *Bacteroidetes* represent the main bacterial phyla, up to 85–90% of total microorganisms, while *Actinobacteria* and *Proteobacteria* are less plentiful, representing up to 10% [12].

In this condition, commensal bacterial species are predominant compared to pathological ones.

Conversely, when this ecosystem balance is perturbed (i.e., by use of antibiotics, motility disorders, diet, host genetic features, etc.) [3], there is a condition called *dysbiosis*, characterized by a lowering in diversity of bacterial species, with abundance of pathogenic ones, and a loss of microbiome physiological functions [13,14]. In some cases, in this dysbiotic environment, there is a reduction of tight junctions between enterocytes, leading to a compromised function of mucosal barrier integrity; this alteration, named leaky gut, sometimes allows bacterial translocation and plays a key role in the development of GI and systemic diseases [11,15].

The composition of gut microbiota may be strongly influenced by both pathological conditions and environmental factors, such as age, diet, drugs, stress [16]. Besides, the abundance and the variety of different species within an individual microbial system (i.e., a single sample) is called α-diversity, while β-diversity refers to differences between microbial communities from different environments (i.e., different samples or different individuals) [17].

In clinical practice, we may manipulate microbiota by administering prebiotics, probiotics or synbiotics, through fecal microbiota transplantation (FMT). Prebiotics are defined as "a substrate that is selectively utilized by host microorganisms conferring a health benefit" [18]; the main prebiotics that have healthy benefits are non-digestible fructooligosaccharides (FOS) and galactans (GOS), preferentially metabolized by *Bifidobacterium* spp. Other examples of prebiotics are polyunsaturated fatty acids (PUFAs) and inulin [19]. Intestinal microorganisms can readily utilize prebiotics, transforming them in metabolic products, such as SCFAs, i.e., propionate, butyrate, acetate. These products are crucial for correct intestinal health. Prebiotics are now largely used in clinical practice for treating many diseases, such as inflammatory bowel disease (IBD) [20], irritable bowel syndrome (IBS) [21], metabolic syndrome [22]. Conversely, probiotics are defined as "live microorganisms that confer a health benefit on the host" [23]. Probiotic foods contain safe live microbes with sufficient evidence for a general beneficial effect in mammals [24]. Synbiotics are a mixed product with a combination of probiotics and prebiotics. Finally, FMT consists of "the infusion of faecal samples from a healthy donor to the GI tract of a recipient patient, in order to cure a specific disease, improving alteration of gut microbiota" [25]. To date, the only indication to perform FMT is the recurrent and refractory (non-responder to conventional antibiotics, i.e., vancomycin, fidaxomicin or metronidazole) *Clostridium difficile* infection with an efficiency rate standing at more than 80–85% [25].

Due to these novelties, microbiota is now a worldwide field of interest and investigations are growing in the recent years. Several studies analyzed the involvement of intestinal dysbiosis in the development of intestinal and extra-intestinal diseases, such as IBD [26], celiac disease [27], IBS [28], multiple sclerosis [29], rheumatologic diseases [30], Alzheimer's disease [31], colorectal and gastric cancer [32]. On the contrary, data about correlation between microbiota and pancreatic diseases are still scarce and controversial.

Few studies described the presence of bacteria in pancreatic tissue; they found bacteria in pancreatic ducts of subjects with chronic pancreatitis or in pancreatic tissue of pancreatic cancer patients. Instead, recently, some authors analyzed microbiome in pancreatic samples and duodenal tissues from patients underwent pancreatectomy, finding a similar bacterial DNA profiles; this may suggest a bacterial translocation from the gut into the pancreas [33]. Due to the impossibility to collect pancreatic tissues routinely, a lot of studies analyzed gut microbiome from fecal samples.

In this review, we analyze the actual available data in literature about microbiota and pancreas in health and disease.

2. Methods

A literature search was performed in PubMed, Scopus, Web of Science, Cochrane Library databases and Embase. The search included papers published from 1 January 1993 to 1 March 2020. Only English studies were considered. All authors participated in the search process and in the critical analysis of selected publications. Keywords used were: "microbiota", "pancreas", "acute pancreatitis", "chronic pancreatitis", "pancreatic cystic neoplasms", "pancreatic ductal adenocarcinoma", "diabetes mellitus", "neuroendocrine tumors", "probiotic", "prebiotic", "synbiotic".

3. Microbiota in Healthy Pancreas

Recently, the pancreatic physiological functions have been shown to have an impact on intestinal microbiota and vice versa [34], by a cross-talking system, in health and disease; hence, it could be possible to talk about "microbiota-pancreas axis" [35].

In an important study, Sun et al. [36] demonstrated that pancreatic β-cells, in mice, produced cathelicidin-related antimicrobial peptide (CRAMP), a protein with antimicrobial activity through bacterial membrane permeabilization [37,38]. They noticed that pancreatic CRAMP expression was induced by SCFAs derived from the gut microbiota, underling the cross-talking system. In a recent study, Ahuja et al. [39] used a mice model with pancreatic acinar cell–specific deletion of Orai1, a Ca^{2+} channel necessary for exocytosis of pancreatic antimicrobials. They found that Orai1-deficient mice showed an altered intestinal microbiota with bacterial overgrowth. In particular, *Proteobacteria* were two-fold increased, including increases in *Succinivibrionaceae* and *Enterobacteriaceae*, and *Prevotella* spp. The authors did not find differences on expression of intestinal antimicrobials in Orai1-deficient mice, proving the role of the pancreas in control of intestinal microbiota. Moreover, Orai1-deficient mice developed spontaneous intestinal inflammation characterized by intestinal CD3+ T-cell infiltration and died after three weeks. This data could be translated on humans, because patients that carry ORAI1 nonsense mutations have susceptibility to GI infection and diarrhea [40]. In an American cohort of patients who underwent a pancreaticoduodenectomy, Rogers et al., studied fecal microbiota composition compared to a group of healthy individuals. Interestingly, surgical patients exhibited fecal dysbiosis and showed an increase in *Klebsiella* and *Bacteroides*, while anaerobic taxa (i.e., *Faecalibacterium prausnitzii* and *Roseburia* species) decreased [41]. After DCP there are several anatomical alterations apart from the pancreatectomy (i.e., partial gastrectomy, the biliary-digestive anastomosis). In this scenario, also the gastric juice changes its composition. These data suggest that both pancreatic and gastric juice, with their antimicrobial activity, are able to modify gut microbiome.

4. Microbiota in Pancreatic Diseases

4.1. Microbiota and Acute Pancreatitis

Acute pancreatitis is caused by gallstones or acute alcoholic intake in the majority of cases. Rare causes of pancreatitis are hypertriglyceridemia, hypercalcemia, genetic causes, smoking, viruses such as cytomegalovirus or herpes simplex virus [42]. The main therapy for acute pancreatitis is early fluid resuscitation; the latter plays a key role by improving the tissue oxygenation and the microcirculation perfusion in order to preserve on the one hand pancreatic function (avoiding further pancreatic necrosis), and on the other hand, renal, cardiac and intestinal perfusion [43,44]. The use of antibiotics is not recommended routinely in severe acute pancreatitis (SAP), but only in the presence of infection, as cholangitis associated to biliary pancreatitis, and suspicion of pancreatic necrosis. In AISP (the Italian Association for the Study of the Pancreas) guidelines [45], the routine use of probiotics is not recommended. Besides, the use of probiotics in clinical practice is not cited in the recent American guidelines addressing the management of pancreatic necrosis [42].

Acute pancreatitis determines hypovolemia that induces splanchnic vasoconstriction to preserve vital organs. Sometimes, this situation favors leaky gut. Indeed, high intestinal permeability promotes bacterial translocation and endotoxemia, with increased risk of infection of necrotic tissues [46]. Moreover, small intestinal bacterial overgrowth (SIBO) and bacterial translocation may be responsible for the majority of the pancreatic complications, but evidences are still scarce. Capurso et al. [44] showed that intestinal ischemia damages gut barrier with bacterial translocation, endotoxemia and rarely multi-organ dysfunction syndrome.

Tan et al. analyzed differences in microbiome in patients with mild acute pancreatitis and SAP and a control group [47] (Table 2). They found fecal dysbiosis characterized by an increase in *Enterococcus* species and a decrease in *Bifidobacterium* species in SAP, when compared with other patients with mild form and control group. These data were in line with other studies [48].

In a recent case control study, Zhang et al. [49] found that fecal samples from 45 patients with acute pancreatitis contained fewer *Actinobacteria* and *Firmicutes* and more *Bacteroidetes* and *Proteobacteria* than those from 44 healthy controls.

The first randomized controlled trial (RCT), assessing the usefulness of probiotics on clinical outcomes of acute pancreatitis (AP), was conducted by Olah et al., in 2002 in Hungary [50] (Table 1).

The results were encouraging. Forty-five patients were recruited, 22 of them received *Lactobacillus plantarum* (*LP*) 299 with a substrate of oat fiber for 1 week by nasojejunal tube; instead, 23 patients were treated with a similar product with *Lactobacillus* inactivated by heat. Only one patient in the first group had pancreatic necrosis versus seven patients in the control group. Similar data was published by Qin et al. [48]. The authors enrolled 74 patients with AP and divided them into two groups: the first was treated with classical parenteral nutrition and the other was treated with enteral feeding and probiotics, containing living *LP*, administered through a nasojejunal tube. Analyzing fecal samples, they found that the second group was colonized with lower number of pathogenic organisms than the first one; besides, the first group had increased permeability with an increase of *Enteroccoccus* spp. and a reduction in *Lactobacteria* and *Bifidobacteria*. Thus, *LP* enteral feeding induced beneficial effects on maintaining the integrity of intestinal mucosal barrier and reducing the risk of septic complications. Olah et al., in 2007, published another RCT [51] with a new synbiotic composition, named "Synbiotic 2000", in the treatment of patients with AP. Sixty-two patients were randomized to probiotics plus prebiotics treatments or to prebiotics treatment alone. Patients in the first group had less complications (i.e., systemic inflammatory response, multiorgan failure) than the control group, but the difference was not statistically significant. In the multi-center, nationwide, double blind placebo-controlled clinical trial called PROPATRIA study [52], 298 patients were enrolled. The probiotic group was treated with *Ecologic 641*, administered twice daily by nasojejunal feeding. It consisted of six strains of microorganisms (four types of *Lactobacilli* and two of *Bifidobacteria*). Instead, the control group received placebo. The authors found [53] that there was no difference in the risk of infections between patients treated with probiotics and the control group (30% versus 28%). However, the data were dramatically different concerning mortality. Indeed, 24 of 152 patients treated with probiotics (16%) died versus 9 of 144 (6%) in the placebo group. In particular, a high risk of mesenteric ischemia was seen in the probiotic group versus the control group. However, Bongaerts et al., made a reassessment of this study eight years later, analyzing the weak points of PROPATRIA trial [54]. One of them was the latency time in the first administration of probiotics; indeed, some patients were treated 24 h after onset of symptoms. Furthermore, there were errors in randomization; in fact, onset of multi-organ failure was already present during admission in more patients in the first group than in the placebo group (41 patients versus 23 patients).

Finally, they suggested, that future studies should evaluate the usefulness of high dose of probiotics, but caution is mandatory to prevent bacterial overgrowth.

Gou et al., in a meta-analysis published in 2014 [55], asserted that probiotics showed neither adverse nor beneficial effects on the clinical conditions of patients with SAP. However, they highlighted a significant heterogeneity in the studies of clinical outcomes. However, they highlighted a significant heterogeneity in the studies of clinical outcomes.

Currently, data are not sufficient to draw a conclusion regarding the effects of probiotics on patients with SAP, since they are controversial and heterogeneous. Future studies should improve the study designs, for example, detecting a peculiar strain of microorganisms (i.e., the type of probiotic), the correct dose of probiotics, or by a standardization of treatment duration.

4.2. Microbiota and Chronic Pancreatitis

Chronic pancreatitis (CP) is a persistent disease characterized by chronic inflammation of the gland with typical findings, such as Wirsung dilatation, intraparenchymal calcifications, gland atrophy, and development of fibrosis [56]. Chronic pancreatitis leads to progressive endocrine and exocrine dysfunction. Data suggest that patients with CP display dysbiosis with growth of pathogenic bacteria. This situation is related to the reduction of antimicrobial peptides in the pancreatic juice [57]. Capurso et al. analyzed by a systematic review and meta-analysis the relationship between SIBO and CP [58]. The authors proved that about 36% (range between 14–92%) of CP patients are affected by SIBO, detected by a glucose or lactulose hydrogen breath test. However, because of high heterogeneity in the results, the relationship is unclear, and further research is needed.

Pancreatic enzyme replacement therapy (PERT) is able to alleviate exocrine pancreatic insufficiency (PEI) related symptoms, helping fat absorption and improving nutritional status of patients [59]. On the other hand, some authors hypothesize that PERT could directly modify gut microbiota, but the mechanism is still unknown. In the study by Nishiyama et al. [60], the authors evaluated the gut microbiota from fecal samples in mice treated with PERT versus controls. Their findings supported the hypothesis that PERT alleviates PEI-associated symptoms by ameliorating digestive activity and by changing the composition of gut microbiota. In particular they found a relative abundance of *Akkermansia muciniphila* and *Latobacillus reuteri* in mice treated with PERT.

In fact, researchers found a relative abundance of two types of microorganisms in fecal samples from pancrelipase-treated mice compared with controls, i.e., *Akkermansia muciniphila* and *Lactobacillus reuteri*. In particular, the first one, found 58-fold higher in the PERT group, is known to enhance intestinal barrier function by promoting mucus thickness and tight junction protein expression reducing the leaky gut [61]; so, this study suggests that PERT may help to maintain *eubiosis*.

Recent studies highlighted the involvement of immune responses against intestinal microbiota in the development of CP [62]. For example, the activation of pattern recognition receptors (PRRs), i.e., toll-like receptors (TLR) and nucleotide-binding oligomerization-like (NOD) receptors that detect pathogen-associated molecular patterns (PAMPs) derived from the intestinal microbiota have been reported to play a critical role in the development of experimental CP [63].

Proton-pump inhibitors (PPI) are not recommended in patients with CP, but in refractory steatorrhea they could be helpful. In fact, patients with severe forms of inflammation can have lower bicarbonate secretion that cannot neutralize the acidity in the duodenum [64].

In a randomized, controlled, double-blinded trial, dos Santos et al., used synbiotics for changing intestinal microenvironment of patients with CP [65]. Synbiotics was composed of 12 g/day of *Lactobacillus casei, Lactobacillus rhamnosus, Lactobacillus acidophilus, Bifidobacterium bifidum* and FOS, and was administered to the intervention group; instead, 12 g/day of medium absorption complex carbohydrate was administered to the control group. The authors found that synbiotics improved clinical and laboratory outcomes in patients with CP. Dylag et al. [66] found that synbiotics may help restoration of the gut microbiota through the fermentation of FOS and the consequent increase in *Bifidobacteria* and the reduction in pathogenic bacteria. The use of prebiotics and synbiotics in patients with CP promotes a reduction in intestinal stool frequency [65], but their clinical relevance role warrants additional investigation.

Collectively, these promising results suggest that manipulation of microbiota, due to low cost and high manageability, may represent a new therapeutic frontier in CP.

Table 1. Randomized clinical trial about the use of probiotics, prebiotics or synbiotics in acute and chronic pancreatitis.

Author, Year, [Ref]	Type of Study	Disease	Patients	Results	Conclusions
1. Olah, 2002, [50]	Randomized clinical trial	Acute pancreatitis (AP)	45 patients with AP: 22 patients with live *Lactobacillus plantarum* (LP) 299 for 1 week by nasojejunal tube 23 with heat-killed LP299	Infected pancreatic necrosis in 1/22 patient in the treatment group vs. 7/23 in the control group ($p = 0.023$)	Number of surgical treatments and pancreatic sepsis could be reduced by Supplementary live LP 299
2. Olah, 2007, [51]	Prospective, randomized, double-blind study	Severe acute pancreatitis (SAP)	62 patients with SAP: 33 patients received four different Lactobacilli preparations + prebiotics by nasojejunal feeding 29 patients received only prebiotics	SIRS and MOF in 8/33 in the first group vs. 14/29 in the second group ($p < 0.05$) Total complications were higher in the second group compared to the first group ($p < 0.05$) Lower rate of organ failure in the first (3.0%) vs. the control group (17.2%)	Early nasojejunal feeding with synbiotics could prevent organ dysfunctions in SAP
3. Qin, 2008, [48]	Prospective, randomized, single-blinded study	AP	74 patients with AP: 36 patients treated with LP enteral feeding (n = 36) 38 patients treated with parenteral nutrition (PN) group	38.9% patients in enteral feeding group were colonized with multiple organisms vs. 73.7% in the PN group ($p < 0.01$) 30.6% patients in the enteral feeding group were colonized with pathogenic organisms vs. 50% patients in PN group ($p < 0.05$)	Disease severity could be reduced by enteral feeding with LP with better clinical outcomes
4. Besselink MG, 2008, [53]	Multicenter, randomized, double-blind, placebo-controlled trial	SAP	296 patients with predicted SAP: 152 patients treated with a multispecies probiotic formulation 144 patients with placebo	Infectious complications in 46/152 patients (30%) in probiotic group vs. 41/144 (28%) in placebo group (RR 1.06; 95% CI 0.75–1.51) 24/152 patients (16%) in first group died versus 9/144 (6%) in placebo group (RR 2.53; 95% CI 1.22–5.25)	Probiotic did not reduce the risk of infectious complications in SAP. Even, probiotics were associated with an increased risk of mortality
5. Gou, 2014, [55]	Systematic review and meta-analysis of randomized controlled trials	SAP	6 trials with an aggregate total of 536 patients	Probiotics did not impact the pancreatic infection rate (RR = 1.19, 95% CI 0.74–1.93; $p = 0.47$), total infections (RR = 1.09; 95% CI 0.80–1.48; $p = 0.57$), operation rate (RR = 1.42, 95% CI = 0.43 to 3.47; $p = 0.71$) and mortality (RR 0.72; 95% CI = 0.42–1.45; $p = 0.25$).	Clinical outcomes of patients with SAP were not modified by probiotics
6. dos Santos, 2017, [65]	Prospective, randomized, controlled, double blind trial	Chronic pancreatitis (CP)	60 patients with chronic pancreatitis: synbiotics administered to the intervention group 12 g/day of maltodextrin (medium absorption complex carbohydrate) to the control group	Important reduction of bowel frequency in treatment group: Average bowel frequency before treatment: 2.33 ($p < 0.153$) 2nd month of treatment: 1.47 ($p = 0.002$) 3rd month: 1.37 ($p = 0.012$) No change in bowel frequency in the control group ($p = 0.157$)	Clinical outcomes of patients with CP could be ameliorated by synbiotics

4.3. Microbiota and Autoimmune Pancreatitis

Autoimmune pancreatitis (AIP), described for the first time in 1995, is a rare fibro-inflammatory form of CP with typical imaging and histological findings, caused by autoimmune abnormality [67,68]. There are two subtypes of AIP: type 1 and type 2. Type 1 is the pancreatic manifestation of a systemic Immunoglobulin G4–related disease (IgG4-RD); it is associated with increased IgG4 serum concentrations, lymphoplasmacytic infiltrate and phlebitis in the pancreas. Instead, type 2 AIP affects only the pancreas, has normal IgG4 serum concentration and, histologically, shows a neutrophilic inflammation [69]. Hereditary and environmental factors together are thought to induce adaptive immune responses to self-antigens [70]. Microbial antigens may underlie the pathogenesis, but the trigger for the autoimmune cascade remains unknown.

At the beginning of the 2000s, several studies have examined the possible association between *Helicobacter pylori* (*H. pylori*) infection and pancreatic diseases, including AIP [71–74].

In 2010, Jesnowski et al., did not isolate *H. pylori* DNA either from samples or pancreatic juice of patients affected by AIP [75], excluding a direct bacterial infection of the gland. Afterwards, it has been proposed that *H. pylori* could cause AIP due to molecular mimicry mechanism. Guarneri et al. [76], found a significant homology between *H. pylori* a-carbonic anhydrase (a-CA) and human CA type II, enzyme highly expressed in pancreatic ductal cells. Moreover, the homologous CA segments contain the binding motif of the HLA molecule DRB1*0405, which confers a risk for AIP development [76]. In 2009, Frulloni et al. [74] reported that 94% of AIP patients exhibited IgG antibodies to *H. pylori* plasminogen-binding protein (PBP), that is homologous to the human protein ubiquitin-protein ligase E3 component n-recognin 2 (UBR2), highly expressed in pancreatic acinar cells. Instead, this finding was found in only 5% of patients with pancreatic cancer adenocarcinoma (PDAC) and none of patients with alcohol-induced CP or intraductal papillary mucinous neoplasms (IPMN) [74]. Unfortunately, to date, these findings have not been confirmed. At first, Buijs et al. in 2016 [77], and then Detlfsen et al. [78] in 2018, did not find significant differences in serum concentrations of anti-PBP antibodies in AIP patients. Furthermore, in the second study the authors investigated the anti-CAII antibodies serum concentration, but no differences were found with the control group. Finally, in a prospective study, Culver et al. [79], found that the prevalence of gastric ulcerations, exposure to *H. pylori*, cytokine response and immunological memory to *H. pylori* PBP did not differ in IgG4-RD patients compared with control group. Hence, they ruled out a role for *H. pylori* PBP as a microbial antigen in IgG4-RD pathogenesis [79].

Watanabe et al., proved that antigens derived from intestinal microflora, through the activation of NOD-2 and TLR pathways, enhance IgG4 responses by peripheral blood mononuclear cells (PBMCs) from AIP patients, showing a possible involvement of innate immune responses against intestinal microflora in the development of AIP [80]. Several AIP-like experimental models have been induced in transgenic mice inoculating microbial agents: C57BL/6 mice infected with the murine leukemia retrovirus LP-BM5, developed histological findings similar to human AIP [81,82]; in MRL/Mp mice the administration of polyinosinic:polycytidylic acid (poly I:C), a synthetic double-stranded RNA and TLR3 ligand, promotes the development of AIP-like pancreatitis [83–86]. After showing in their first study that repeated inoculations with heat-killed non-pathogenic *Escherichia coli* (*E. coli*) (ATCC 25922), a common commensal bacterium from gut microbiota, into C57BL/6 mice induced AIP-like pathological alterations accompanied by an elevation in serum IgG [87], Yanagisawa et al. identified [88] the *E. coli* antigen capable of these alterations: FliC, the major component of the flagella, an important cell surface structure of Gram-negative bacteria. In murine model, when injected intraperitoneally, FliC was able to induce AIP-like pancreatitis. Moreover, serum concentration of anti-FliC antibodies was found to be significantly higher in AIP patients than in those with CP, pancreatic cancer, and pancreatic disease-free controls. These findings indicate that FliC from *E. coli* may be involved in the pathogenesis of AIP [88]. Finally, Kamata et al. [89], investigated in a murine model of AIP the role of immune response against intestinal microflora, via plasmacytoid dendritic cells (pDCs) activation, whose products, interferon (IFN)-α and interleukin (IL)-33, are responsible for chronic inflammation and pancreatic fibrosis [89–92]. They proved that bowel sterilization by broad spectrum antibiotics decreased pancreatic accumulation of pDCs, and consequently IFN-α and interleukin (IL)-33 levels, halting AIP development. They observed a reduction in the microbial diversity as well as alteration in the microbial composition in the feces of mice with AIP, with the abundance of *Bifidobacterium* spp. in the gut of AIP mice. Lastly, they proved that intestinal dysbiosis, due to transmission of intestinal microflora by co-housing or by FMT, makes mice more sensitive to develop experimental AIP when they were injected with a lower dose of an inducing agent [89]. If these data are confirmed in the human form of AIP, patients with this condition might be efficiently treated with a blockade of IFN-α and IL-33, in combination with the normalization of the intestinal microflora.

4.4. Microbiota and Type 1 Diabetes Mellitus

Type 1 diabetes (T1D) is an autoimmune disease characterized by the destruction of pancreatic insulin-producing β cells. Susceptibility to T1D is influenced by both genetic and environmental factors that act on immune system dysregulation [93]. The risk of developing T1D, in fact, has been related to viral infections, dietetic factors, and vitamin D deficiency, while the role of antibiotics is still controversial [94].

The impact of intestinal microbiota in T1D predisposition and pathogenesis has been studied in human subjects and in murine models, such as non-obese diabetic mice [95,96]. Early-life events, such as delivery mode, breastfeeding, solid food introduction and antibiotics, strongly influenced the microbiota composition and its interaction with mucosal and systemic immunity [95]. Diabetes resulted to be associated with higher *Bacteroidetes/Firmicutes* ratio and lower α-diversity in fecal samples [95,96]. Moreover, subjects affected by T1D showed an increase in levels of *Clostridium*, *Bacteroides dorei* and *vulgatus*, *Blautia*, *Rikenellaceae*, *Ruminococcus* and *Streptococcus*, while *Lactobacillus*, *Bifidobacterium* and SCFAs-producing bacteria were reduced [94,95].

Microbiota dysregulation affects the risk of T1D through different mechanisms, including intestinal permeability [97,98], molecular mimicry [99] and immune system modulation [100–103].

The intestinal barrier prevents the translocation of toxins, food antigens and infectious factors, which can activate the immune system. Specific microorganisms of gut microbiota, including *Dialister invisus*, *Bifidobacterium longum*, *Gemella sanguinis* and *Clostridium perfringens*, can compromise the intestinal barrier, leading to an increased risk of T1D [94]. Alterations of the barrier function, in fact, are associated with activation and proliferation of islet-autoantigen specific CD8+ T cells, with pro-diabetogenic effect [98].

Moreover, children affected by T1D showed a significantly higher intestinal permeability [98].

The molecular mimicry is an important pathogenetic mechanism not only for diabetes but also for other autoimmune diseases. The molecular structure of some bacterial proteins showed to be similar to pancreatic self-antigens. Monofunctional glycosyltransferase protein (MGT) of *Leptotrichia goodfellowii*, for example, showed similarity to islet specific glucose-6-phosphatase related protein and could cause immune cross-reactions [94,104,105].

Innate immunity involves macrophages, granulocytes and natural killer cells, and a key role in the antigen recognition is played by TLRs, which are activated by PAMPs. Many components of intestinal bacteria, such as lipopolysaccharides (LPS), lipoproteins, peptidoglycan and nucleic acids, act like PAMPs and can activate TLRs, with pro-diabetogenic or anti-diabetogenic effects [101]. Different TLRs, in fact, can promote or inhibit autoimmune processes: TLR2-pathway showed to facilitate T1D, while TLR4-signaling resulted to be protective against diabetes development [101]. In addition, some microorganisms can modulate T-cells of B-cells functions. Even if the exact mechanism is still unknown, *Listeria* can induce Th1 response [102], while *Clostridia* can induce regulatory T cells [102]. SCFAs are associated with reduced serum levels of pro-inflammatory cytokines which promote T1D development, such as interleukin-21 (IL-21). They preserve the intestinal barrier function and promote B cells differentiation into plasma-cells and memory cells [103]. Even if there is no current evidence-based treatment for preventing or delaying T1D onset by acting on gut microbiome, the above-mentioned data suggest some possible therapeutic approaches. The immune dysregulation, for instance, can be modulated through the administration of *Escherichia coli Nissle* (*EcN*), which is associated with reduced pathogenic bacteria colonization, decreased serum levels of IL-2 and TNFα and increased IL-10 [95]. Other possible strategies include the correction of dysbiosis and the improvement of microbial diversity through probiotics and prebiotics, such as inulin and oligosaccharides [95]. These treatments have been tested in mouse models, but further studies are needed to prove their efficacy in humans.

4.5. Microbiota and Pancreatic Cystic Neoplasms

Pancreatic cystic neoplasms (PCN) represent up to 5% of the total amount of pancreatic cancerous neoplasms [106]. Frequently, the discovery of pancreatic cysts is casual, and these are found during screening or diagnostic procedures for other problems. Diagnostic refinement by computed tomography (CT) and magnetic resonance imaging (MRI) have allowed us to define PCN, undetected in the past. PCN are divided into various types, such as serous cystadenomas (SCA), mucinous cystic neoplasm (MCN) and IPMN; other forms of PCN are very unusual [107]. IPMN can be divided into three types: IPMN main duct, IPMN branch duct and the mixed form [108]. In recent years, researchers tried to find a connection between gut microbiota and cystic pancreatic lesions, but some questions have not been answered yet. Following data reporting the correlation between poor oral health and PDAC [109,110]. Olson et al., in a pilot study, assessed the difference between oral microbiota in patients with PDAC, IPMN and controls [111]. The authors evaluated the characteristics of the oral microbiota of 40 PDAC patients, 39 of whom with IPMN and 58 patients included as control group. Eligible participants were age 21 or over, had not smoked tobacco products in the past year, had not taken antibiotics in the past 30 days, had not been treated for any cancer (other than non-melanoma skin cancer) in the past two years. The 16s rRNA microbiota screening was performed in saliva samples. Patients with PDAC had a higher mean relative proportion of *Firmicutes/Bacteroidetes* ratio, while *Proteobacteria* were predominant in controls; in fact, the first group had high levels of *Firmicutes* and *Lactobacillae*. However, differences were observed only in the main relative proportion of some Operational taxonomic unit (OTU). No differences were detected between PDAC and IPMN groups about alpha diversity [111]. Gaiser et al., have reported a prospective study about the harbor of intracystic microbiome in PCN [112]. Patients, undergoing pancreatectomy, were enrolled. Cystic fluid samples were collected at the day of surgery. The authors found that 16s DNA copy number were higher in IPMN with high grade of risk malignancy than benign neoplasms. Moreover, IL-1 beta protein was higher in IPMN and cancer. In particular, *Proteobacteria* were predominant in benign cystic forms, while *Firmicutes* in IPMN with high grade dysplasia (HGD) and PDAC. A sub-analysis was performed to investigate the potential role of invasive endoscopic procedures [i.e., endoscopic ultrasonography-fine needle agoaspiration (EUS-FNA) or endoscopic retrograde cholangiopancreatography (ERCP) or percutaneous transhepatic cholangiography (PTC)] in the microbiota composition. *Fusobacterium nucleatum* (*F. nucleatum*) was one of the predominant pathogens in cystic specimens. qPCR assay confirmed that *F. nucleatum* were increased in IPMN HGD and in PDAC. Previous procedures had no impact on microbiota composition, as well as the previous use of PPI [112]. It is now believed that *F. nucleatum* have an oncogenic role in some cancers, such as colorectal cancer [113] and PDAC itself [114].

Li et al. [115] studied pancreatic cyst fluid (PCF) to determine the genera of bacteria present. Sixty-nine pancreatic fluid samples were collected. Twenty-seven were IPMN, 13 MCN, nine pseudocysts and nine SCA; the rest were classified as "other". Predominant microorganisms in the cysts were *Bacteroides* spp. and *Escherichia* spp., and even less *Fusobacterium* spp. and *Bacillus* spp. The authors found that PCF contained their bacterial microenvironment with a unique ecosystem. Finally, *Helicobacter* were marginally detected in pancreatic cyst fluid. In this case, more studies are necessary as may be further warranted.

4.6. Microbiota and Pancreatic Ductal Adenocarcinoma

Pancreatic ductal adenocarcinoma is the 12th most common cancer worldwide [116] and the fourth most fatal cancer in both men and women [117]. The incidence of PDAC is higher in North America and in Western Europe and it is more common in men than in women [116].

Risk factors for PDAC include cigarette smoking, obesity and CP. Some chemical compounds, nickel-based, chromium-based, and silica dust have been reported to increase the risk of PDAC too [117]. Moreover, the development of PDAC has been related to dietary factors, *H. pylori* infection, oral, gut and pancreatic microbiota [117]. The mechanisms by which microbiota influences carcinogenesis involve innate and adaptive immune suppression [118,119] and stimulation of pro-carcinogenic cellular pathways [118,120]. In preclinical mice models, in fact, microbial ablation with broad-spectrum antibiotics has been associated with increased presence of intratumoral T cells [117], while the administration of cell-free extracts from fecal samples of gut bacteria from PDAC-bearing mice or cell-free extracts from *Bifidobacterium pseudolongum* were associated with lower expression of MHC II and up-regulation of IL-10 [118]. Moreover, bacteria-associated PAMPs bind to specific TLRs, such as TLR4, thus activating MAP (mitogen-activated protein) Kinase and NF-kB (nuclear-factor kappa-light-chain-enhancer of activated B cells) pathways, which are potent promoter of carcinogenesis [121].

The etiologic relationship between gut microbiota and PDAC has been initially studied in mice models. In these studies, germ-free mice and those treated with oral antibiotics showed a lower incidence of pancreatic cancer, while fecal transplant from PDAC-bearing mice resulted in an increased risk of tumor [118].

In murine models, the presence of PDAC has been related to increased number of gut bacteria from fecal samples belonging to *Bacteroides*, *Firmicutes* and selected genera associated to *Actinobacteria* and *Deferribacteres*. Moreover, different microbiota composition has been related to a different rate of pancreatic carcinoma progression [118]. *Elizabethkingia*, *Enterobacteriaceae* and *Mycoplasmacetaceae* resulted to be associated with slower progression, while aggressive PDAC was associated with *Helicobacteriaceae*, *Bacteroidales* and *Mogibacteriaceae* [118]. In humans, *Proteobacteria*, *Actinobacteria*, *Fusobacteria* and *Verrucomicrobia*, which normally represent a minor proportion of human intestinal microbiome [122], were present in abundance in the gut of PDAC patients if compared to controls [118].

Table 2. Microbial changes in the pancreatic diseases.

Author, Year, [Ref.]	Study Population	Material	Disease	Microbial Changes
Tan, 2015, [47]	Humans	Fecal samples	SAP and MAP	↑*Enterococci* and ↓*Bifidobacteria* in patients with SAP versus patients with MAP
Zhang, 2018, [49]	Humans	Fecal samples	AP	↑*Proteobacteria* and *Bacteroidetes* ↓*Actinobacteria* and *Firmicutes*
Capurso, 2016, [58]	Humans	Breath tests	CP	1/3 of CP patients show SIBO
Nishiyama, 2018, [60]	Mouse	Cecum, transverse colon and fecal samples	CP	↑*Akkermansia muciniphila* and ↑*Lactobacillus reuteri* in mice treated with PERT
Li, 2017, [115]	Humans	Pancreatic cystic fluid	PCN	↑↑*Bacteroides* spp. and *Escherichia/Shigella* spp. + ↑*Fusobacterium* spp. and *Bacillus* spp. in PCN *Helicobacter* were marginally detected in pancreatic cyst fluid
Knip, 2017, [95]	Humans	Fecal samples	T1D	↑*Bacteroidetes/Firmicutes* ratio + ↑*Clostridium*, *Bacteroides dorei* and *vulgatus*, *Blautia*, *Rikenellaceae*, *Ruminococcus* and *Streptococcus* ↓*Lactobacillus*, *Bifidobacterium* and short-chain fatty acids-producing bacteria
Pushalkar, 2018, [118]	Humans	PDAC specimens and fecal samples	PDAC	↑*Proteobacteria*, *Actinobacteria*, *Fusobacteria* and *Verrucomicrobia* in PDAC
Fan, 2018, [110]	Humans	Oral samples	PDAC	↑*Porphyromonas gingivalis* and *Aggregatibacter actinomycetemcomitans* and ↓*Fusobacteria* and its genus *Leptotrichia*: high risk of PDAC development
Mitsuhashi, 2015, [114]	Humans	PDAC specimens	PDAC	*Fusobacterium* spp. observed in 8.8% of PDAC specimens
Olson, 2017, [111]	Humans	Oral samples	PDAC e IPMN	↑*Firmicutes/Bacteroidetes* ratio + ↑*Lactobacillae* in PDAC and IPMN (mean relative proportion) ↑*Proteobacteria* in healthy controls (mean relative proportion)
Gaiser, 2019, [112]	Humans	Cystic fluid samples from resected pancreas	PDAC and PCN	↑*Firmicutes* in IPMN-HGD and PDAC ↑*Fusobacterium nucleatum* in IPMN-HGD and PDAC ↑*Proteobacteria* in benign cystic neoplasms

AP: acute pancreatitis; CP: chronic pancreatitis; IPMN-HGD: intraductal papillary mucinous neoplasm with high grade dysplasia; LP: Lactobacillus plantarum; MAP: moderate acute pancreatitis; PCN: pancreatic cystic neoplasms PDAC: pancreatic ductal adenocarcinoma; PERT: pancreatic enzyme replacement therapy; SAP: severe acute pancreatitis; SIBO: small intestine bacterial overgrowth; T1D: type 1 diabetes.

In epidemiological studies, poor oral health and periodontal diseases have been related to PDAC incidence [121]: these data suggest a possible relationship between oral microbiome and pancreatic cancer, as mentioned above. In human studies, in fact, the carriage of *Porphyromonas gengivalis* and *Aggregatibacter actinomycetemcomitans* and a decreased proportion of *Fusobacteria* and its genus *Leptotrichia* resulted to be associated with higher risk of PDAC development [110]. Many studies have demonstrated the role of *Porphyromonas gingivalis*, an oral pathogen that causes periodontitis and gingivitis, in the PDAC. Smoking and alcohol consumption are recognized risk factors for pancreatic cancer, but at the same time they can affect oral microbiome composition. Therefore, the association between oral bacteria and PDAC has been studied in ever and never-smokers and in ever and never-drinkers: the results suggest that the association between oral microbiota and PDAC are not likely due to these potential confounders [110]. The presence and composition of pancreatic microbiota have been associated to PDAC development: cancerous pancreas showed a more abundant microbiota compared to normal pancreas in both murine models and human subjects [118]. Translocation of gut bacteria and their migration into the pancreas have been demonstrated by Pushalkar et al. [118], through comparison between fecal samples and pancreatic microbiota and through oral administration of fluorescently labelled *Enterococcus faecalis* and Green Fluorescent Protein (GFP)-labeled *Escherichia coli*. Thus, gut microbiota could influence pancreatic microenvironment. The composition of pancreatic microbiota in PDAC resulted to be different from normal human pancreas. Thirteen phyla were detected in tumor tissue. The most abundant were *Proteobacteria*, *Bacteroidetes* and *Firmicutes* [118]. Interestingly, *Proteobacteria* only amount for about 8% of gut bacteria from fecal samples in PDAC patients, while they were one of the most represented bacteria in their pancreatic tissue [118]; this suggests a differentially increased translocation of these Gram-negative bacteria to the pancreas. Nowadays, it is believed that *F. nucleatum*, an inhabitant of the oral mucosa, is important in the colon rectal dysplasia and cancer. Similar results were found on PDAC. In a landmark study, Mitsuhashi et al. [114] studied the correlation between PDAC and oral microbiota; they analyzed a database of 283 patients with PDAC who underwent surgery and found *Fusobacterium* spp. in 8.8% of pancreatic cancer samples; the presence of tumor *Fusobacterium* was not associated with any molecular and clinical features, but with worse prognosis. Mitsuhashi et al. suggested that *Fusobacterium* could be a negative prognostic negative independent biomarker for PDAC.

This data about intestinal, oral and pancreatic microbiota can represent useful screening and prevention tools. In fact, they suggest that the analysis of oral and gut microbiota composition could be used for risk stratification and early diagnosis of PDAC. Moreover, oral antibiotics could be proposed as a preventive therapy for high-risk patients or in association with chemotherapy with a synergic effect [118]. Both these diagnostic and therapeutic implications, however, need further studies to be confirmed.

4.7. Microbiota and Pancreatic Neuroendocrine Tumors

Evidences about a link between pancreatic neuroendocrine tumors (pNET) and microbiota are very poor. Currently, therapies for pNET are surgery for not invasive neoplasms, somatostatin analogues (SSA), peptide receptor radionuclide therapy (PRRT), target therapy with Everolimus and Sunitinib and chemotherapy (for advanced NET) [123]. In this scenario, immunotherapy could have a futuristic role; in particular, PD-1 inhibitors and PD-1 ligands are a group of checkpoint inhibitors that have been developed for treatment of some cancers (i.e., melanoma, squamous cell lung cancer, advanced cell renal carcinoma, Merkel-cell carcinoma, a cutaneous neuroendocrine tumor) [124,125]. Specific clinical trials are looking for a role of immune checkpoint inhibitors in pNETs [126], that may conduct to more personalized target therapy; in particular researchers are testing pembrolizumab in NET with advanced stage. In a landmark study of Nghiem et al. [125], they used pembrolizumab as first-line therapy in patients with advanced Merkel-cell carcinoma (a type of skin neuroendocrine tumor) with an objective response rate of 56%.

Recent data support a role for the commensal microbiota in the efficacy of immunotherapy itself. Indeed, gut microbiota may have a "mechanistic impact" on antitumor immunity in the cancer [127]. Matson et al., collected 38 stool samples from metastatic melanoma patients on anti-PD-1 treatment and, after 16S RNA sequencing and quantitative PCR analysis, they identified *Bifidobacterium* spp., *Colinsella aerofaciens*, *Enterococcus faecium* as bacteria associated with beneficial response [127]. They transplanted fecal material from responding patients in a germ-free mice model of melanoma. They observed that FMT could lead to improve tumor control, augmenting T cell responses, and greater efficacy of anti-PD-L1 therapy.

The commensal microbiota composition might be useful as a biomarker to predict response to checkpoint blockade therapy, and in the future, it could be possible to translate this research for the pNET. However, data are very poor now, and the relationship between immunotherapy and microbiota, in NET patients, is still unclear.

5. Conclusions

Although the relationship between microbiota and pancreatic diseases is an innovative and inspiring field of research, several points warrant further clarification. At present, the association between pancreatic diseases and microbiota is not well established. Hence, the correlation between microbiota and pancreas remains fraught with challenges. Given the potential role of microbiota in the pancreatic diseases, technological improvement in microbiota manipulation as well as randomized controlled trials could represent a powerful therapeutic strategy for their prevention and treatment.

Author Contributions: Conceptualization, C.G.D.A.; methodology, M.G. and F.R.; literature search, S.R. and F.C.; writing—original draft preparation, M.G., F.R., S.B.; writing—review and editing, M.G. and F.R., C.G.D.A.; supervision, G.M.S. and C.G.D.A. All authors have read and agreed to the published version of the manuscript.

Funding: This research received no external funding.

Conflicts of Interest: The authors declare no conflict of interest.

References

1. Thaiss, C.A.; Zmora, N.; Levy, M.; Elinav, E. The microbiome and innate immunity. *Nature* **2016**, *535*, 65–74. [CrossRef] [PubMed]
2. Marchesi, J.R.; Adams, D.H.; Fava, F.; Hermes, G.D.A.; Hirschfield, G.M.; Hold, G.; Quraishi, M.N.; Kinross, J.; Smidt, H.; Tuohy, K.M.; et al. The gut microbiota and host health: A new clinical frontier. *Gut* **2016**, *65*, 330–339. [CrossRef] [PubMed]
3. Lynch, S.V.; Pedersen, O. The human intestinal microbiome in health and disease. *N. Engl. J. Med.* **2016**, *375*, 2369–2379. [CrossRef] [PubMed]
4. Charbonneau, M.R.; Blanton, L.V.; Di Giulio, D.B.; Relman, D.A.; Lebrilla, C.B.; Mills, D.A.; Gordon, J.I. A microbial perspective of human developmental biology. *Nature* **2016**, *535*, 48–55. [CrossRef] [PubMed]
5. Qin, J.; Li, R.; Raes, J.; Arumugam, M.; Burgdorf, K.S.; Manichanh, C.; Nielsen, T.; Pons, N.; Levenez, F.; Yamada, T.; et al. A human gut microbial gene catalogue established by metagenomic sequencing. *Nature* **2010**, *464*, 59–65. [CrossRef]
6. Sonnenburg, J.L.; Bäckhed, F. Diet–microbiota interactions as moderators of human metabolism. *Nature* **2016**, *535*, 56–64. [CrossRef]
7. Le Gall, M.; Gallois, M.; Sève, B.; Louveau, I.; Holst, J.J.; Oswald, I.P.; Lallès, J.P.; Guilloteau, P. Comparative effect of orally administered sodium butyrate before or after weaning on growth and several indices of gastrointestinal biology of piglets. *Br. J. Nutr.* **2009**, *102*, 1285–1296. [CrossRef]
8. Pagliari, D.; Piccirillo, C.A.; Larbi, A.; Cianci, R. The interactions between innate immunity and microbiota in gastrointestinal diseases. *J. Immunol. Res.* **2015**, *2015*, 898297. [CrossRef]
9. Hooper, L.V.; Macpherson, A.J. Immune adaptations that maintain homeostasis with the intestinal microbiota. *Nat. Rev. Immunol.* **2010**, *10*, 159–169. [CrossRef]
10. Macpherson, A.J.; Geuking, M.B.; McCoy, K.D. Innate and adaptive immunity in host-microbiota mutualism. *Front. Biosci.* **2012**, *4*, 685–698. [CrossRef]

11. Caviglia, G.P.; Rosso, C.; Ribaldone, D.G.; Dughera, F.; Fagoonee, S.; Astegiano, M.; Pellicano, R. Physiopathology of intestinal barrier and the role of zonulin. *Minerva Biotecnol.* **2019**, *31*, 83–92. [CrossRef]
12. Rinninella, E.; Raoul, P.; Cintoni, M.; Franceschi, F.; Miggiano, G.A.D.; Gasbarrini, A.; Mele, M.C. What is the healthy gut microbiota composition? A changing ecosystem across age, environment, diet, and diseases. *Microorganisms* **2019**, *7*, 14. [CrossRef] [PubMed]
13. Zhang, Y.J.; Li, S.; Gan, R.Y.; Zhou, T.; Xu, D.P.; Li, H.B. Impacts of Gut Bacteria on Human Health and Diseases. *Int. J. Mol. Sci.* **2015**, *16*, 7493–7519. [CrossRef] [PubMed]
14. Forbes, J.D.; Van Domselaar, G.; Bernstein, C.N. The gut microbiota in immune-mediated inflammatory diseases. *Front. Microbiol.* **2016**, *7*, 1081. [CrossRef] [PubMed]
15. Camilleri, M. Leaky gut: Mechanisms, measurement and clinical implications in humans. *Gut* **2019**, *68*, 1516–1526. [CrossRef]
16. Rawls, J.F.; Mahowald, M.A.; Ley, R.E.; Gordon, J.I. Reciprocal gut microbiota transplants from zebrafish and mice to germ-free recipients reveal host habitat selection. *Cell* **2006**, *127*, 423–433. [CrossRef]
17. Ammer-Herrmenau, C.; Pfisterer, N.; Weingarten, M.F.; Neesse, A. The microbiome in pancreatic diseases: Recent advances and future perspectives. *United Eur. Gastroenterol. J.* **2020**, *8*, 878–885. [CrossRef]
18. Pineiro, M.; Asp, N.G.; Reid, G.; Macfarlane, S.; Morelli, L.; Brunser, O.; Tuohy, K. FAO Technical meeting on prebiotics. *J. Clin. Gastroenterol.* **2008**, *42*, S156–S159. [CrossRef]
19. Gibson, G.R.; Hutkins, R.; Sanders, M.E.; Prescott, S.L.; Reimer, R.A.; Salminen, S.J.; Scott, K.; Stanton, C.; Swanson, K.S.; Cani, P.D.; et al. The International Scientific Association for Probiotics and Prebiotics (ISAPP) consensus statement on the definition and scope of prebiotics. *Nat. Rev. Gastroenterol. Hepatol.* **2017**, *14*, 491–502. [CrossRef]
20. Ghouri, Y.A.; Richards, D.M.; Rahimi, E.F.; Krill, J.T.; Jelinek, K.; DuPont, A.W. Systematic review of randomized controlled trials of probiotics, prebiotics and synbiotics in inflammatory bowel disease. *Clin. Exp. Gastroenterol.* **2014**, *7*, 473–487.
21. Mari, A.; Baker, F.A.; Mahamid, M.; Sbeit, W.; Khoury, T. The evolving role of gut microbiota in the management of irritable bowel syndrome: An overview of the current knowledge. *J. Clin. Med.* **2020**, *9*, 685. [CrossRef] [PubMed]
22. Dewulf, E.M.; Cani, P.D.; Claus, S.P.; Fuentes, S.; Puylaert, P.G.B.; Neyrinck, A.M.; Bindels, L.B.; de Vos, W.M.; Gibson, G.R.; Thissen, J.P.; et al. Insight into the prebiotic concept: Lessons from an exploratory, double blind intervention study with inulin-type fructans in obese women. *Gut* **2013**, *62*, 1112–1121. [CrossRef]
23. Guarner, F.; Khan, A.G.; Garisch, J.; Eliakim, R.; Gangl, A.; Thomson, A.; Krabshuis, J.; Lemair, T.; Kaufmann, P.; de Paula, J.A.; et al. World Gastroenterology Organisation Global Guidelines: Probiotics and prebiotics October 2011. *J. Clin. Gastroenterol.* **2012**, *46*, 468–481. [CrossRef]
24. Hill, C.; Guarner, F.; Reid, G.; Gibson, G.R.; Merenstein, D.J.; Pot, B.; Morelli, L.; Canani, R.B.; Flint, H.J.; Salminem, S.; et al. Expert consensus document. The International Scientific Association for Probiotics and Prebiotics consensus statement on the scope and appropriate use of the term probiotic. *Nat. Rev. Gastroenterol. Hepatol.* **2014**, *11*, 506–514. [CrossRef] [PubMed]
25. Cammarota, G.; Ianiro, G.; Kelly, C.R.; Mullish, B.H.; Allegretti, J.R.; Kassam, Z.; Putignani, L.; Fischer, M.; Keller, J.J.; Paul, S.; et al. International consensus conference on stool banking for faecal microbiota transplantation in clinical practice. *Gut* **2019**, *68*, 2111–2121. [CrossRef]
26. Ribaldone, D.G.; Caviglia, G.P.; Abdulle, A.; Pellicano, R.; Ditto, M.C.; Morino, M.; Fusaro, E.; Saracco, G.M.; Bugianesi, E.; Astegiano, M. Adalimumab Therapy Improves Intestinal Dysbiosis in Crohn's Disease. *J. Clin. Med.* **2019**, *8*, 1646. [CrossRef]
27. Panelli, S.; Capelli, E.; Lupo, G.F.D.; Schiepatti, A.; Betti, E.; Sauta, E.; Marini, S.; Bellazzi, R.; Vanoli, A.; Pasi, A.; et al. Comparative Study of Salivary, Duodenal, and Fecal Microbiota Composition Across Adult Celiac Disease. *J. Clin. Med.* **2020**, *9*, E1109. [CrossRef]
28. Mayer, E.A.; Savidge, T.; Shulman, R.J. Brain-gut microbiome interactions and functional bowel disorders. *Gastroenterology* **2014**, *146*, 1500–1512. [CrossRef]
29. Yadav, S.K.; Boppana, S.; Ito, N.; Mindur, J.E.; Mathay, M.T.; Patel, A.; Dhib-Jalbut, S.; Ito, K. Gut dysbiosis breaks immunological tolerance toward the central nervous system during young adulthood. *Proc. Natl. Acad. Sci. USA* **2017**, *114*, E9318–E9327. [CrossRef]

30. Korotkyi, O.H.; Vovk, A.A.; Dranitsina, A.S.; Falalyeyeva, T.M.; Dvorshchenko, K.O.; Fagoonee, S.; Ostapchenko, L.I. The influence of probiotic diet and chondroitin sulfate administration on Ptgs2, Tgfb1 and Col2a1 expression in rat knee cartilage during monoiodoacetate-induced osteoarthritis. *Minerva Med.* **2019**, *110*, 419–424. [CrossRef]
31. Li, Z.; Zhu, H.; Zhang, L.; Qin, C. The intestinal microbiome and Alzheimer's disease: A review. *Animal Model. Exp. Med.* **2018**, *1*, 180–188. [CrossRef]
32. Wroblewski, L.E.; Peek, R.M., Jr.; Coburn, L.A. The Role of the Microbiome in Gastrointestinal Cancer. *Gastroenterol. Clin. N. Am.* **2016**, *45*, 543–556. [CrossRef] [PubMed]
33. Del Castillo, E.; Meier, R.; Chung, M.; Koestler, D.C.; Chen, T.; Paster, B.J.; Charpentier, K.P.; Kelsey, K.T.; Izard, J.; Michaud, D.S. The Microbiomes of Pancreatic and Duodenum Tissue Overlap and Are Highly Subject Specific but Differ between Pancreatic Cancer and Noncancer Subjects. *Cancer Epidemiol. Biomark. Prev.* **2019**, *28*, 370–383. [CrossRef] [PubMed]
34. Pagliari, D.; Saviano, A.; Newton, E.E.; Serricchio, M.L.; Dal Lago, A.A.; Gasbarrini, A.; Cianci, R. Gut microbiota–immune system crosstalk and pancreatic disorders. *Mediat. Inflamm.* **2018**, *2018*, 7946431. [CrossRef]
35. Thomas, R.M.; Jobin, C. Microbiota in pancreatic health and disease: The next frontier in microbiome research. *Nat. Rev. Gastroenterol. Hepatol.* **2020**, *17*, 53–64. [CrossRef]
36. Sun, J.; Furio, L.; Mecheri, R.; van der Does, A.M.; Lundeberg, E.; Saveanu, L.; Chen, Y.; van Endert, P.; Agerberth, B.; Diana, J. Pancreatic β-cells limit autoimmune diabetes via an immunoregulatory antimicrobial peptide expressed under the influence of the gut microbiota. *Immunity* **2015**, *43*, 304–317. [CrossRef]
37. Kościuczuk, E.M.; Lisowski, P.; Jarczak, J.; Strzałkowska, N.; Jóźwik, A.; Horbańczuk, J.; Krzyżewski, J.; Zwierzchowski, L.; Bagnicka, E. Cathelicidins: Family of antimicrobial peptides. A review. *Mol. Biol. Rep.* **2012**, *39*, 10957–10970. [CrossRef]
38. Gallo, R.L.; Kim, K.J.; Bernfield, M.; Kozak, C.A.; Zanetti, M.; Merluzzi, L.; Gennaro, R. Identification of CRAMP, a cathelin-related antimicrobial peptide expressed in the embryonic and adult mouse. *J. Biol. Chem.* **1997**, *272*, 13088–13093. [CrossRef]
39. Ahuja, M.; Schwartz, D.M.; Tandon, M.; Son, A.; Zeng, M.; Swaim, W.; Eckhaus, M.; Hoffman, V.; Cui, Y.; Xiao, B.; et al. Orai1-mediated antimicrobial secretion from pancreatic acini shapes the gut microbiome and regulates gut innate immunity. *Cell Metab.* **2017**, *25*, 635–646. [CrossRef]
40. McCarl, C.A.; Picard, C.; Khalil, S.; Kawasaki, T.; Rother, J.; Papolos, A.; Kutok, J.; Hivroz, C.; Ledeist, F.; Plogmann, K.; et al. ORAI1 deficiency and lack of store-operated Ca2+ entry cause immunodeficiency, myopathy, and ectodermal dysplasia. *J. Allergy Clin. Immunol.* **2009**, *124*, 1311–1318. [CrossRef]
41. Rogers, M.B.; Aveson, V.; Firek, B.; Yeh, A.; Brooks, B.; Brower-Sinning, R.; Steve, J.; Banfield, J.F.; Zureikat, A.; Hogg, M.; et al. Disturbances of the perioperative microbiome across multiple body sites in patients undergoing pancreaticoduodenectomy. *Pancreas* **2017**, *46*, 260–267. [CrossRef]
42. Baron, T.H.; DiMaio, C.J.; Wang, A.Y.; Morgan, K.A. American gastroenterological association clinical practice update: Management of pancreatic necrosis. *Gastroenterology* **2020**, *158*, 67–75. [CrossRef] [PubMed]
43. Liu, H.; Li, W.; Wang, X.; Li, J.; Yu, W. Early gut mucosal dysfunction in patients with acute pancreatitis. *Pancreas* **2008**, *36*, 192–196. [CrossRef]
44. Capurso, G.; Zerboni, G.; Signoretti, M.; Valente, R.; Stigliano, S.; Piciucchi, M.; Fave, G.D. Role of the gut barrier in acute pancreatitis. *J. Clin. Gastroenterol.* **2012**, *46*, S46–S51. [CrossRef] [PubMed]
45. Italian Association for the study of Pancreas (AISP); Pezzilli, R.; Zerbi, A.; Campra, D.; Capurso, G.; Golfieri, R.; Arcidiacono, P.G.; Billi, P.; Butturini, G.; Calculli, L.; et al. Consensus guidelines on severe acute pancreatitis. *Dig. Liver Dis.* **2015**, *47*, 532–543.
46. Signoretti, M.; Roggiolani, R.; Stornello, C.; Delle Fave, G.; Capurso, G. Gut microbiota and pancreatic diseases. *Minerva Gastroenterol. Dietol.* **2017**, *63*, 399–410. [PubMed]
47. Tan, C.; Ling, Z.; Huang, Y.; Cao, Y.; Liu, Q.; Cai, T.; Yuan, H.; Liu, C.; Li, Y.; Xu, K. Dysbiosis of intestinal microbiota associated with inflammation involved in the progression of acute pancreatitis. *Pancreas* **2015**, *44*, 868–875. [CrossRef] [PubMed]
48. Qin, H.-L.; Zheng, J.-J.; Tong, D.-N.; Chen, W.-X.; Fan, X.-B.; Hang, X.-M.; Jiang, Y.-Q. Effect of Lactobacillus plantarum enteral feeding on the gut permeability and septic complications in the patients with acute pancreatitis. *Eur. J. Clin. Nutr.* **2008**, *62*, 923–930. [CrossRef]

49. Zhang, X.M.; Zhang, Z.Y.; Zhang, C.H.; Wu, J.; Wang, Y.X.; Zhang, G.X. Intestinal Microbial Community Differs between Acute Pancreatitis Patients and Healthy Volunteers. *Biomed. Environ. Sci.* **2018**, *31*, 81–86. [PubMed]
50. Oláh, A.; Belágyi, T.; Issekutz, A.; Gamal, M.E.; Bengmark, S. Randomized clinical trial of specific lactobacillus and fibre supplement to early enteral nutrition in patients with acute pancreatitis. *Br. J. Surg.* **2002**, *89*, 1103–1107. [CrossRef]
51. Oláh, A.; Belágyi, T.; Pótó, L.; Romics, L., Jr.; Bengmark, S. Synbiotic control of inflammation and infection in severe acute pancreatitis: A prospective, randomized, double blind study. *Hepatogastroenterology* **2007**, *54*, 590–594. [PubMed]
52. Besselink, M.G.; Timmerman, H.M.; Buskens, E.; Niwuwenhuijs, V.B.; Akkermans, L.M.A.; Gooszen, H.G. Probiotic prophylaxis in patients with predicted severe acute pancreatitis (PROPATRIA): Design and rationale of a double-blind, placebo-controlled randomized multicenter trial. *BMC Surg.* **2004**, *4*, 12. [CrossRef]
53. Besselink, M.G.; van Santvoort, H.C.; Buskens, E.; Boermeester, M.A.; van Goor, H.; Timmerman, H.M.; Nieuwenhuijs, V.B.; Bollen, T.L.; van Ramshorst, B.; Witteman, B.J.; et al. Probiotic prophylaxis in predicted severe acute pancreatitis: A randomised, double-blind, placebo-controlled trial. *Lancet* **2008**, *371*, 651–659. [CrossRef]
54. Bongaerts, G.P.; Severijnen, R.S. A reassessment of the PROPATRIA study and its implication for probiotic therapy. *Nat. Biotechnol.* **2016**, *34*, 55–63. [CrossRef]
55. Gou, S.; Yang, Z.; Liu, T.; Wu, H.; Wang, C. Use of probiotics in the treatment of severe acute pancreatitis: A systematic review and meta-analysis of randomized controlled trials. *Crit. Care* **2014**, *18*, R57. [CrossRef]
56. Dumonceau, J.M.; Delhaye, M.; Tringali, A.; Arvanitakis, M.; Sanchez-Yague, A.; Vaysse, T.; Aithal, G.P.; Andreloni, A.; Bruno, M.; Cantù, P.; et al. Endoscopic treatment of chronic pancreatitis: European society of Gastrointestinal Endoscopy (ESGE) Guideline-updated August 2018. *Endoscopy* **2019**, *51*, 179–193. [CrossRef]
57. Witt, H.; Apte, M.V.; Keim, V.; Wilson, J.S. Chronic pancreatitis: Challenges and advances in pathogenesis, genetics, diagnosis, and therapy. *Gastroenterology* **2007**, *132*, 1557–1573. [CrossRef] [PubMed]
58. Capurso, G.; Signoretti, M.; Archibugi, L.; Stigliano, S.; Delle Fave, G. Systematic review and meta-analysis: Small intestinal bacterial overgrowth in chronic pancreatitis. *United Eur. Gastroenterol. J.* **2016**, *4*, 697–705. [CrossRef] [PubMed]
59. D'Haese, J.G.; Ceyhan, G.O.; Demir, I.E.; Layer, P.; Uhl, W.; Löhr, M.; Rychlik, R.; Pirilis, K.; Zöllner, Y.; Gradl, B.; et al. Pancreatic enzyme replacement therapy in patients with exocrine pancreatic insufficiency due to chronic pancreatitis: A 1-year disease management study on symptom control and quality of life. *Pancreas* **2014**, *43*, 834–841. [CrossRef]
60. Nishiyama, H.; Nagai, T.; Kudo, M.; Okazaki, Y.; Azuma, Y.; Watanabe, T.; Goto, S.; Ogata, H.; Sakurai, T. Supplementation of pancreatic digestive enzymes alters the composition of intestinal microbiota in mice. *Biochem. Biophys. Res. Commun.* **2018**, *495*, 273–279. [CrossRef]
61. Grander, C.; Adolph, T.E.; Wieser, V.; Lowe, P.; Wrzosek, L.; Gyongyosi, B.; Ward, D.V.; Grabherr, F.; Gerner, R.R.; Pfister, A.; et al. Recovery of ethanol-induced Akkermansia muciniphila depletion ameliorates alcoholic liver disease. *Gut* **2018**, *67*, 891–901. [CrossRef]
62. Jandhyala, S.M.; Madhulika, A.; Deepika, G.; Rao, G.V.; Reddy, D.N.; Subramanyam, C.; Sasikala, M.; Talukdar, R. Altered intestinal microbiota in patients with chronic pancreatitis: Implications in diabetes and metabolic abnormalities. *Sci. Rep.* **2017**, *7*, 43640. [CrossRef] [PubMed]
63. Watanabe, T.; Kudo, M.; Strober, W. Immunopathogenesis of pancreatitis. *Mucosal Immunol.* **2017**, *10*, 283–298. [CrossRef] [PubMed]
64. Domínguez-Munoz, J.E.; Iglesias-Garcia, J.; Iglesias-Rey, M.; Vilarino-Insua, M. Optimising the therapy of exocrine pancreatic insufficiency by the association of a proton pump inhibitor to enteric coated pancreatic extracts. *Gut* **2006**, *55*, 1056–1057. [CrossRef] [PubMed]
65. dos Santos, P.Q.; Guedes, J.C.; de Jesus, R.P.; Santos, R.R.D.; Fiaconne, R.L. Effects of using synbiotics in the clinical nutritional evolution of patients with chronic pancreatitis: Study prospective, randomized, controlled, double blind. *Clin. Nutr. ESPEN* **2017**, *18*, 9–15. [CrossRef]
66. Dylag, K.; Hubalewska-Mazgaj, M.; Surmiak, M.; Szmyd, J.; Brzozowski, T. Probiotics in the mechanism of protection against gut inflammation and therapy of gastrointestinal disorders. *Curr. Pharm. Des.* **2014**, *20*, 1149–1155. [CrossRef]

67. Okazaki, K.; Chari, S.T.; Frulloni, L.; Lerch, M.M.; Kamisawa, T.; Kawa, S.; Kim, M.-H.; Lévy, P.; Masamune, A.; Webster, G.; et al. International consensus for the treatment of autoimmune pancreatitis. *Pancreatology* **2017**, *17*, 1–6. [CrossRef]
68. Yoshida, K.; Toki, F.; Takeuchi, T.; Watanabe, S.; Shiratori, K.; Hayashi, N. Chronic pancreatitis caused by an autoimmune abnormality. Proposal of the concept of autoimmune pancreatitis. *Dig. Dis. Sci.* **1995**, *40*, 1561–1568. [CrossRef]
69. Sureka, B.; Rastogi, A. Autoimmune Pancreatitis. *Pol. J. Radiol.* **2017**, *82*, 233–239. [CrossRef]
70. Mills, K.H. TLR-dependent T cell activation in autoimmunity. *Nat. Rev. Immunol.* **2011**, *11*, 807–822. [CrossRef]
71. Raderer, M.; Wrba, F.; Kornek, G.; Maca, T.; Koller, D.Y.; Weinlaender, G.; Hejna, M.; Scheithauer, W. Association between Helicobacter pylori infection and pancreatic cancer. *Oncology* **1998**, *55*, 16–19. [CrossRef]
72. Risch, H.A.; Lu, L.; Kidd, M.S.; Wang, J.; Zhang, W.; Ni, Q.; Gao, Y.T.; Yu, H. Helicobacter pylori seropositivities and risk of pancreatic carcinoma. *Cancer Epidemiol. Biomark. Prev.* **2014**, *23*, 172–178. [CrossRef]
73. Khan, J.; Pelli, H.; Lappalainen-Lehto, R.; Järvinen, S.; Sand, J.; Nordback, I. Helicobacter pylori in alcohol induced acute pancreatitis. *Scand. J. Surg.* **2009**, *98*, 221–224. [CrossRef] [PubMed]
74. Frulloni, L.; Lunardi, C.; Simone, R.; Dolcino, M.; Scattolini, C.; Falconi, M.; Benini, L.; Vantini, I.; Corrocher, R.; Puccetti, A. Identification of a novel antibody associated with autoimmune pancreatitis. *N. Engl. J. Med.* **2009**, *361*, 2135–2142. [CrossRef]
75. Jesnowski, R.; Isaksson, B.; Möhrcke, C.; Bertsch, C.; Bulajic, M.; Schneider-Brachert, W.; Klöppel, G.; Lowenfels, A.B.; Maisonneuve, P.; Löhr, J.M. Helicobacter pylori in autoimmune pancreatitis and pancreatic carcinoma. *Pancreatology* **2010**, *10*, 462–466. [CrossRef]
76. Guarneri, F.; Guarneri, C.; Benvenga, S. Helicobacter pylori and autoimmune pancreatitis: Role of carbonic anhydrase via molecular mimicry? *J. Cell. Mol. Med.* **2005**, *9*, 741–744. [CrossRef] [PubMed]
77. Buijs, J.; Cahen, D.L.; van Heerde, M.J.; Hansen, B.E.; van Buuren, H.R.; Peppelenbosch, M.P.; Fuhler, G.M.; Bruno, M.J. Testing for Anti-PBP Antibody Is Not Useful in Diagnosing Autoimmune Pancreatitis. *Am. J. Gastroenterol.* **2016**, *111*, 1650–1654. [CrossRef]
78. Detlefsen, S.; de Vos, J.D.; Tanassi, J.T.; Heegaard, N.H.H.; Fristrup, C.; de Muckadell, O.B.S. Value of anti-plasminogen binding peptide, anti-carbonic anhydrase II, immunoglobulin G4, and other serological markers for the differentiation of autoimmune pancreatitis and pancreatic cancer. *Medicine* **2018**, *97*, e11641. [CrossRef]
79. Culver, E.L.; Smit, W.L.; Evans, C.; Sadler, R.; Cargill, T.; Makuch, M.; Wang, L.M.; Ferry, B.; Klenerman, P.; Barnes, E. No evidence to support a role for Helicobacter pylori infection and plasminogen binding protein in autoimmune pancreatitis and IgG4-related disease in a UK cohort. *Pancreatology* **2017**, *17*, 395–402. [CrossRef] [PubMed]
80. Watanabe, T.; Yamashita, K.; Fujikawa, S.; Sakurai, T.; Kudo, M.; Shiokawa, M.; Kodama, Y.; Uchida, K.; Okazaki, K.; Chiba, T. Activation of Toll-like receptors and NOD-like receptors is involved in enhanced IgG4 responses in autoimmune pancreatitis. *Arthritis Rheum.* **2012**, *64*, 914–924. [CrossRef] [PubMed]
81. Suzuki, K.; Makino, M.; Okada, Y.; Kinoshita, J.; Yui, R.; Kanazawa, H.; Asakura, H.; Fujiwara, M.; Mizouchi, T.; Komuro, K. Exocrinopathy resembling Sjogren's syndrome induced by a murine retrovirus. *Lab. Investig.* **1993**, *69*, 430–435. [PubMed]
82. Watanabe, S.; Suzuki, K.; Kawauchi, Y.; Yamagiwa, S.; Yoneyama, H.; Kawachi, H.; Okada, Y.; Shimizu, F.; Asakura, H.; Aoyagi, Y. Kinetic analysis of the development of pancreatic lesions in mice infected with a murine retrovirus. *Clin. Immunol.* **2003**, *109*, 212–223. [CrossRef]
83. Qu, W.M.; Miyazaki, T.; Terada, M.; Okada, K.; Mori, S.; Kanno, H.; Nose, M. A novel autoimmune pancreatitis model in MRL mice treated with polyinosinic: Polycytidylic acid. *Clin. Exp. Immunol.* **2002**, *129*, 27–34. [CrossRef] [PubMed]
84. Soga, Y.; Komori, H.; Miyazaki, T.; Arita, N.; Terada, M.; Kamada, K.; Tanaka, Y.; Fujino, T.; Hiasa, Y.; Matsuura, B.; et al. Toll-like receptor 3 signaling induces chronic pancreatitis through the Fas/Fas ligand-mediated cytotoxicity. *Tohoku J. Exp. Med.* **2009**, *217*, 175–184. [CrossRef] [PubMed]
85. Asada, M.; Nishio, A.; Akamatsu, T.; Tanaka, J.; Saga, K.; Kido, M.; Watanabe, N.; Uchida, K.; Fukui, T.; Okazaki, K.; et al. Analysis of humoral immune response in experimental autoimmune pancreatitis in mice. *Pancreas* **2010**, *39*, 224–231. [CrossRef] [PubMed]

86. Nishio, A.; Asada, M.; Uchida, K.; Fukui, T.; Chiba, T.; Okazaki, K. The role of innate immunity in the pathogenesis of experimental autoimmune pancreatitis in mice. *Pancreas* **2011**, *40*, 95–102. [CrossRef]
87. Haruta, I.; Yanagisawa, N.; Kawamura, S.; Furukawa, T.; Shimizu, K.; Kato, H.; Kobayashi, M.; Shiratori, K.; Yagi, J. A mouse model of autoimmune pancreatitis with salivary gland involvement triggered by innate immunity via persistent exposure to avirulent bacteria. *Lab. Investig.* **2010**, *90*, 1757–1769. [CrossRef]
88. Yanagisawa, N.; Haruta, I.; Shimizu, K.; Furukawa, T.; Higuchi, T.; Shibata, N.; Shiratori, K.; Yagi, J. Identification of commensal flora-associated antigen as a pathogenetic factor of autoimmune pancreatitis. *Pancreatology* **2014**, *14*, 100–106. [CrossRef]
89. Kamata, K.; Watanabe, T.; Minaga, K.; Hara, A.; Yoshikawa, T.; Okamoto, A.; Yamao, K.; Takenaka, M.; Park, A.M.; Kudo, M. Intestinal dysbiosis mediates experimental autoimmune pancreatitis via activation of plasmacytoid dendritic cells. *Int. Immunol.* **2019**, *31*, 795–809. [CrossRef]
90. Arai, Y.; Yamashita, K.; Kuriyama, K.; Shiokawa, M.; Kodama, Y.; Sakurai, T.; Mizugishi, K.; Uchida, K.; Kadowaki, N.; Takaori-Kondo, A.; et al. Plasmacytoid dendritic cell activation and IFN-α production are prominent features of murine autoimmune pancreatitis and human IgG4-related autoimmune pancreatitis. *J. Immunol.* **2015**, *195*, 3033–3044. [CrossRef]
91. Watanabe, T.; Yamashita, K.; Arai, Y.; Minaga, K.; Kamata, K.; Nagai, T.; Komeda, Y.; Takenaka, M.; Hagiwara, S.; Ida, H.; et al. Chronic fibro-inflammatory responses in autoimmune pancreatitis depend on IFN-α and IL-33 produced by plasmacytoid dendritic cells. *J. Immunol.* **2017**, *198*, 3886–3896. [CrossRef]
92. Watanabe, T.; Minaga, K.; Kamata, K.; Kudo, M.; Strober, W. Mechanistic insights into autoimmune pancreatitis and IgG4-related disease. *Trends Immunol.* **2018**, *39*, 874–889. [CrossRef] [PubMed]
93. Bluestone, J.A.; Herold, K.; Eisenbarth, G. Genetics, pathogenesis and clinical interventions in type 1 diabetes. *Nature* **2010**, *464*, 1293–1300. [CrossRef] [PubMed]
94. Zheng, P.; Li, Z.; Zhou, Z. Gut microbiome in type 1 diabetes: A comprehensive review. *Diabetes Metab. Res. Rev.* **2018**, *34*, e3043. [CrossRef]
95. Knip, M.; Honkanen, J. Modulation of Type 1 Diabetes Risk by the Intestinal Microbiome. *Curr. Diab. Rep.* **2017**, *17*, 105. [CrossRef]
96. Giongo, A.; Gano, K.A.; Crabb, D.B.; Mukherjee, N.; Novelo, L.L.; Casella, G.; Drew, J.C.; Ilonen, J.; Knip, M.; Hyoty, H.; et al. Toward defining the autoimmune microbiome for type 1 diabetes. *ISME J.* **2011**, *5*, 82–91. [CrossRef]
97. Bibbò, S.; Dore, M.P.; Pes, G.M.; Delitala, G.; Delitala, A.P. Is there a role for gut microbiota in type 1 diabetes pathogenesis? *Ann. Med.* **2017**, *49*, 11–22. [CrossRef]
98. Li, X.; Atkinson, M.A. The role for gut permeability in the pathogenesis of type 1 diabetes—A solid or leaky concept? *Pediatr Diabetes* **2015**, *16*, 485–492. [CrossRef]
99. Tai, N.; Peng, J.; Liu, F.; Gulden, E.; Hu, Y.; Zhang, X.; Chen, L.; Wong, F.S.; Wen, L. Microbial antigen mimics activate diabetogenic CD8 T cells in NOD mice. *J. Exp. Med.* **2016**, *213*, 2129–2146. [CrossRef]
100. Ferris, S.T.; Zakharov, P.N.; Wan, X.; Calderon, B.; Artyomov, M.N.; Unanue, E.R.; Carrero, J.A. The islet-resident macrophage is in an inflammatory state and senses microbial products in blood. *J. Exp. Med.* **2017**, *214*, 2369–2385. [CrossRef] [PubMed]
101. Burrows, M.P.; Volchkov, P.; Kobayashi, K.S.; Chervonsky, A.V. Microbiota regulates type 1 diabetes through Toll-like receptors. *Proc. Natl. Acad. Sci. USA* **2015**, *112*, 9973–9977. [CrossRef]
102. Legaria, M.C.; Lumelsky, G.; Rodriguez, V.; Rosetti, S. Clindamycin-resistant Fusobacterium Varium bacteremia and decubitus ulcer infection. *J. Clin. Microbiol.* **2005**, *43*, 4293–4295. [CrossRef]
103. Mariño, E.; Richards, J.L.; McLeod, K.H.; Stanley, D.; Yap, Y.A.; Knight, J.; McKenzie, C.; Kranich, J.; Oliveira, A.C.; Rossello, F.J.; et al. Gut microbial metabolites limit the frequency of autoimmune T cells and protect against type 1 diabetes. *Nat. Immunol.* **2017**, *18*, 552–562. [CrossRef]
104. Janeway, C.A., Jr. Pillars article: Approaching the asymptote? Evolution and revolution in immunology. Cold spring harb symp quant biol. 1989. 54: 1–13. *J. Immunol.* **2013**, *191*, 4475–4487.
105. McCoy, K.D.; Ronchi, F.; Geuking, M.B. Host-microbiota interactions and adaptive immunity. *Immunol. Rev.* **2017**, *279*, 63–69. [CrossRef]
106. Wu, B.U.; Sampath, K.; Berberian, C.E.; Kwok, K.K.; Lim, B.S.; Kao, K.T.; Giap, A.Q.; Kosco, A.E.; Akmal, Y.M.; Difronzo, A.L.; et al. Prediction of malignancy in cystic neoplasms of the pancreas: A population-based cohort study. *Am. J. Gastroenterol.* **2014**, *109*, 121–130. [CrossRef]

107. Del Chiaro, M.; Verbeke, C.; Salvia, R.; Kloppel, G.; Werner, J.; McKay, C.; Friess, H.; Manfredi, R.; van Cutsem, E.; Lohr, M.; et al. European experts consensus statement on cystic tumours of the pancreas. *Dig. Liver Dis.* **2013**, *45*, 703–711. [CrossRef] [PubMed]
108. Tanaka, M.; Fernández-Del Castillo, C.; Kamisawa, T.; Jang, J.Y.; Levy, P.; Ohtsuka, T.; Salvia, R.; Shimizu, Y.; Tada, M.; Wolfgang, C.L. Revisions of international consensus Fukuoka guidelines for the management of IPMN of the pancreas. *Pancreatology* **2017**, *17*, 738–753. [CrossRef]
109. Michaud, D.S.; Izard, J. Microbiota, oral microbiome, and pancreatic cancer. *Cancer J.* **2014**, *20*, 203–206. [CrossRef]
110. Fan, X.; Alekseyenko, A.V.; Wu, J.; Peters, B.A.; Jacobs, E.J.; Gapstur, S.M.; Purdue, M.P.; Abnet, C.C.; Stolzenberg-Solomon, R.; Miller, G.; et al. Human oral microbiome and prospective risk for pancreatic cancer: A population-based nested case-control study. *Gut* **2018**, *67*, 120–127. [CrossRef]
111. Olson, S.H.; Satagopan, J.; Xu, Y.; Ling, L.; Leong, S.; Orlow, I.; Saldia, A.; Li, P.; Nunes, P.; Madonia, V.; et al. The Oral Microbiota in Patients with Pancreatic Cancer, Patients with IPMNs, and Controls—A Pilot Study. *Cancer Causes Control.* **2017**, *28*, 959–969. [CrossRef] [PubMed]
112. Gaiser, R.A.; Halimi, A.; Alkharaan, H.; Lu, L.; Davanian, H.; Healy, K.; Hugerth, L.W.; Ateeb, Z.; Valente, R.; Moro, C.F.; et al. Enrichment of oral microbiota in early cystic precursors to invasive pancreatic cancer. *Gut* **2019**, *68*, 2186–2194. [CrossRef] [PubMed]
113. Liu, X.; Cheng, Y.; Shao, L.; Ling, Z. Alterations of the Predominant Fecal Microbiota and Disruption of the Gut Mucosal Barrier in Patients with Early-Stage Colorectal Cancer. *Biomed. Res. Int.* **2020**, *2020*, 2948282. [CrossRef]
114. Mitsuhashi, K.; Nosho, K.; Sukawa, Y.; Matsunaga, Y.; Ito, M.; Kurihara, H.; Kanno, S.; Igarashi, H.; Naito, T.; Adachi, A.; et al. Association of Fusobacterium species in pancreatic cancer tissues with molecular features and prognosis. *Oncotarget* **2015**, *6*, 7209–7220. [CrossRef]
115. Li, S.; Fulher, G.M.; Bn, N.; Jose, T.; Bruno, M.J.; Peppelenbosch, M.P.; Konstantinov, S.R. Pancreatic cyst fluid harbor a unique microbiome. *Microbiome* **2017**, *5*, 147. [CrossRef]
116. Simoes, P.K.; Olson, S.H.; Saldia, A.; Kurtz, R.C. Epidemiology of pancreatic adenocarcinoma. *Chin. Clin. Oncol.* **2017**, *6*, 24. [CrossRef]
117. Ducreux, M.; Cuhna, A.S.; Caramella, C.; Hollebecque, A.; Burtin, P.; Goere, D.; Seufferlein, T.; Haustermans, K.; van Laethem, J.L.; Conroy, T.; et al. Cancer of the pancreas: ESMO Clinical Practice Guidelines for diagnosis, treatment and follow-up. *Ann. Oncol.* **2015**, *26* (Suppl. 5), v56–v68. [CrossRef]
118. Pushalkar, S.; Hundeyin, M.; Daley, D.; Zambirinis, C.P.; Kurz, E.; Mishra, A.; Mohan, N.; Aykut, B.; Usyk, M.; Torres, L.E.; et al. The Pancreatic Cancer Microbiome Promotes Oncogenesis by Induction of Innate and Adaptive Immune Suppression. *Cancer Discov.* **2018**, *8*, 403–416. [CrossRef]
119. Zheng, L.; Xue, J.; Jaffee, E.M.; Habtezion, A. Role of immune cells and immune-based therapies in pancreatitis and pancreatic ductal adenocarcinoma. *Gastroenterology* **2013**, *144*, 1230–1240. [CrossRef] [PubMed]
120. Zambirinis, C.P.; Ochi, A.; Barilla, R.; Greco, S.; Deutsch, M.; Miller, G. Induction of TRIF- or MYD88-dependent pathways perturbs cell cycle regulation in pancreatic cancer. *Cell Cycle* **2013**, *12*, 1153–1154.
121. Leal Lopes, C.; Velloso, F.J.; Campopiano, J.C.; Sogayar, M.C.; Correa, R.G. Roles of Commensal Microbiota in Pancreas Homeostasis and Pancreatic Pathologies. *J. Diabetes Res.* **2015**, *2015*, 284680. [CrossRef] [PubMed]
122. Tojo, R.; Suárez, A.; Clemente, M.G.; de los Reyes-Gavilan, C.G.; Margolles, A.; Gueimonde, M.; Ruas-Madiedo, P. Intestinal microbiota in health and disease: Role of bifidobacteria in gut homeostasis. *World J. Gastroenterol.* **2014**, *20*, 15163–15176. [CrossRef] [PubMed]
123. Delle Fave, G.; O'Toole, D.; Sundin, A.; Taal, B.; Ferolla, P.; Ramage, J.K.; Ferone, D.; Ito, T.; Weber, W.; Zheng-Pei, Z.; et al. ENETS Consensus Guidelines Update for gastroduodenal neuroendocrine neoplasms. *Neuroendocrinology* **2016**, *103*, 119–124. [CrossRef] [PubMed]
124. Gopalakrishnan, V.; Spencer, C.N.; Nezi, L.; Reuben, A.; Andrews, M.C.; Karpinets, T.V.; Prieto, P.A.; Vicente, D.; Hoffman, K.; Wei, S.C.; et al. Gut microbiome modulates response to anti–PD-1 immunotherapy in melanoma patients. *Science* **2018**, *359*, 97–103. [CrossRef]
125. Nghiem, P.T.; Bhatia, S.; Lipson, E.J.; Kudchadkar, R.R.; Miller, N.J.; Annamalai, L.; Berry, S.; Chartash, E.K.; Daud, A.; Fling, S.P.; et al. PD-1 blockade with Pembrolizumab in advanced Merckel-cell carcinoma. *N. Engl. J. Med.* **2016**, *374*, 2542–2552. [CrossRef]

126. Chauhan, A.; Horn, M.; Magee, G.; Hodges, K.; Evers, M.; Arnold, S.; Anthony, L. Immune checkpoint inhibitors in neuroendocrine tumors: A single institution experience with review of literature. *Oncotarget* **2017**, *9*, 8801–8809. [CrossRef]

127. Matson, V.; Fessler, J.; Bao, R.; Chongsuwat, T.; Zha, Y.; Alegre, M.L.; Luke, J.J.; Gajewski, T.F. The commensal microbiome is associated with anti-PD-1 efficacy in metastatic melanoma patients. *Science* **2018**, *359*, 104–108. [CrossRef]

Publisher's Note: MDPI stays neutral with regard to jurisdictional claims in published maps and institutional affiliations.

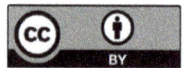

© 2020 by the authors. Licensee MDPI, Basel, Switzerland. This article is an open access article distributed under the terms and conditions of the Creative Commons Attribution (CC BY) license (http://creativecommons.org/licenses/by/4.0/).

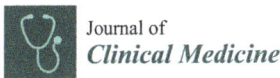

Review

Gastrointestinal Microbiota and Type 1 Diabetes Mellitus: The State of Art

Marilena Durazzo *, Arianna Ferro and Gabriella Gruden

Department of Medical Sciences, University of Turin, C.so A.M. Dogliotti 14, 10126 Turin, Italy; arianna.ferro@unito.it (A.F.); gabriella.gruden@unito.it (G.G.)
* Correspondence: marilena.durazzo@unito.it; Tel.: +39-0110918473

Received: 14 October 2019; Accepted: 29 October 2019; Published: 2 November 2019

Abstract: The incidence of autoimmune type 1 diabetes (T1DM) is increasing worldwide and disease onset tends to occur at a younger age. Unfortunately, clinical trials aiming to detect predictive factors of disease, in individuals with a high risk of T1DM, reported negative results. Hence, actually there are no tools or strategies to prevent T1DM onset. The importance of the gut microbiome in autoimmune diseases is increasingly recognized and recent data suggest that intestinal dysbiosis has a pathogenic role in T1DM by affecting both intestinal immunostasis and the permeability of the gut barrier. An improved understanding of the mechanisms whereby dysbiosis in the gut favors T1DM development may help develop new intervention strategies to reduce both the incidence and burden of T1DM. This review summarizes available data on the associations between gut microbiota and T1DM in both experimental animals and humans and discusses future perspectives in this novel and exciting area of research.

Keywords: type 1 diabetes; microbiota; microbiome; auto-immunity; gut permeability

1. Introduction

In the last decade, the gut microbiota has gained increasing interest because of a major shift in our way of thinking: the microbiota is no longer considered a passive collection of microbes hosted in the gut, but an integral part of the body, providing important functions to the host. Landmark studies have significantly improved our understanding of microbiota function, dynamic, and interactions. Today, we know that the gut microbiota is involved in both the development and progression of many pathological conditions and targeting the microbiota has become a novel promising intervention strategy. Recent data suggest that an imbalance in gut microbiota (dysbiosis) could be involved in the pathogenesis of autoimmune type 1 diabetes (T1DM) and may contribute to explaining the global rise in T1DM incidence, particularly in childhood [1–3]. Indeed, a dysfunctional microbiota can favor the development of autoimmune diseases by altering the maturation of the immune system in early infancy and by increasing both intestinal permeability and inflammation. Despite major research effort, clinical trials in individuals with high T1DM risk reported negative results and there is no effective strategy for the primary prevention of T1DM. Hopefully, studying the role of the intestinal microbiota in T1DM may provide insights into developing new strategies to reduce T1DM incidence.

2. Type 1 Diabetes Mellitus

T1DM accounts for 5–10% of all diagnosed cases of diabetes and onset of the disease usually occurs during childhood or adolescence [4]. The International Diabetes Federation (IDF) estimated that more than a million subjects (<20 years) were affected by T1DM in 2017 and approximately 86,000 children develop T1DM every year; however, the incidence varies among countries and even in different areas within the same country [5]. In Europe, there is a north–south gradient, with Scandinavian countries exhibiting the highest incidence rate. The incidence is much lower in the Mediterranean area, though Sardinia has the second highest incidence in the world after Finland [6]. T1DM incidence has increased over the last 50–60 years in many countries, with an approximate 3% rise in incidence rate per year [6,7]. In some countries, the disease is also occurring at a much earlier age, with a marked increase in the 0–4 years age range [8], indicating a lowered threshold for T1DM development.

T1DM is characterized by absolute insulin deficiency due to pancreatic β cell loss. This process, occurring in genetically susceptible individuals, may be triggered by environmental factors, and progresses over many months or years, during which the subject is asymptomatic and euglycemic. Indeed, autoimmune β cell destruction by autoimmune T cells progresses slowly and hyperglycemia and symptomatic diabetes only develops when a critical mass of β cells (~80%) is lost. Therefore, clinical T1DM is preceded by a silent phase in which the presence of autoantibodies (insulin, glutamic acid decarboxylase, insulinoma-2-associated, and zinc transporter 8 autoantibodies), which are biomarkers of T1DM-associated autoimmunity, is the only detectable abnormality [9,10].

Clinical onset is characterized by polyuria, thirst, polydipsia, weight loss, hunger, polyphagia, and fatigue. Early recognition is important to prevent the development of diabetic ketoacidosis (DKA), a severe condition characterized by hyperglycemia, acidosis, ketonemia, and ketonuria. DKA occurs at the time of T1DM diagnosis in approximately 30% of children in the United States and the incidence rate in children with established diabetes is approximately 6–8% per year. DKA is the leading cause of morbidity and mortality in pediatric T1DM. Indeed, in children, cerebral injury occurs in 0.3 to 0.9 percent of DKA episodes and has a mortality of 20–25% [11].

In the absence of DKA, T1DM diagnosis is based on one of the following criteria: (1) random plasma glucose ≥ 200 mg/dL in a patient with classic symptoms of hyperglycemia, (2) fasting plasma glucose ≥ 126 mg/dL, (3) plasma glucose ≥ 200 mg/dL two hours after a glucose load of 1.75 g/kg (oGTT), and (4) glycated hemoglobin (HbA1C) ≥ 6.5%. Unless symptomatic hyperglycemia is present, the diagnosis should be confirmed by repeat testing [4]. Because of the rapid T1DM onset, HbA1C may not be markedly elevated; therefore, an HbA1C level below 6.5% does not exclude the diagnosis of diabetes in pediatric patients.

Once it is diagnosed, T1DM requires immediate treatment with insulin replacement therapy. Intensive insulin therapy combines the administration of long-acting basal insulin together with pre-meal boluses of rapid-acting insulin to mimic the physiological secretion of insulin by the β cells. This can be achieved by either Multiple Daily insulin Injections (MDI) or Continuous Subcutaneous Insulin Infusion (CSII). The general aim of T1DM therapy is to maintain glucose control as near to normal as possible without causing hypoglycemia. In addition, T1DM care should also include diabetes education, self-management training, patient-tailored plans on healthy nutrition and exercise, and psychosocial support [4].

To prevent the burden of T1DM care, the best approach would be the primary prevention of T1DM in subjects at risk of developing the disease [12]. However, clinical trials focusing on primary prevention failed to prove benefit so far and there is no effective tool to block the development of the disease [12]. This is, at least in part, due to our poor understanding of T1DM pathogenesis. *HLA-DR* and *-DQ* genes account for 40–50% of the susceptibility to the disease [13]. Moreover, recent studies suggest an important role of gene polymorphisms, such as Toll-like receptor exon polymorphisms and polymorphisms in genes critical for vitamin D metabolism [14–17]. However, genetics alone cannot explain T1DM onset, as less than 10% of the children, who are genetically predisposed, develop the disease. Thus, environmental factors that affect the immune response, changing the probability of an autoimmune reaction against β cells in genetically susceptible subjects, play a crucial role. Environmental influences implicated in the pathogenesis of T1DM include pregnancy-related and perinatal factors, viruses, ingestion of cow's milk and cereals, and use of both antibiotics and probiotics [18]. These factors also affect the microbiota, adding to the hypothesis of a role of the gut microbiome in linking environment influences with the development of T1DM.

3. The Microbiota

The microbiota is defined as the set of microorganisms living in symbiosis with their human/animal host [19]. The human microbiota consists of symbiotic microbial cells harbored on skin, respiratory and urogenital systems and gastrointestinal tract. In the latter, microbial populations reach the highest density and form a complex microbial community of ~4×10^{13} cells [19,20]. Although the gut microbiota includes different types of microorganisms, bacteria are the best studied. Sequencing the 16S rRNA is a key methodology to identify and classify these bacterial populations [21,22]. Furthermore, new metagenomic methods can precisely identify functional and strain-specific differences in the microbiome [23]. Healthy adults share most gut bacterial populations, which constitute a "core microbiota". In fact, even if thousands of bacterial species have been isolated from human intestine, most of them belong to just four phyla: Bacteroidetes and Firmicutes are predominant (90%), while Actinobacteria and Proteobacteria are less abundant [24]. However, the concept of the "core microbiota" has been challenged by data showing a vast microbial diversity both over time and across human populations [25].

Colonization of the gut starts at birth, though recent studies questioned the dogma that the womb is a sterile environment, and is markedly affected by the mode of delivery. Vaginally delivered infants acquire microbial communities resembling maternal vaginal microbiota, predominantly Lactobacillus. In contrast, C-section infants harbor bacterial strains similar to those found on the skin, such as Staphylococcus and Clostridium genera [26,27]. Fecal microbiota resembles that of the mothers in 72% of vaginally delivered infants, while this percentage is reduced to 41% in babies delivered by C-section [26]. However, recent evidence shows that maternal skin and vaginal strains only transiently colonize the infant and that mother-to-infant transmission of gut strains, which occurs after birth via unclear mechanisms, is more relevant and persistent [28].

The intestinal microbiota of newborns is generally low in diversity and is dominated by two main phyla: Actinobacteria and Proteobacteria. Later, the gut microbiota becomes more diverse, with the predominance of Firmicutes and Bacteroidetes. By approximately 2–3 years of age, the composition, diversity and function of the microbiota are very similar to that of adult subjects.

Although the gut microbiota is relatively stable in adults compared to infants, it can undergo major changes in response to environmental influences, such as diet composition, the use of drugs, the lifestyle, environment hygiene standards and geographical location [29]. For instance, diet composition can modulate gut bacteria composition since childhood [26,30]. In breastfed infants, the gut microbiota is characterized by higher levels of probiotic genera, such as Lactobacillus and Bifidobacterium, and shows a lower microbial diversity compared to that of formula-fed babies [26,30]. Moreover, the consumption of animal proteins is positively associated with the presence of Bacteroides and Alistipes genera, while fiber intake is linked to increased Bifidobacterium and Lactobacillium genera, both in childhood and adulthood [31,32]. These genera are also enhanced by supplementation with probiotics [31,33]. Other environmental factors that greatly influence the gut microbiota composition are the use of drugs, particularly antibiotics, and geographical location [25]. Although it is well established that antibiotic therapy can reshape the gut microbiota, it remains unclear whether the microbial community can fully recover following antibiotic treatment [34,35].

The gut microbiota becomes unstable and less diverse with aging and the centenarian microbiota shows an increase in facultative anaerobe species, such as Escherichia coli, and a rearrangement of the profile of butyrate producers, such as a decrease in Faecalibacterium prausnitzii [36]. These events are closely associated with both an age-related decline in immunocompetence and coexisting illnesses [36].

4. Importance of the Microbiota to the Host

The human gut microbiota plays a multitude of important functions. It provides protection against pathogen overgrowth, preventing their colonization via the inhibition of adherence, production of bacteriocins, and both site and nutrient competition. It metabolizes specific drugs and eliminates exogenous toxins, thus playing an important detoxifying role. It is involved in the synthesis of essential vitamins, such as B1, B2, B5, B6, B12, K, folic acid, and performs biliary acid deconjugation. In addition, fermentation of indigestible carbohydrates by intestinal bacteria allows their use as a source of energy and provides 5–10% of daily energy requirement [37,38]. Furthermore, in the normal colon, the gut microbiota contributes to intestinal repair by promoting cellular proliferation and differentiation and it is of paramount importance in maintaining the integrity of the gut barrier [37]. Growing evidence points to a key role of the gut microbiota in both maturation and continued education of the host immune system [39]. Indeed, the immune system learns to discriminate between commensal and pathogenic bacteria and, following education, commensal bacteria triggers an anti-inflammatory response, while pathogenic bacteria a pro-inflammatory reaction. Moreover, the gut microbiota modulates both the migration and function of neutrophils and affects T cell differentiation, favoring both the differentiation and expansion of regulatory T cells (Tregs), which are key mediators of immune tolerance. An important mechanism by which the gut microbiota controls the immune system is through the formation of short-chain fatty acids (SCFAs), such as butyrate, acetate, and propionate [38,40]. SCFAs are mainly generated by bacterial fermentation of non-digestible carbohydrates, such as dietary fiber [40]. In T lymphocytes, SCFAs activate G protein-coupled receptors (GPR41/GPR43) signaling pathways, inhibit histone deacetylases, and induce metabolic alterations by enhancing the activity of the mammalian target of rapamycin (mTOR) complex. This results in the inhibition of inflammatory cascades, the expansion of mucosal Tregs, and the decreased production of inflammatory cytokines, such as interleukin-10 (IL-10) and interferon-γ (IFN-γ) [40].

Given the key role of the gut microbiota in maintaining the host health, it is not surprising that alterations in the microbiota (dysbiosis) could be implicated in the pathogenesis of a growing number of extraintestinal diseases including T1DM [41,42].

The term "dysbiosis" refers to an imbalance of the gut microbiota due to the loss of beneficial microbial organisms, the expansion of potentially harmful microorganisms and/or lower microbial diversity [43,44]. Although this term has been widely used in the field of microbiota research, the concept of gut microbiota dysbiosis, which is predominantly based on early microbiome taxonomic studies, is poorly defined and has been recently questioned [45]. Given the complexity and great variability of the human microbiota, changes in the microbiota may be irrelevant to the host health and there is an increasing quest for more rigorous criteria, such as modified Koch criteria, to identify abnormalities pertinent to the microbiota that can be of clinical relevance.

5. Microbiota and Type 1 Diabetes Mellitus

5.1. The Microbiota in Experimental T1DM

The possible role of the gut microbiota in the pathogenesis of autoimmune diabetes was first suggested in the 1980s, but scientific interest on this topic has dramatically increased in the last two decades. Experimental studies have been predominantly performed in animal models of autoimmune diabetes such as Non-Obese Diabetic (NOD) mice and BioBreeding diabetes-prone rats. Consistent with the hypothesis that dysbiosis occurs in T1DM, most of the studies in experimental autoimmune diabetes reported changes in both diversity and composition of gut microbiota. Moreover, fecal transplantation from NOD to Non-Obese Diabetes-Resistant (NOR) mice caused insulitis, indicating a diabetogenic effect of the NOD microbiota [46]. Cross fostering is another effective mean to induce a sustained microbial shift. Cross fostering of NOD mice by NOR mice was capable to protect from diabetes. Specifically, no development of diabetes was observed in NOD male mice nursed by a NOR mother, compared to an 80% incidence of T1DM in male NOD mice nursed by NOD mothers [47].

The link between microbiota-induced innate immunity alterations and T1DM risk was highlighted by studies performed in animals lacking Myeloid differentiation primary response 88 (MyD88), an adaptor protein for the toll-like receptors that recognize microbial patterns and regulate the innate immune response [48]. NOD mice lacking MyD88 were protected from T1DM, indicating that MyD88 is important in T1DM development [48]. However, MyD88 deletion in germ-free NOD mice increased the risk of T1DM [48]. Therefore, the protective effect of MyD88 deficiency is microbiota-dependent, confirming that interactions between the microbiota and innate immunity are important in the development of the disease. In addition, inflammatory lymphocytes, such as T helper 17 and type 3 innate lymphoid cells, are increased in the intestinal lamina propria of NOD mice, while tolerogenic dendritic cells and Treg are reduced in the lymph nodes draining the gut [49]. These changes in adaptive immunity may favor the activation of auto-reactive T cells against β cell antigens and thus T1DM development.

Dysbiosis can also affect the integrity of the gut barrier, resulting in enhanced permeability and the transit of antigens. Tight junctions, sealing the gap between adjacent intestinal epithelial cells, control gut permeability, allowing nutrient absorption, while preventing the transit of dietary, bacterial, and viral antigens. The mucus layer covering the epithelium represents another important barrier and controls the type of commensal bacteria residing in the epithelium [50]. In early experimental autoimmune diabetes prior to the development of insulitis, dysbiosis and altered immunostasis are paralleled by abnormalities of the gut barrier, such as decreased numbers of goblet cells and diminished mucus production [49], leading to enhanced intestinal permeability [51–53]. Cross fostering of NOD mice by NOR mothers corrected the defect in mucus production, indicating a key role of NOD microbiota in the dysfunction of the gut barrier [49].

How the loss of gut barrier integrity triggers β cell autoimmunity remains unclear. It has been proposed that the entrance of antigenic bacterial components into the systemic circulation can directly induce β cell damage and/or activate β cell autoimmunity in the pancreatic lymph nodes. Consistent with this hypothesis, translocation of the microbiota to the pancreatic lymph nodes has been observed in the NOD model [49]. Alternatively, T cells recognizing β cell antigens can be activated by bacterial products in the gut and then travel to the pancreatic lymph nodes to induce β cell injury [54]. In line with this, the induction of chronic colitis, which alters both gut barrier integrity and mucus layer composition, triggered the activation of islet-reactive T cells in the gut mucosa and led to autoimmune diabetes in BDC2.5XNOD mice, an animal model mimicking subjects at high risk of T1DM. Moreover, treatment of these mice with antibiotics prevented T1DM, confirming that the microbiota was required to induce β cell autoimmunity [55]

Taken together, results from experimental animals support the hypothesis that the microbiota may play a role in the pathogenesis of T1DM by affecting both the immune response and the gut barrier integrity. However, the mechanisms leading to β cell autoimmunity are still unclear and require further investigations.

5.2. Intervention Studies in Experimental Autoimmune Diabetes

Several studies in susceptible experimental animals have explored whether intervention strategies affecting the microbiota can modulate the risk of developing T1DM. Probiotic supplementation [56–58], prebiotic assumption [59], antibiotic therapy [46,60–64], and SCFA supplementation [65,66] has been shown to reduce the risk of T1DM onset. NOD pups born to mothers treated with broad-spectrum antibiotics showed increased T1DM incidence together with changes in the microbiota and inflammatory alterations in the intestinal mucosa [67]. Similarly, NOD mice intermittently treated with a macrolide in early life showed increased insulitis, enhanced T1DM incidence, and abnormalities in both innate immunity and T cell differentiation [63]. More recently, a study has shown that a single early-life antibiotic course accelerated T1DM development in male NOD mice and this was paralleled by persistent changes in the gut microbiome and altered the expression of genes controlling both innate and adaptive immunity [68]. On the contrary, supplementation with VSL#3, a probiotic preparation containing eight different strains, decreased T1DM incidence in NOD mice [56]. Similarly, high doses of butyrate in the diet significantly reduced T1DM incidence in NOD mice through the expansion of Treg cells [65]. Recently, supplementation with low-methoxyl pectin (LMP) dietary fiber has been shown to reduce T1DM incidence and fasting glucose levels in NOD mice. This was paralleled by the enrichment of bacterial species producing SCFAs, reduced inflammation, the amelioration of gut barrier integrity and an increase in Treg cells. Antibiotic treatment worsened T1DM autoimmunity in this model, but the transfer of feces from LMP-fed mice reversed the effect of antibiotics [69], confirming the key role of the microbiome in mediating the beneficial effects of LMP. Treatment of NOD mice with the probiotic bacteria Clostridium butyricum increased Tregs in both mesenteric and pancreatic lymph nodes, enhanced expression of microbial genes important in butyrate production, and delayed the onset of T1DM [70].

Taken together, these findings support the hypothesis of a causal link between changes in the microbiota composition and the risk of T1DM onset and they also suggest potential therapeutic strategies to restore a healthy microbiome. However, inbred mouse strains are genetically homogenous, and thus they cannot capture the inherent genetic variations of humans. Moreover, a number of factors (i.e., mode of delivery, diet, social activity) that shape human microbiota are absent in mice. Therefore, results from animal models are not easily translatable to humans and conclusions in experimental models should be taken with caution (Figure 1).

5.3. The Microbiota in Human T1DM

Table 1 summarizes both the design and results of a selection of recent studies performed in humans [1]. Studies exploring the role of the microbiota in human T1DM have been performed in different stages of the disease, ranging from genetic predisposition to clinical diabetes [71–82]. To support the hypothesis of a microbiota contribution to T1DM pathogenesis, studies carried out in the preclinical stage of the disease, identified by the appearance of one or more T1DM-specific autoantibodies in the circulation (seroconversion), are of particular relevance [71–73,76–80,82]. Longitudinal studies in large series of children are also of paramount importance as they can prove that microbiome abnormalities precede seroconversion and/or clinical T1DM onset [71,73,76–78,80,82].

However, establishing a causal relationship between microbiome alterations and T1DM in humans is very challenging because of the complexity of the microbiota immune system cross talk. It is also difficult to identify microbiota abnormalities consistently associated with diabetes, because seroconversion occurs in early life when the microbiota is unstable and it undergoes substantial changes over time [25,26]. Furthermore, factors as delivery mode, diet, geographical location, and lifestyle dramatically affect the microbiota and, besides being potential causes of dysbiosis, they can also act as relevant confounders [27,29,32]. Although causality between dysbiosis and T1DM has not yet been proven in humans, as there are no placebo-controlled trials showing that long-term changes in the intestinal microbiota modify the risk of T1DM, there are data suggesting a role of the gut microbiota in the development of human T1DM.

Children diagnosed with T1DM have reduced gut microbiota diversity in fecal samples. A lower microbial diversity was also shown in children with at least two positive disease-associated autoantibodies compared to autoantibody-negative children. Moreover, longitudinal studies in children at risk of T1DM have shown that the decrease in microbial diversity occurs after seroconversion, but prior to T1DM onset [71–73].

Several studies on the microbiota composition in T1DM reported an increase in Bacteroidetes (Gram negative) and a decrease in Firmicutes (Gram positive) [72–75]. The prevalent species from the Firmicutes phylum produce protective SCFAs, including butyrate [83], suggesting that the reduction in Firmicutes seen in T1DM may be deleterious because of diminished butyrate production. On the other hand, the Bacteroidetes phylum is dominated by Bacteroides and Prevotella [19]. In T1DM, the quantity of Bacteroides is significantly higher, whereas that of Prevotella is significantly lower than in healthy controls and this is of relevance, as Bacteroides have been associated with gastrointestinal inflammation and increased intestinal permeability, while Prevotella appear protective. In a cross-sectional study an increased abundance of Bacteroides characterized the microbiota of children who seroconverted compared with non-converters [72]. Similarly, a study performed in 76 Finnish children found increased Bacteroides dorei and Bacteroides vulgatus species in seroconverted T1DM patients. Of interest, longitudinal data from this study showed that the increase in Bacteroides dorei peaked at 7.6 months of age in autoantibody-positive children and preceded the appearance of the first anti-islet autoantibodies, suggesting that early dysbiosis may predict T1DM in genetically predisposal subjects [76]. The increased abundance of Bacteroides species in Finnish and Estonian compared to Russian children has been even proposed as a possible explanation for their higher incidence of T1DM [84]. Bifidobacterium species were also reduced in autoantibody-positive compared to autoantibodies negative children [72] and this may be of functional relevance as Bifidobacteria contribute to the production of butyrate and inhibit bacterial translocation through the gut barrier.

However, recent metagenomic studies suggest that changes in microbiome function are more relevant and consistently associated with the risk of seroconversion and/or T1DM onset than changes in specific taxa. The Environmental Determinants of Diabetes in the Young (TEDDY) study did not find important taxonomic differences in the gut microbiome of children who seroconverted or developed T1DM. However, metagenomic analysis revealed that the microbiome of these children contained significantly lower numbers of genes involved in the production of SCFAs [77]. This finding is in line with a previous study by de Goffau et al., reporting that β cell autoimmunity prior to T1DM onset is associated with a reduction in butyrate-producing species [72]. Dietary factors may induce changes in the composition of the gut microbiome, leading to both reduced butyrate production and enhanced risk of autoantibodies associated to the development of T1DM [78]. A recent metaproteomic analysis has also shown that microbial taxa associated with host proteins involved in maintaining function of the mucous barrier and microvilli adhesion were depleted in patients with new-onset T1DM [79]. Moreover, intestinal permeability was increased in children at risk of developing T1DM and correlated with microbiota alterations [85,86]. These findings support the notion that increased gut permeability is important in linking the microbiome to T1DM in humans as previously demonstrated in animal model of autoimmune diabetes.

Adding a further layer of complexity to the field, a recent study has shown that *HLA* can influence the composition of the human gut microbiome [80]. Indeed, genetic risk for developing T1DM autoimmunity was associated with distinct changes in the gut microbiome. Therefore, in T1DM genetic susceptibility can not only synergically interact with, but also contribute to shape the microbiome [80]. This finding may also be relevant for the design of future clinical studies as recruitment of children at high genetic risk for T1DM is less desirable than we previously thought because it can mask the effect of *HLA* on the microbiome.

Overall data in humans are more conflicting than in experimental animals. Most of the available data in humans come from underpowered case-control studies and this may partially explain inconsistencies. Moreover, human studies mainly prove associations between dysbiosis and T1DM rather than a causal relationship and they explored taxonomic rather than functional changes in the microbiota. New approaches such as metagenomics and metaproteomics applied to large cohort of patients and intervention studies may provide better insights on this topic in the future and move this area of research from a description of abnormalities to translational applications.

Table 1. Type 1 Diabetes and the Microbiota: Human Studies.

Study Design	Study Sample	Main Findings	Ref.
Prospective	In total, 33 genetically predisposed infants	Microbial diversity in T1DM progressors in the time window between seroconversion and T1DM onset and inflammation-favoring organisms	[71]
Case Control	In total, 18 Ab (+) vs. 18 Ab (−) children matched for HLA	Ab-positive children: microbial diversity, *Bacteroidetes* (*Bacteroides* and *Prevotella*), *Bifidobacterium* species, short-chain fatty acid (SCFA)-producing bacteria	[72]
Case Control (longitudinal data)	In total, four HLA-matched case (Ab+) –control (Ab−) pairs (three time points)	*Bacteroidetes* (Bacteroidales) and *Firmicutes* (Clostriales) in cases vs. controls at all time points. Children progressing T1DM: microbial diversity	[73]
Case Control	In total, 28 newly diagnosed type 1 diabetes (T1DM) (average duration 4.8 years) vs. 27 age-matched control children	In children < 3 years: *Bacteroidetes* in cases and *Clostridium clusters IV* and *XIVa* in controls	[74]
Case Control	In total, 16 T1DM vs. 16 healthy children	Cases: Bacteroidetes, Firmicutes and Actinobacteria	[75]
Case Control (longitudinal data)	In total, 29 Ab (+) cases vs. 47 Ab (−) healthy controls	*B. dorei* and *B. vulgatus* in cases prior to seroconversion	[76]
Prospective	In total, 783 genetically predisposed children	SCFA-producing bacteria genes in children who seroconverted or developed T1DM	[77]
Prospective	In total, 19 Ab (+) and 21 Ab (−) children	*Bacteroides Akkermansia* SCFA-producing bacteria genes. A functional association between diet (early introduction of non-milk diet), gut microbiome (*Bacteroides*), metagenomic changes (genes for the production of butyrate) and development of islet Ab	[78]
Case Control	In total, 33 recent-onset T1DM, 17 Ab (+), 29 Ab (−), and 22 healthy subjects	T1DM: microbial taxa associated with host proteins involved in maintaining the function of the mucous barrier, microvilli adhesion, and exocrine pancreas	[79]
Cohort Study	In total, 403 children (age = 1 year)	Genetic risk for developing T1DM autoimmunity is associated with distinct changes in the gut microbiome	[80]
RCT	T1DM children (8–17 years) randomized to prebiotic oligofructose-enriched inulin (n = 17) or placebo (n = 21) for 12 weeks	At 3 months, C-peptide was significantly higher in the group that received prebiotics	[81]
Prospective Cohort	In total, 7473 children (4–10 years)	Early probiotic supplementation (at the age of 0–27 days) associated with a decreased risk of islet autoimmunity in children with the *HLADR3/4* genotype	[82]

T1DM: type 1 diabetes, RCT: randomized control trial, HLA: human leukocyte antigen, Ab (+): islet auto-antibodies positive, and Ab (−): islet auto-antibodies negative.

6. Future perspective

Research on the microbiome in T1DM has expanded dramatically in recent years; however, a causal relationship between dysbiosis and the risk of T1DM has not yet been established in humans. Even though intervention studies in susceptible animals have provided evidence that strategies ameliorating/reversing dysbiosis reduce the incidence of T1DM, this evidence is still lacking in humans. However, tailored changes in the intestinal microbiome may represent a novel therapeutic approach for the primary prevention of T1DM and various strategies have been proposed to reshape the gut microbiota in children at high risk of T1DM. Infants delivered by C-section can be exposed to maternal vaginal fluids at birth to make their microbiota composition comparable to that of vaginally born babies [87]. Supplementation with LMP dietary fiber may be beneficial in humans as recently proven in mice. Prebiotics, such as inulin, lactulose, and in particular human milk oligosaccharides, can promote the growth of Bifidobacteria and a recent pilot study showed that treatment for 3 months with the prebiotic oligofructose-enriched inulin in children with T1DM significantly increased C-peptide levels [81]. Clinical trials are currently testing the efficacy of supplementation with probiotics in human T1DM [88]. Notably, a recent study demonstrated that the administration of probiotics in the first month of life was associated with a 60% reduction in the autoimmunity risk in children with the high-risk *HLA-DR3/4* genotype [82]. Moreover, a clinical trial with the probiotics Lactobacillus rhamnosus GG and Bifidobacterium lactis Bb12L is currently ongoing in children with new-onset T1DM [89]. In the era of precision medicine, personalized diets, tailored in accordance with both the host's genetic background and individual microbiome may hopefully correct dysbiosis and reduce the risk of developing T1DM.

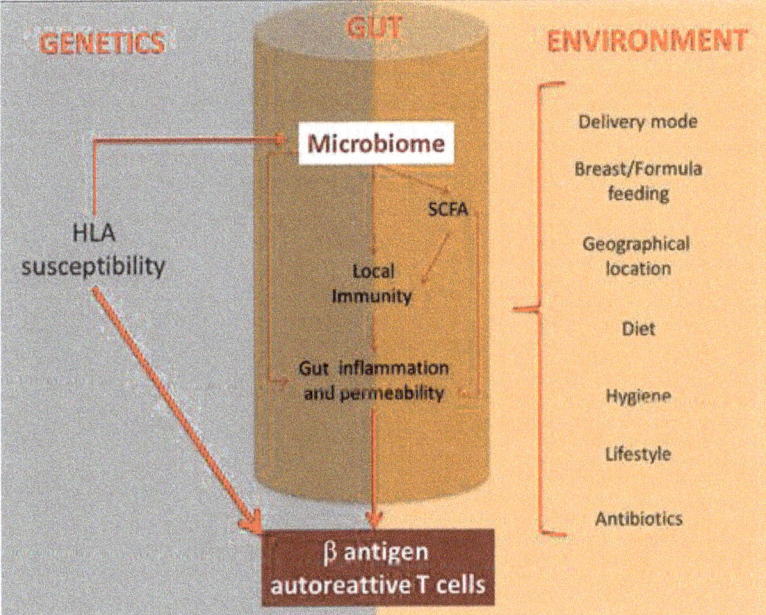

Figure 1. Interplay between genetics, environment, and gut microbiota in T1DM pathogenesis. Specific *HLA* allele can increase susceptibility to the development of type 1 diabetes and influence the composition of the gut microbiota. Many environmental factors can also shape the gut microbiota. Abnormalities in the gut microbiome are believed to favor autoimmunity against pancreatic b-cells by modulating the gut immune/inflammatory response and by enhancing the gut barrier permeability both directly and indirectly through reduced production of short-chain fatty acids (SCFAs).

Author Contributions: M.D. designed the review and critically revised the work; A.F. performed the research; M.D. and A.F. wrote the paper; G.G. revised the text.

Funding: This research received no external funding.

Acknowledgments: We apologize to all the investigators whose important works have not been cited due to space restrictions.

Conflicts of Interest: The authors declare no conflict of interest.

References

1. Gülden, E.; Wong, F.S.; Wen, L. The gut microbiota and type 1 diabetes. *Clin. Immunol.* **2015**, *159*, 143–153. [CrossRef] [PubMed]
2. Paun, A.; Yau, C.; Danska, J.S. The influence of the microbiome on type 1 diabetes. *J. Immunol.* **2017**, *198*, 590–595. [CrossRef] [PubMed]
3. Hu, C.; Wong, F.S.; Wen, L. Type 1 diabetes and gut microbiota: Friend or foe? *Pharmacol. Res.* **2015**, *98*, 9–15. [CrossRef] [PubMed]
4. American Diabetes Association. Classification and diagnosis of diabetes: Standards of medical care in diabetes. *Diabetes Care* **2019**, *4*, S13–S28. [CrossRef]
5. International Diabetes Federation. *IDF Diabetes Atlas*, 8th ed. 2017. Available online: http://www.diabetesatlas.org (accessed on 1 November 2019).
6. Soltesz, G.; Patterson, C.C.; Dahlquist, G.; EURODIAB Study Group. Worldwide childhood type 1 diabetes incidence–what can we learn from epidemiology? *Pediatric Diabetes* **2007**, *8*, 6–14. [CrossRef]
7. Patterson, C.C.; Gyürüs, E.; Rosenbauer, J.; Cinek, O.; Neu, A.; Schober, E.; Parslow, R.C.; Joner, G.; Svensson, J.; Castell, C. Trends in childhood type 1 diabetes incidence in Europe during 1989–2008: Evidence of non-uniformity over time in rates of increase. *Diabetologia* **2012**, *55*, 2142–2147. [CrossRef]
8. Harjutsalo, V.; Sjöberg, L.; Tuomilehto, J. Time trends in the incidence of type 1 diabetes in Finnish children: A cohort study. *Lancet* **2008**, *371*, 1777–1782. [CrossRef]
9. Knip, M.; Korhonen, S.; Kulmala, P.; Veijola, R.; Reunanen, A.; Raitakari, O.T.; Viikari, J.; Åkerblom, H.K. Prediction of type 1 diabetes in the general population. *Diabetes Care* **2010**, *33*, 1206–1212. [CrossRef]
10. Regnell, S.E.; Lernmark, Å. Early prediction of autoimmune (type 1) diabetes. *Diabetologia* **2017**, *60*, 1370–1381. [CrossRef]
11. Wolfsdorf, J.; Glaser, N.; Sperling, M.A. Diabetic ketoacidosis in infants, children, and adolescents: A consensus statement from the American Diabetes Association. *Diabetes care* **2006**, *29*, 1150–1159. [CrossRef]
12. Dayan, C.M.; Korah, M.; Tatovic, D.; Bundy, B.N.; Herold, K.C. Changing the landscape for type 1 diabetes: The first step to prevention. *Lancet* **2019**. [CrossRef]
13. Pociot, F.; Lernmark, Å. Genetic risk factors for type 1 diabetes. *Lancet* **2016**, *387*, 2331–2339. [CrossRef]
14. Sun, C.; Zhi, D.; Shen, S.; Luo, F.; Sanjeevi, C.B. SNPs in the exons of Toll-like receptors are associated with susceptibility to type 1 diabetes in Chinese population. *Hum. Immunol.* **2014**, *75*, 1084–1088. [CrossRef] [PubMed]
15. Infante, M.; Ricordi, C.; Sanchez, J.; Clare-Salzler, M.J.; Padilla, N.; Fuenmayor, V.; Chavez, C.; Alvarez, A.; Baidal, D.; Alejandro, R.; et al. Influence of Vitamin D on Islet Autoimmunity and Beta-Cell Function in Type 1 Diabetes. *Nutrients* **2019**, *11*, 2185. [CrossRef] [PubMed]
16. Nam, H.K.; Rhie, Y.J.; Lee, K.H. Vitamin D level and gene polymorphisms in Korean children with type 1 diabetes. *Pediatric Diabetes* **2019**, *20*, 750–758. [CrossRef] [PubMed]
17. Ahmed, A.E.A.; Sakhr, H.M.; Hassan, M.H.; El-Amir, M.I.; Ameen, H.H. Vitamin D receptor rs7975232, rs731236 and rs1544410 single nucleotide polymorphisms, and 25-hydroxyvitamin D levels in Egyptian children with type 1 diabetes mellitus: Effect of vitamin D co-therapy. *Diabetes Metab. Syndr. Obes.* **2019**, *12*, 703. [CrossRef] [PubMed]
18. Rewers, M.; Ludvigsson, J. Environmental risk factors for type 1 diabetes. *Lancet* **2016**, *387*, 2340–2348. [CrossRef]
19. Bäckhed, F.; Ley, R.E.; Sonnenburg, J.L.; Peterson, D.A.; Gordon, J.I. Host-bacterial mutualism in the human intestine. *Science* **2005**, *307*, 1915–1920. [CrossRef]
20. Sender, R.; Fuchs, S.; Milo, R. Are we really vastly outnumbered? Revisiting the ratio of bacterial to host cells in humans. *Cell* **2016**, *164*, 337–340. [CrossRef]

21. Fuks, G.; Elgart, M.; Amir, A.; Zeisel, A.; Turnbaugh, P.J.; Soen, Y.; Shental, N. Combining 16S rRNA gene variable regions enables high-resolution microbial community profiling. *Microbiome* **2018**, *6*, 17. [CrossRef]
22. Poretsky, R.; Rodriguez-R, L.M.; Luo, C.; Tsementzi, D.; Konstantinidis, K.T. Strengths and limitations of 16S rRNA gene amplicon sequencing in revealing temporal microbial community dynamics. *PLoS ONE* **2014**, *9*, e93827. [CrossRef] [PubMed]
23. Qin, J.; Li, R.; Raes, J.; Arumugam, M.; Burgdorf, K.S.; Manichanh, C.; Nielsen, T.; Pons, N.; Levenez, F.; Yamada, T.; et al. A human gut microbial gene catalogue established by metagenomic sequencing. *Nature* **2010**, *464*, 59. [CrossRef] [PubMed]
24. Eckburg, P.B.; Bik, E.M.; Bernstein, C.N.; Purdom, E.; Dethlefsen, L.; Sargent, M.; Gill, S.R.; Nelson, K.E.; Relman, D.A. Diversity of the human intestinal microbial flora. *Science* **2005**, *308*, 1635–1638. [CrossRef] [PubMed]
25. Yatsunenko, T.; Rey, F.E.; Manary, M.J.; Trehan, I.; Dominguez-Bello, M.G.; Contreras, M.; Magris, M.; Hidalgo, G.; Baldassano, R.N.; Anokhin, A.P.; et al. Human gut microbiome viewed across age and geography. *Nature* **2012**, *486*, 222. [CrossRef]
26. Bäckhed, F.; Roswall, J.; Peng, Y.; Feng, Q.; Jia, H.; Kovatcheva-Datchary, P.; Li, Y.; Xia, Y.; Xie, H.; Zhong, H.; et al. Dynamics and stabilization of the human gut microbiome during the first year of life. *Cell Host Microbe* **2015**, *17*, 690–703. [CrossRef]
27. Dominguez-Bello, M.G.; Costello, E.K.; Contreras, M.; Magris, M.; Hidalgo, G.; Fierer, N.; Knight, R. Delivery mode shapes the acquisition and structure of the initial microbiota across multiple body habitats in newborns. *Proc. Natl. Acad. Sci. USA* **2010**, *107*, 11971–11975. [CrossRef]
28. Ferretti, P.; Pasolli, E.; Tett, A.; Asnicar, F.; Gorfer, V.; Fedi, S.; Armanini, F.; Truong, D.T.; Manara, S.; Zolfo, M.; et al. Mother-to-infant microbial transmission from different body sites shapes the developing infant gut microbiome. *Cell Host Microbe* **2018**, *24*, 133–145. [CrossRef]
29. Rinninella, E.; Raoul, P.; Cintoni, M.; Franceschi, F.; Miggiano, G.A.D.; Gasbarrini, A.; Mele, M.C. What is the healthy gut microbiota composition? a changing ecosystem across age, environment, diet, and diseases. *Microorganisms* **2019**, *7*, 14. [CrossRef]
30. Praveen, P.; Jordan, F.; Priami, C.; Morine, M.J. The role of breast-feeding in infant immune system: A systems perspective on the intestinal microbiome. *Microbiome* **2015**, *3*, 41. [CrossRef]
31. Singh, R.K.; Chang, H.W.; Yan, D.; Lee, K.M.; Ucmak, D.; Wong, K.; Abrouk, M.; Farahnik, B.; Nakamura, M.; Zhu, T.H.; et al. Influence of diet on the gut microbiome and implications for human health. *J. Transl. Med.* **2017**, *15*, 73. [CrossRef]
32. De Filippo, C.; Cavalieri, D.; Di Paola, M.; Ramazzotti, M.; Poullet, J.B.; Massart, S.; Collini, S.; Pieraccini, G.; Lionetti, P. Impact of diet in shaping gut microbiota revealed by a comparative study in children from Europe and rural Africa. *Proc. Natl. Acad. Sci. USA* **2010**, *107*, 14691–14696. [CrossRef] [PubMed]
33. Venkataraman, R.; Juwal, J.; Princy, J. The effect of probiotics on glycemic index. *Panminerva Med.* **2018**, *60*, 234–235. [CrossRef] [PubMed]
34. Fjalstad, J.W.; Esaiassen, E.; Juvet, L.K.; van den Anker, J.N.; Klingenberg, C. Antibiotic therapy in neonates and impact on gut microbiota and antibiotic resistance development: A systematic review. *J. Antimicrob. Chemother.* **2017**, *73*, 569–580. [CrossRef] [PubMed]
35. Antonopoulos, D.A.; Huse, S.M.; Morrison, H.G.; Schmidt, T.M.; Sogin, M.L.; Young, V.B. Reproducible community dynamics of the gastrointestinal microbiota following antibiotic perturbation. *Infect. Immun.* **2009**, *77*, 2367–2375. [CrossRef] [PubMed]
36. Claesson, M.J.; Jeffery, I.B.; Conde, S.; Power, S.E.; O'connor, E.M.; Cusack, S.; Harris, H.M.; Coakley, M.; Lakshminarayanan, B.; O'Sullivan, O.; et al. Gut microbiota composition correlates with diet and health in the elderly. *Nature* **2012**, *488*, 178. [CrossRef] [PubMed]
37. Krishnan, S.; Alden, N.; Lee, K. Pathways and functions of gut microbiota metabolism impacting host physiology. *Curr. Opin. Biotechnol.* **2015**, *36*, 137–145. [CrossRef]
38. LeBlanc, J.G.; Chain, F.; Martín, R.; Bermúdez-Humarán, L.G.; Courau, S.; Langella, P. Beneficial effects on host energy metabolism of short-chain fatty acids and vitamins produced by commensal and probiotic bacteria. *Microb. Cell Fact* **2017**, *16*, 79. [CrossRef]
39. Thaiss, C.A.; Zmora, N.; Levy, M.; Elinav, E. The microbiome and innate immunity. *Nature* **2016**, *535*, 65. [CrossRef]

40. Luu, M.; Visekruna, A. Short-Chain fatty acids: Bacterial messengers modulating the immunometabolism of T cells. *Eur. J. Immunol.* **2019**, *49*, 842–848. [CrossRef]
41. Lazar, V.; Ditu, L.; Pircalabioru, G.; Gheorghe, I.; Curutiu, C.; Holban, A.M.; Chifiriuc, C.M. Aspects of gut microbiota and immune system interactions in infectious diseases, immunopathology and cancer. *Front. Immunol.* **2018**, *9*, 1830. [CrossRef]
42. Skonieczna-Żydecka, K.; Marlicz, W.; Misera, A.; Koulaouzidis, A.; Łoniewski, I. Microbiome—The Missing Link in the Gut-Brain Axis: Focus on Its Role in Gastrointestinal and Mental Health. *J. Clin. Med.* **2018**, *7*, 521. [CrossRef] [PubMed]
43. Petersen, C.; Round, J.L. Defining dysbiosis and its influence on host immunity and disease. *Cell Microbiol.* **2014**, *16*, 1024–1033. [CrossRef] [PubMed]
44. Vangay, P.; Ward, T.; Gerber, J.S.; Knights, D. Antibiotics, pediatric dysbiosis, and disease. *Cell Host Microbe* **2015**, *17*, 553–564. [CrossRef] [PubMed]
45. Brüssow, H. Problems with the concept of gut microbiota dysbiosis. *Microb. Biotechnol.* **2019**, 1–12. [CrossRef] [PubMed]
46. Brown, K.; Godovannyi, A.; Ma, C.; Zhang, Y.; Ahmadi-Vand, Z.; Dai, C.; Gorzelak, M.A.; Chan, Y.; Chan, J.M.; Lochner, A.; et al. Prolonged antibiotic treatment induces a diabetogenic intestinal microbiome that accelerates diabetes in NOD mice. *ISME J.* **2016**, *10*, 321. [CrossRef]
47. Daft, J.G.; Ptacek, T.; Kumar, R.; Morrow, C.; Lorenz, R.G. Cross-fostering immediately after birth induces a permanent microbiota shift that is shaped by the nursing mother. *Microbiome* **2015**, *3*, 17. [CrossRef]
48. Wen, L.; Ley, R.E.; Volchkov, P.Y.; Stranges, P.B.; Avanesyan, L.; Stonebraker, A.C.; Hu, C.; Wong, F.S.; Szot, G.L.; Bluestone, J.A.; et al. Innate immunity and intestinal microbiota in the development of Type 1 diabetes. *Nature* **2008**, *455*, 1109. [CrossRef]
49. Miranda, M.C.G.; Oliveira, R.P.; Torres, L.; Aguiar, S.L.F.; Pinheiro Rosa, N.; Lemos, L.; Guimarães, M.A.; Reis, D.; Silveira, T.; Ferreira, Ê.; et al. Frontline Science: Abnormalities in the gut mucosa of non-obese diabetic mice precede the onset of type 1 diabetes. *J. Leukoc. Biol.* **2019**, *106*, 513–529. [CrossRef]
50. Caviglia, G.P.; Rosso, C.; Ribaldone, D.G.; Dughera, F.; Fagoonee, S.; Astegiano, M.; Pellicano, R. Physiopathology of intestinal barrier and the role of zonulin. *Minerva Biotecnol.* **2019**, *31*, 83–92. [CrossRef]
51. Neu, J.; Reverte, C.M.; Mackey, A.D.; Liboni, K.; Tuhacek-Tenace, L.M.; Hatch, M.; Li, N.; Caicedo, R.A.; Schatz, D.A.; Atkinson, M. Changes in intestinal morphology and permeability in the biobreeding rat before the onset of type 1 diabetes. *J. Pediatric Gastroenterol. Nutr.* **2005**, *40*, 589–595. [CrossRef]
52. Vaarala, O.; Atkinson, M.A.; Neu, J. The "perfect storm" for type 1 diabetes: The complex interplay between intestinal microbiota, gut permeability, and mucosal immunity. *Diabetes* **2008**, *57*, 2555–2562. [CrossRef] [PubMed]
53. Lee, A.S.; Gibson, D.L.; Zhang, Y.; Sham, H.P.; Vallance, B.A.; Dutz, J.P. Gut barrier disruption by an enteric bacterial pathogen accelerates insulitis in NOD mice. *Diabetologia* **2010**, *53*, 741–748. [CrossRef] [PubMed]
54. Turley, S.J.; Lee, J.W.; Dutton-Swain, N.; Mathis, D.; Benoist, C. Endocrine self and gut non-self intersect in the pancreatic lymph nodes. *Proc. Natl. Acad. Sci. USA* **2005**, *102*, 17729–17733. [CrossRef] [PubMed]
55. Sorini, C.; Cosorich, I.; Conte, M.L.; De Giorgi, L.; Facciotti, F.; Lucianò, R.; Rocchi, M.; Ferrarese, R.; Sanvito, F.; Canducci, F.; et al. Loss of gut barrier integrity triggers activation of islet-reactive T cells and autoimmune diabetes. *Proc. Natl. Acad. Sci. USA* **2019**, *116*, 15140–15149. [CrossRef] [PubMed]
56. Calcinaro, F.; Dionisi, S.; Marinaro, M.; Candeloro, P.; Bonato, V.; Marzotti, S.; Corneli, R.B.; Ferretti, E.; Gulino, A.; Grasso, F.; et al. Oral probiotic administration induces interleukin-10 production and prevents spontaneous autoimmune diabetes in the non-obese diabetic mouse. *Diabetologia* **2005**, *48*, 1565–1575. [CrossRef] [PubMed]
57. Dolpady, J.; Sorini, C.; Di Pietro, C.; Cosorich, I.; Ferrarese, R.; Saita, D.; Clementi, M.; Canducci, F.; Falcone, M. Oral probiotic VSL# 3 prevents autoimmune diabetes by modulating microbiota and promoting indoleamine 2, 3-dioxygenase-enriched tolerogenic intestinal environment. *J. Diabetes Res.* **2016**, *2016*, 7569431. [CrossRef] [PubMed]
58. Valladares, R.; Sankar, D.; Li, N.; Williams, E.; Lai, K.K.; Abdelgeliel, A.S.; Gonzalez, C.F.; Wasserfall, C.H.; Larkin, J.; Schatz, D.; et al. Lactobacillus johnsonii N6. 2 mitigates the development of type 1 diabetes in BB-DP rats. *PLoS ONE* **2010**, *5*, e10507. [CrossRef]

59. Chen, K.; Chen, H.; Faas, M.M.; de Haan, B.J.; Li, J.; Xiao, P.; Zhang, H.; Diana, J.; de Vos, P.; Sun, J. Specific inulin-type fructan fibers protect against autoimmune diabetes by modulating gut immunity, barrier function, and microbiota homeostasis. *Mol. Nutr. Food Res.* **2017**, *61*, 1601006. [CrossRef]
60. Hansen, C.H.F.; Krych, L.; Nielsen, D.S.; Vogensen, F.K.; Hansen, L.H.; Sørensen, S.J.; Buschard, K.; Hansen, A.K. Early life treatment with vancomycin propagates Akkermansia muciniphila and reduces diabetes incidence in the NOD mouse. *Diabetologia* **2012**, *55*, 2285–2294. [CrossRef]
61. Brugman, S.; Klatter, F.A.; Visser, J.T.J.; Wildeboer-Veloo, A.C.M.; Harmsen, H.J.M.; Rozing, J.; Bos, N.A. Antibiotic treatment partially protects against type 1 diabetes in the Bio-Breeding diabetes-prone rat. Is the gut flora involved in the development of type 1 diabetes? *Diabetologia* **2006**, *49*, 2105–2108. [CrossRef]
62. Hu, Y.; Jin, P.; Peng, J.; Zhang, X.; Wong, F.S.; Wen, L. Different immunological responses to early-life antibiotic exposure affecting autoimmune diabetes development in NOD mice. *J. Autoimmun.* **2016**, *72*, 47–56. [CrossRef] [PubMed]
63. Livanos, A.E.; Greiner, T.U.; Vangay, P.; Pathmasiri, W.; Stewart, D.; McRitchie, S.; Li, H.; Chung, J.; Sohn, J.; Kim, S.; et al. Antibiotic-Mediated gut microbiome perturbation accelerates development of type 1 diabetes in mice. *Nat. Microbiol.* **2016**, *1*, 16140. [CrossRef] [PubMed]
64. Hara, N.; Alkanani, A.K.; Ir, D.; Robertson, C.E.; Wagner, B.D.; Frank, D.N.; Zipris, D. Prevention of virus-induced type 1 diabetes with antibiotic therapy. *J. Immunol.* **2012**, *189*, 3805–3814. [CrossRef] [PubMed]
65. Mariño, E.; Richards, J.L.; McLeod, K.H.; Stanley, D.; Yap, Y.A.; Knight, J.; McKenzie, C.; Kranich, J.; Oliveira, A.C.; Rossello, F.J.; et al. Gut microbial metabolites limit the frequency of autoimmune T cells and protect against type 1 diabetes. *Nat. Immunol.* **2017**, *18*, 552. [CrossRef] [PubMed]
66. Needell, J.C.; Ir, D.; Robertson, C.E.; Kroehl, M.E.; Frank, D.N.; Zipris, D. Maternal treatment with short-chain fatty acids modulates the intestinal microbiota and immunity and ameliorates type 1 diabetes in the offspring. *PLoS ONE* **2017**, *12*, e0183786. [CrossRef] [PubMed]
67. Candon, S.; Perez-Arroyo, A.; Marquet, C.; Valette, F.; Foray, A.P.; Pelletier, B.; Milani, C.; Ventura, M.; Bach, J.F.; Chatenoud, L. Antibiotics in early life alter the gut microbiome and increase disease incidence in a spontaneous mouse model of autoimmune insulin-dependent diabetes. *PLoS ONE* **2015**, *10*, e0125448. [CrossRef] [PubMed]
68. Zhang, X.S.; Li, J.; Krautkramer, K.A.; Badri, M.; Battaglia, T.; Borbet, T.C.; Koh, H.; Ng, S.; Sibley, R.A.; Li, Y.; et al. Antibiotic-induced acceleration of type 1 diabetes alters maturation of innate intestinal immunity. *Elife* **2018**, *7*, e37816. [CrossRef]
69. Wu, C.; Pan, L.L.; Niu, W.; Fang, X.; Liang, W.; Li, J.; Li, H.; Pan, X.; Chen, W.; Zhang, H.; et al. Modulation of gut microbiota by low methoxyl pectin attenuates type 1 diabetes in non-obese diabetic mice. *Front. Immunol.* **2019**, *10*, 1733. [CrossRef]
70. Jia, L.; Shan, K.; Pan, L.L.; Feng, N.; Lv, Z.; Sun, Y.; Li, J.; Wu, C.; Zhang, H.; Chen, W.; et al. Clostridium butyricum CGMCC0313.1 protects against autoimmune diabetes by modulating intestinal immune homeostasis and inducing pancreatic regulatory T cells. *Front. Immunol.* **2017**, *8*, 1345. [CrossRef]
71. Kostic, A.D.; Gevers, D.; Siljander, H.; Vatanen, T.; Hyötyläinen, T.; Hämäläinen, A.M.; Peet, A.; Tillmann, V.; Pöhö, P.; Mattila, I.; et al. The dynamics of the human infant gut microbiome in development and in progression toward type 1 diabetes. *Cell Host Microbe* **2015**, *17*, 260–273. [CrossRef]
72. De Goffau, M.C.; Luopajärvi, K.; Knip, M.; Ilonen, J.; Ruohtula, T.; Härkönen, T.; Orivuori, L.; Hakala, S.; Welling, G.W.; Harmsen, H.J.; et al. Fecal microbiota composition differs between children with β-cell autoimmunity and those without. *Diabetes* **2012**, *62*, 1238–1244. [CrossRef] [PubMed]
73. Giongo, A.; Gano, K.A.; Crabb, D.B.; Mukherjee, N.; Novelo, L.L.; Casella, G.; Drew, J.C.; Ilonen, J.; Knip, M.; Hyöty, H.; et al. Toward defining the autoimmune microbiome for type 1 diabetes. *ISME J.* **2011**, *5*, 82. [CrossRef] [PubMed]
74. De Goffau, M.C.; Fuentes, S.; van den Bogert, B.; Honkanen, H.; de Vos, W.M.; Welling, G.W.; Hyöty, H.; Harmsen, H.J. Aberrant gut microbiota composition at the onset of type 1 diabetes in young children. *Diabetologia* **2014**, *57*, 1569–1577. [CrossRef] [PubMed]
75. Murri, M.; Leiva, I.; Gomez-Zumaquero, J.M.; Tinahones, F.J.; Cardona, F.; Soriguer, F.; Queipo-Ortuño, M.I. Gut microbiota in children with type 1 diabetes differs from that in healthy children: A case-control study. *BMC Med.* **2013**, *11*, 46. [CrossRef] [PubMed]

76. Davis-Richardson, A.G.; Ardissone, A.N.; Dias, R.; Simell, V.; Leonard, M.T.; Kemppainen, K.M.; Drew, J.C.; Schatz, D.; Atkinson, M.A.; Kolaczkowski, B.; et al. Bacteroides dorei dominates gut microbiome prior to autoimmunity in Finnish children at high risk for type 1 diabetes. *Front. Microbiol.* **2014**, *5*, 678. [CrossRef]
77. Vatanen, T.; Franzosa, E.A.; Schwager, R.; Tripathi, S.; Arthur, T.D.; Vehik, K.; Lernmark, Å.; Hagopian, W.A.; Rewers, M.J.; She, J.X.; et al. The human gut microbiome in early-onset type 1 diabetes from the TEDDY study. *Nature* **2018**, *562*, 589. [CrossRef]
78. Endesfelder, D.; Engel, M.; Davis-Richardson, A.G.; Ardissone, A.N.; Achenbach, P.; Hummel, S.; Winkler, C.; Atkinson, M.; Schatz, D.; Triplett, E.; et al. Towards a functional hypothesis relating anti-islet cell autoimmunity to the dietary impact on microbial communities and butyrate production. *Microbiome* **2016**, *4*, 17. [CrossRef]
79. Gavin, P.G.; Mullaney, J.A.; Loo, D.; Lê Cao, K.A.; Gottlieb, P.A.; Hill, M.M.; Zipris, D.; Hamilton-Williams, E.E. Intestinal metaproteomics reveals host-microbiota interactions in subjects at risk for type 1 diabetes. *Diabetes Care* **2018**, *41*, 2178–2186. [CrossRef]
80. Russell, J.T.; Roesch, L.F.; Ördberg, M.; Ilonen, J.; Atkinson, M.A.; Schatz, D.A.; Triplett, E.W.; Ludvigsson, J. Genetic risk for autoimmunity is associated with distinct changes in the human gut microbiome. *Nat. Commun.* **2019**, *10*, 1–12. [CrossRef]
81. Ho, J.; Nicolucci, A.C.; Virtanen, H.; Schick, A.; Meddings, J.; Reimer, R.A.; Huang, C. Effect of prebiotic on microbiota, intestinal permeability and glycemic control in children with type 1 diabetes. *J. Clin. Endocrinol. Metab.* **2019**, *104*, 4427–4440. [CrossRef]
82. Uusitalo, U.; Liu, X.; Yang, J.; Aronsson, C.A.; Hummel, S.; Butterworth, M.; Lernmark, Å.; Rewers, M.; Hagopian, W.; She, J.X.; et al. Association of early exposure of probiotics and islet autoimmunity in the TEDDY study. *JAMA Pediatric* **2016**, *170*, 20–28. [CrossRef] [PubMed]
83. Canani, R.B.; Di Costanzo, M.; Leone, L.; Pedata, M.; Meli, R.; Calignano, A. Potential beneficial effects of butyrate in intestinal and extraintestinal diseases. *World J. Gastroenterol.* **2011**, *17*, 1519. [CrossRef] [PubMed]
84. Vatanen, T.; Kostic, A.D.; d'Hennezel, E.; Siljander, H.; Franzosa, E.A.; Yassour, M.; Kolde, R.; Vlamakis, H.; Arthur, T.D.; Hämäläinen, A.M.; et al. Variation in microbiome LPS immunogenicity contributes to autoimmunity in humans. *Cell* **2016**, *165*, 842–853. [CrossRef] [PubMed]
85. Maffeis, C.; Martina, A.; Corradi, M.; Quarella, S.; Nori, N.; Torriani, S.; Plebani, M.; Contreas, G.; Felis, G.E. Association between intestinal permeability and faecal microbiota composition in Italian children with beta cell autoimmunity at risk for type 1 diabetes. *Diabetes Metab. Res. Rev.* **2016**, *32*, 700–709. [CrossRef] [PubMed]
86. Harbison, J.E.; Roth-Schulze, A.J.; Giles, L.C.; Tran, C.D.; Ngui, K.M.; Penno, M.A.; Thomson, R.L.; Wentworth, J.M.; Colman, P.G.; Craig, M.E.; et al. Gut microbiome dysbiosis and increased intestinal permeability in children with islet autoimmunity and type 1 diabetes: A prospective cohort study. *Pediatric Diabetes* **2019**, *20*, 574–583. [CrossRef]
87. Dominguez-Bello, M.G.; De Jesus-Laboy, K.M.; Shen, N.; Cox, L.M.; Amir, A.; Gonzalez, A.; Bokulich, N.A.; Song, S.J.; Hoashi, M.; Rivera-Vinas, J.I.; et al. Partial restoration of the microbiota of cesarean-born infants via vaginal microbial transfer. *Nat. Med.* **2016**, *22*, 250. [CrossRef]
88. Mishra, S.; Wang, S.; Nagpal, R.; Miller, B.; Singh, R.; Taraphder, S.; Yadav, H. Probiotics and prebiotics for the amelioration of type 1 diabetes: Present and future perspectives. *Microorganisms* **2019**, *7*, 67. [CrossRef]
89. Groele, L.; Szajewska, H.; Szypowska, A. Effects of Lactobacillus rhamnosus GG and Bifidobacterium lactis Bb12 on beta-cell function in children with newly diagnosed type 1 diabetes: Protocol of a randomised controlled trial. *BMJ Open* **2017**, *7*, e017178. [CrossRef]

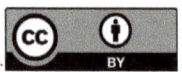

© 2019 by the authors. Licensee MDPI, Basel, Switzerland. This article is an open access article distributed under the terms and conditions of the Creative Commons Attribution (CC BY) license (http://creativecommons.org/licenses/by/4.0/).

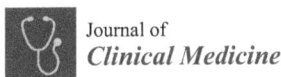

Review

Gut Microbiota and Liver Interaction through Immune System Cross-Talk: A Comprehensive Review at the Time of the SARS-CoV-2 Pandemic

Emidio Scarpellini [1,2,*], Sharmila Fagoonee [3], Emanuele Rinninella [4,5], Carlo Rasetti [1], Isabella Aquila [6], Tiziana Larussa [7], Pietrantonio Ricci [6], Francesco Luzza [7] and Ludovico Abenavoli [7,*]

1. Internal Medicine Unit, "Madonna del Soccorso" General Hospital, San Benedetto del, 63074 Tronto, Italy; bonimv@libero.it
2. Department of Biomedical Sciences, KU Leuven, Gasthuisberg University Hospital, TARGID, 3000 Leuven, Belgium
3. Institute for Biostructure and Bioimaging, National Research Council, Molecular Biotechnology Center, 10121 Turin, Italy; sharmila.fagoonee@unito.it
4. Nephrology and Urology Department, Gastroenterology, Endocrinology, Fondazione Policlinico A, Clinical Nutrition Unit, Gemelli IRCCS, 00168 Rome, Italy; e.rinninella@gmail.com
5. Institute of Medical Pathology, Catholic University of the Sacred Heart, 00168 Rome, Italy
6. Institute of Legal Medicine and Department of Surgical and Medical Sciences, University "Magna Graecia" of Catanzaro (UMG), 88100 Viale Europa, Italy; isabella.aquila@hotmail.it (I.A.); ricci@unicz.it (P.R.)
7. Department of Health Sciences, University "Magna Græcia", 88100 Catanzaro, Italy; tiziana.larussa@gmail.com (T.L.); luzza@unicz.it (F.L.)
* Correspondence: scarpidio@gmail.com (E.S.); l.abenavoli@unicz.it (L.A.); Tel.: +39-0735-793304 or +39-0735-793306 (E.S.); +39-0961-3694387 (L.A.); Fax: +39-0961-754220 (L.A.)

Received: 2 July 2020; Accepted: 28 July 2020; Published: 3 August 2020

Abstract: Background and aims: The gut microbiota is a complex ecosystem containing bacteria, viruses, fungi, yeasts and other single-celled organisms. It is involved in the development and maintenance of both innate and systemic immunity of the body. Emerging evidence has shown its role in liver diseases through the immune system cross-talk. We review herein literature data regarding the triangular interaction between gut microbiota, immune system and liver in health and disease. Methods: We conducted a search on the main medical databases for original articles, reviews, meta-analyses, randomized clinical trials and case series using the following keywords and acronyms and their associations: gut microbiota, microbiome, gut virome, immunity, gastrointestinal-associated lymphoid tissue (GALT), non-alcoholic fatty liver disease (NAFLD), non-alcoholic steato hepatitis (NASH), alcoholic liver disease, liver cirrhosis, hepatocellular carcinoma. Results: The gut microbiota consists of microorganisms that educate our systemic immunity through GALT and non-GALT interactions. The latter maintain health but are also involved in the pathophysiology and in the outcome of several liver diseases, particularly those with metabolic, toxic or immune-mediated etiology. In this context, gut virome has an emerging role in liver diseases and needs to be further investigated, especially due to the link reported between severe acute respiratory syndrome-coronavirus-2 (SARS-CoV-2) infection and hepatic dysfunctions. Conclusions: Changes in gut microbiota composition and alterations in the immune system response are involved in the pathogenesis of metabolic and immune-mediated liver diseases.

Keywords: gut microbiota; gut virome; steatosis; cirrhosis; hepatocellular carcinoma

1. Introduction

The human microbiota, now considered as a functional organ in se, consists of a complex community of microorganisms (bacteria, yeasts, fungi, archea, protozoa and virus), living on our skin and mucosal tissues, hence forming an efficient ecosystem with the body [1,2].

Despite the apparent alliance between gut microbiota and its host, this intimate relationship poses a permanent threat to the host's health, requiring constant control. Thus, the role of the human immune system in fine-tuning and shaping the microbiota is of paramount importance [3].

The function of microbiota can be further extrapolated and considered beneficial or pathological beyond the gastrointestinal (GI) tract, for example in the liver. In fact, venous blood flow from the gut reaches the liver via the portal vein, carrying microbial products and inducing the host's immunological responses to these. On the other hand, the liver produces bile that flows to the gut directly and influences the resident microbial environment [4]. This circulatory loop between liver and gut is an explicative tale of how changes in the gut flora can have both beneficial and/or harmful consequences for the host [5].

This review summarizes the evidences on the triangular interaction between gut microbiota, immune system and liver, in health and disease. Since the epidemiology of chronic liver diseases is changing, due to the decreasing rate of viral hepatitis and the increasing new epidemic of a wide spectrum of alcoholic and non-alcoholic fatty liver disease (NAFLD) [6,7], we focus our attention on non-viral hepatitis. Furthermore, due to the link reported between severe acute respiratory syndrome-coronavirus 2 (SARS-CoV-2) infection and hepatic dysfunctions, we outline the emerging role of the gut virome in liver diseases.

2. Methods

We conducted a PubMed and Medline search for original articles, reviews, meta-analyses and case series using the following keywords, their acronyms and their associations: gut microbiota, microbiome, gut virome, immunity, gastrointestinal associated lymphoid tissue (GALT), liver disease, non-alcoholic fatty liver disease, non-alcoholic steato-hepatitis (NASH), alcoholic liver disease, liver cirrhosis and hepatocellular carcinoma. When appropriate, preliminary evidences from abstracts belonging to main national and international gastroenterological meetings (e.g., United European Gastroenterology Week, Digestive Disease Week) were also included. The papers found from the above mentioned sources were reviewed by two of the authors (L.A. and E.S.) according to PRISMA guidelines [8]. The last MEDLINE search was performed on 30th April 2020.

3. Gut Microbiota, Immune System and Liver Diseases

3.1. Gut Microbiota Composition and Main Functions

The human GI tract hosts over 100 trillion microbes, predominantly bacteria. Intriguingly, the total number of microbes outnumbers by about ten times that of the cells of the human body [3]. Taxonomically, bacteria harbouring human gut microbiota are divided in phyla, classes, orders, families, genera, and species. A few phyla include more than 160 species [9]. The main gut microbial phyla are: *Firmicutes, Bacteroidetes, Actinobacteria, Proteobacteria, Fusobacteria,* and *Verrucomicrobia*. The two phyla *Firmicutes* and *Bacteroidetes* account for almost 90% of the entire gut microbiota with the former being composed of more than 200 different genera (e.g., *Lactobacillus, Bacillus, Clostridium, Enterococcus, Ruminicoccus* and *Clostridium*) and *Bacteroidetes* having two predominant genera (namely, *Bacteroides* and *Prevotella*) [1,9].

The collective genome of the gut microbiota (called microbiome) tends to be 150-fold bigger than that of human cells. This may explain the fact that gut microbiota composition variability inter-subjects is almost infinite [10]. Around one-tenth of the total colonizing bacterial species per individual constitute a plastic "microbial fingerprint" varying through life, starting from delivery to ageing, and subject to dietary changes and exposure to antibiotics, prebiotics and probiotics [11].

Indeed, a microbial 'core' intestinal microbiota includes 66 species conserved in over 50% of the general population. Nevertheless, the majority of species are individual-specific [12]. The use of culture-based methods has limited the study of gut microbiome. On the contrary, the use of new metagenomic technologies has unravelled the limitless potential for inter/intra-individual variability of gut microbiome [11].

Microbial life starts with a limited and unstable repertoire of microorganisms amenable to changes to allow evolution of a stable ecosystem. Thus, caesarean-born neonates acquire the dominant bacterial phyla, *Firmicutes* and *Bacteroidetes*, at a later stage than those born transvaginally. On the other hand, infants born transvaginally have a more precocious skin and oral microbiota colonization [13].

The first year of neonatal life frames a critical window, shaping the composition of the microbiota, influenced primarily by maternal-neonate interactions [14]. Changes in gut microbiota ensue through adolescence until a stable asset is reached in adulthood. This setup is variably modulated by diet, lifestyle, drugs/substances/food use and abuse until another shift in the elderly and very ultra-elderly occurs [15].

Gut microbiota is crucial for nutrients absorption and fermentation, regulation of intestinal permeability (IP), host metabolism (e.g., carbohydrates absorption and processing, proteins putrefaction, bile acids formation, insulin sensitivity) and last but not least, modulation of intestinal and systemic immunity, thus maintaining antigen tolerance and avoiding pathogen expansion [16]. Thousands of years of microbial and immune bidirectional evolution have created a harmonious co-existence that can be disrupted and re-established in a continuous manner both in health and disease in humans [3,17].

3.2. GALT and Non-GALT Systems and Their Interactions with Gut Microbiota

The small intestine itself is a barrier towards the environment. In fact, it consists of one mucosal layer with epithelial cell-derived antimicrobial peptides (RegIIIγ) that prevent bacterial penetration through the mucus layer [18,19] (Figure 1).

Gut microbiota composition changes throughout the entire GI tract. This variation depends on different environmental conditions of the diverse tracts. More specifically, one of these environmental conditions is represented by changes in IP, resembled by alterations in the tight junctions (TJ). TJ are plastic gates for the translocation of microbial antigens and drive systemic inflammation. In fact, changes in the expression of claudin (one of the proteins constituting the TJ) have been associated with the development of colitis in animal models [20,21]. On the other hand, tight junctions closing is impaired by various inflammatory cytokines [22]. There is also a putative role for modified claudin expression in mucosal immunity dysfunctions [22]. More recently, it has been shown that activation of myosin light chain kinase (MLCK), by the cytokines tumor necrosis factor (TNF) and interferon (IFN)-γ, may affect mucosal permeability through the endocytosis of occludin proteins belonging to TJ [23]. Furthermore, MLCK can also be activated by *Escherichia coli* (*E. coli*) bacterial lipopolysaccharide (LPS) and interleukin (IL)-1β [22].

The role and behaviour of gut microbiota in the modulation of GALT has been clarified by experiments on germ-free animals [24]. GALT is composed by Peyer's patches and mesenteric lymph nodes [25]. Although GALT tolerance is genetically programmed, its maturation and development (e.g., isolated lymphoid follicles—ILFs) are dependent on the environment [26]. Indeed, germ-free mice have hypoplastic Peyer's patches/mesenteric lymph nodes but no ILFs in the small intestine [27]. Prenatal Peyer's patches and mesenteric lymph nodes functioning is driven by pro-inflammatory lymphoid tissue inducers (LTi), innate lymphoid cells able to recruit and send B and T lymphocytes into B-cell follicles and T-cell zones, respectively, in the absence of microbiota [27]. Postnatally, ILFs are also driven by LTi cells but only after microbiota colonization of the GI tract. Therefore, ILFs are able to control gut homeostasis through microbes. In fact, mice with LTi cells dysfunction have an overgrowth of anaerobic, Gram-negative bacteria in the gut [28].

GALT is able to inform and educate both the innate and adaptive immune system through antigen-sampling of gut microbiota via specialized M cells [28,29]. Microbe-associated molecular patterns (MAMPs) (e.g., peptidoglycan, LPS) can be recognized by several pattern recognition receptors present on enterocytes' surface (namely, toll-like receptor (TLR) and cytosolic nucleotide-binding oligomerization domain (NOD)-like receptor), resulting in ILFs development and production of other antibacterial proteins [29]. On the other hand, gut microbiota is also able to modulate signal transduction through interaction with enterocytes. This process helps in maintaining a microbial balance, hence preserving host health [3].

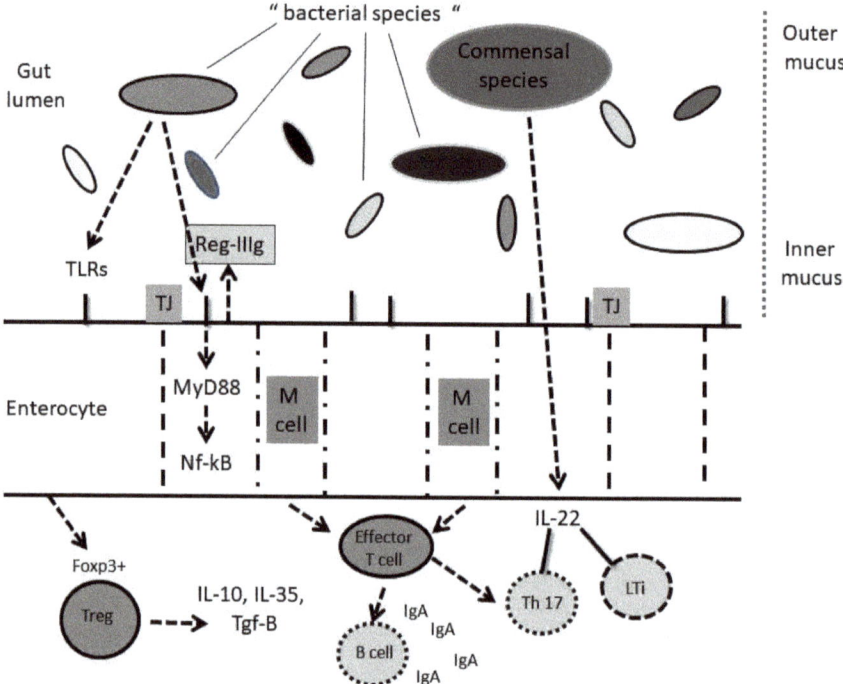

Figure 1. Example of microbial-immune interplay through intestine in hepatic diseases. M cells "sense" gut microbiota and educate mucosal immunity. In particular; Toll Like receptors (TLRs) on the enterocytes' surface sense microbe associated molecular patterns (MAMPs) and pathogen associated molecular patterns (PAMPs) are allowed to pass through tight juctions (TJ) among cells with production of nuclear factor (NF)k-B via the MY-D88 pathway. This results in anti-microbial peptides production (namely, RegIIIy) that regulate the resident gut microbiota.

3.3. The Immune System

3.3.1. Innate Immunity

TLRs activate downstream signals primarily facilitated by the adaptor protein MyD88. This process seems to be crucial for survival as indicated by MyD88 deficient control animals [30]. This step helps immune system to recognize commensal from pathogenic bacteria [3].

When commensal bacteria are recognized by TLRs, they induce a significant production of cytoprotective cytokines, heat-shock and anti-microbial proteins. In fact, Biswas et al. showed that TLR signalling downregulation by protein IRAK-M is able to protect from colitis development by maintaining intestinal microbiota homeostasis [31].

Moreover, innate NOD-like receptors (NLRs) help in the maintenance of gut microbial homeostasis. Similar to TLRs, these are intracellular proteins able to activate nuclear factor (NF)-κB and other transcriptional factors, the mutations of which are implicated in the pathogenesis of inflammatory bowel diseases (IBD) [32–34]. Importantly, a subset of NLRs can activate caspase-1 through the assembly of the inflammasome, a multiprotein complex associated with the production of interleukin IL-1β and IL-1, which are protective against colitis development [35].

3.3.2. Adaptive Immunity

Adaptive immunity involves both T and B cells. T cells' highly diverse receptors are able to recognize distinct molecular sequences; B cells have other receptors generated by somatic hypermutations. Altogether, these receptors allow a highly specific, direct immune response and generate the well-known immunological memory that is the core of adaptive immunity [36].

T and B cells interact via a continuous crosstalk (Figure 1). Gut microbiota educate and stimulate T lymphocyte subsets in the intestinal lamina propria. This has been shown in germ-free animals with T cell deficiencies that are partially restored by gut microbiota reshuffling [37]. These features are typical of immune-mediated allergies and hypersensitivities [38].

Gut colonization with single filamentous bacteria can lead to the induction of IL-17 and IL-22 secreting CD4+ lymphocytes (Th17 cells) [39], formerly associated with *Helicobacter pylori*-induced gastritis [40]. However, the induction of these effector T cells is crucial in lowering the number of pathogenic bacteria. Indeed, mice lacking single filamentous bacteria colonization cannot counteract the growth of the pathogenic *Citrobacter rodentium*, a strain very similar to the human-associated pathogen *E. coli* [39,40]. Not only the single filamentous bacteria but also typical dendritic resident intestinal CD70^{high}CD11c^{low} antigen-presenting cells interacting with adenosine triphosphate (ATP) are able to regulate Th17 differentiation [41].

Finally, the quick shift towards a pathogenetic immunological environment may affect gut microbiota. For example, non-pathogenic *E. coli* and *Enterococcus faecalis* (*E. faecalis*) are capable of inducing an aggressive Th1/Th17 pancolitis in IL-10 knockout mice, thus further altering the gut microbiota [41].

Regulatory T cells (namely, T$_{regs}$) can suppress the intestinal inflammation and maintain commensal microbiota tolerance through a mutual interaction [42]. These cells represent 1–3% of circulating CD4+T cells and have a high expression of CD25 as well as of intracellular transcription factor forkhead box P3 (FOXP3) [43,44]. Notably, their concentration is higher in the gut [45,46]. They inhibit the effector T lymphocytes (Th1, Th2 and Th17) and antigen-presenting cells [46,47], mainly through the production of IL-10 [47]. Indeed, germ-free mice show reduced levels of T$_{regs}$ in the colon [48].

From an evolutionistic point of view, it is conceivable that gut microbiota has evolved enhancing these natural anti-inflammatory T cells components (namely T$_{regs}$). DNA sequencing has unravelled the microbial-immune system interactions. For instance, polysaccharide A, a bacterial component of the commensal bug *Bacteroides fragilis*, is able to promote the differentiation of IL-10-producing T$_{regs}$ through an interaction with TLR2 expressed on T cells [49,50]. In addition, Gram-positive *Clostridia* colonization prevents the development of dextran sulphate sodium (DSS)-induced colitis through a T-reg-mediated mechanism [50,51]. Furthermore, fermentation of complex carbohydrates by the microbiota leads to the production of short chain fatty acids (namely, acetic acid, propionic acid and butyric acid) in the colon. These products also induce T$_{reg}$ proliferation [51]. On the contrary, the recently recognized microbial TLR ligand, cytosine–guanine (CpG)-containing DNA, can have both direct and indirect suppressive effects on T$_{regs}$ [52].

A recent paper by Wesemann et al. has shown that the very first B cells can develop in the intestinal mucosa with the production of modulating immunoglobulins (Ig) [53]. Germ-free mice colonization with commensals gut bacteria are able to increase recombination activating gene (RAG) endonucleases, involved in the production of both heavy and light Ig chains [53]. This microbial-dependent maturation of B cells is crucial for removing autoreactive B cells responsible for autoimmunity. In fact, in systemic lupus erythematosus, B cells are deficient in gut homing receptors [54,55].

All the evidences considered so far support the ability of the gut microbiota in educating our GALT- and non-GALT-associated immune systems. Within this chain of events, gut microbiota helps

GALT to produce B cells. In particular, the production of IgA involves CD40-CD40L interactions among B and activated T cells. Thus, the strict and complex interplay between B cells and gut microbiota supports the hypothesis that microbial diversity is responsible for regulatory B cells formation [56].

More in particular; commensal (e.g., single filamentous bacteria) and/or probiotic strains are able to induce the development of T helper 17 cells (Th17); regulatory T cells (Tregs) can produce immunoregulatory cytokines (e.g., IL-10 TGF-β and IL-35) balancing the mutual coexistence of the microbial species. Th17 cells and lymphoid tissue inducers (LTi) through IL-22 production, and the consequent step-down in RegIIIγ production, further reshape the gut microbiota. Finally, B cells produce secretory IgA (sIgA) following CD40-CD40L T cell interactions with another immuno-mediated balancing effect on gut microbiota.

3.4. Gut Microbiota Derangements in Liver Diseases through Immune System Alterations

The gut microbiota has a clear role in the physiopathology of liver diseases. Small quantities of intestinal bacterial antigens can, through increased IP, enter the portal venous blood flow and trigger GALT- and non-GALT-based immune responses. Bacterial translocation is harmful for NAFLD pathogenesis, hepatic encephalopathy and spontaneous bacterial peritonitis development in liver cirrhosis patients [57]. The liver, however, can maintain a sensitive balance between protective immune response against exogenous antigens and immune tolerance through the large number of immune cells belonging to both innate and adaptive immune systems [58–60].

The strict association between gut microbiota imbalance or dysbiosis and hepatic encephalopathy was first reported in humans in the 1950s by Phillips et al. They found that nitrogenous-compounds, such as ammonia, produced by microbial-ingested proteins putrefaction, could escape hepatic detoxification, resulting in accumulation of these across the blood-brain barrier until coma develops [61].

3.4.1. Alcoholic Liver Disease

Although the hepato-toxicity of alcohol is well-known, its disruptive effects cannot be attributed to toxicity only. Increased bacterial endotoxin and DNA levels are found in the systemic circulation of alcoholic liver disease patients. Bacterial LPS can activate both systemic and resident immune cells through TLR4 signalling with the induction of pro-inflammatory cytokines, forming a positive feedback loop [62]. Bacterial DNA is recognised by TLR9 that triggers the liver LPS-related inflammatory cascade [63].

However, alcoholic liver disease natural history also regards another pathophysiological mechanism involving gut microbiota. Chronic excessive alcohol consumption can lead to a significant increase in the total number of Gram-negative anaerobic bacteria of faecal origin within the jejunum [64]. Another study reported that mice chronically exposed to alcohol showed increased presence of species belonging to the *Bacteroides versus Firmicutes* phyla [65]. Finally, chronic excess alcohol intake can also lead to deregulated intestinal mycobiosis (with reduced fungi diversity and richness) and hepatic inflammation in mice [66]. In humans, marked intestinal fungal dysbiosis was also observed in alcohol-dependent patients with a significant difference among alcoholic liver disease, alcoholic steatohepatitis and liver cirrhosis [67] (Table 1).

Table 1. Liver diseases and gut microbiota derangements.

Liver Disease	Gut Microbial Derangement
ALD	↓Butyrate-producing *Clostridiales* spp. ↓*Bacteroides* and *Lactobacillus* ↓*Lachnospiracea* and *Ruminococceae* ↑pro-inflammatory *Enterobacteriaceae* ↑*Fusobacteria*
NAFLD/NASH	↓*Prevotella* ↑*Firmicutes/Nacteroides* ratio ↑*Bacteroides* and *Ruminococcus* ↑*Escherichia coli, Bacteroides vulgatus* (namely, in liver cirrhosis stage)
Autoimmune Hepatitis	UC typical gut microbiota derangement (PSC) [68] ↑*E.coli rough form* (PBC)
Liver cirrhosis	↓*Bacteroidetes* and *Firmicutes* ↓*Lachnospiraceae, Ruminococceae* ↑*Enterobacteriaceae* ↑*Streptococcus* spp., *Veilonella* species ↑*Veilonella, Megasphera, Dialister, Atobium, Prevotella*
HCC	↓*Lactobacillus* spp. *Bifidobacterium* spp., *Enterococcus* spp. ↑*Escherichia coli* ↑*Clostridium*

Abbreviations: ALD: alcoholic liver disease; NAFLD: non-alcoholic liver disease; NASH: non-alcoholic steato-hepatitis; UC: ulcerative colitis; PSC: primary sclerosing cholangitis; PBC: primary biliry cholangitis; HCC: hepatocellular carcinoma; ↓: reduced; ↑: increased.

Chronic alcohol consumption also impairs barrier immunity as ethanol inhibits natural killer cell responses with contemporary depletion of other types of lymphoid cells. Therefore, alcohol-related dysbiosis increases the susceptibility to infections which is a very severe complication in alcoholic liver disease patients with liver cirrhosis [69].

3.4.2. Non-Alcoholic Fatty Liver Disease

The rapid and even more consistent epidemic of obesity in the Westernized societies, has occurred during the last 40 years and has recalled our attention on its terrible implications for health in terms of morbidity and mortality [70]. NAFLD includes a spectrum of hepatic manifestations ranging from steatosis to liver cirrhosis and, sometimes, leading directly from NASH to hepatocellular carcinoma development [71]. NAFLD is a peculiar condition associated with obesity, type 2 diabetes and insulin resistance, in the absence of significant alcohol consumption. Its histopathology is somehow indistinguishable from the alcoholic steato-hepatitis [72]. More unexpectedly, NALFD pathogenesis is similar to those of alcoholic liver disease. LPS triggering of systemic micro-inflammation is the hallmark of the triangular relationship between obesity, insulin resistance and liver steatosis/hepatitis [73]. Another peculiarity of this physiopathology is represented by the bi-directional changes occurring in obesity and gut microbiota [73]. In fact, obesity itself, with or without a high fat-diet intake, can shape the gut microbiota. On the other hand, this "obese" microbiota can reprogram the gut as well as the entire body to maximize nutrient absorption and an accumulative metabolism [74]. Furthermore, this shift in microbial populations has been associated with a metabolic endotoxaemia due to higher LPS passage through an impaired IP [75]. Who is responsible for this altered IP remains an open question in NAFLD physiopathology. An altered "dysmetabolic" gut microbiota could be the answer [76–78]. This obesogenic intestinal microbiota has been linked to the development of insulin resistance through the LPS/TLR4/CD14 systems [79]. Once again, the immune response is crucial to close the physiopathologic ring between diet, microbiota and diabetes/insulin resistance [80] (Table 1).

3.4.3. Autoimmune Diseases

Autoimmune hepatic diseases include several pathological entities, named autoimmune hepatitis (AIH), primary biliary cholangitis (PBC) and primary sclerosing cholangitis (PSC), characterized by antibody formation to self-antigens. These diseases do not have a selective hepatic manifestation but are systemic with phenotypic diversity and grading [81].

Recently, convincing data on the association between the influence of gut microbiota and the diffusion of these diseases have been presented. In fact, almost 20% of chronic hepatitis in the Caucasian population have hypergammaglobulinaemia and liver-directed autoantibodies. The consequent histopathological feature is the hepatic lymphocytic infiltration and subsequent hepatocellular injury as revealed in murine liver where significant TLR4 signalling correlates with the consequent trapping of CD8+ T cells [82]. TLR9 was also shown to mediate the process of homing and activation of hepatic natural killer (NK) T cells via the hepatic immune guardians, namely Kupffer cells [34]. IL-10 is another cytokine crucial for autoimmune hepatic damage regulation according to data on animals. In fact, lack of IL-10 abolishes the induction of T_{regs} and the consequent suppression of autoimmune colitis in mice via TLR4 expression on intestinal CD4+ T cells [83]. These data suggest that gut-derived products such as pathogen associated molecular patterns (PAMPs) are able to regulate T cell function within the liver.

PBC is an immune-mediated liver disease caused by immune cell activation with direct damage of intrahepatic bile ducts; almost 95% of these patients present with anti-mitochondrial antibodies at the biochemical check [84]. Hopf et al. showed a significant association between *E. coli* rough form and the presence of lipid A, a lipid component of the endotoxin responsible for germ's toxicity, within the liver of PBC patients but not in healthy subjects. This association seems to be disease-specific [85]. Thus, pharmacological modulation of *E. coli* subpopulations might be a treatment option in PBC patients.

PSC is a progressive autoimmune disease, characterized by the complete destruction of intrahepatic and extrahepatic bile ducts, inhibition of bile acid secretion and chronic hepatocellular injury until liver cirrhosis develops [68]. In PSC patients, the pathophysiological link between gut microbiota, bowel and liver is more evident. Indeed, almost 75% of PSC patients show signs of IBD, mainly ulcerative colitis (UC). In addition, experimental models of IBD bearing pathogenic gut microflora have shown hepatic periportal inflammation [86]. These reports confirmed that intestinal microbial factors may initiate the immune response which leads to liver damage, even in the absence of underlying immune cell disease (Table 1).

3.4.4. Liver Cirrhosis

In patients with liver cirrhosis, the advanced stage of chronic hepatitis that may evolve to hepatocellular carcinoma, an altered gut microbiota might play an important role [87,88] under several aspects.

Delayed bowel motility, reported during cirrhosis and potentially responsible for small bowel bacterial overgrowth, increases the time of contact of faeces with the enterocytes. Moreover, altered IP allows bacterial translocation to the systemic venous blood circulation and finally to the liver [89,90].

Recently, impaired bile secretion has been shown to be another source of bacterial translocation. In liver cirrhosis, the level of bile salts is significantly reduced, thus lowering the stability of the gut microbiota. The load of bacteria belonging to the *Clostridiales* order and responsible for the metabolism of bile salts, was found significantly reduced [91] while a higher number of the potentially pathogenic *Enterobacteriaceae* were detected in liver cirrhosis patients *versus* controls [92].

Furthermore, urease-producing bacteria (e.g., *Klebsiella* and *Proteus* species) have been associated with increased production of ammonia and LPS, both involved in the pathogenesis of hepatic encephalopathy and spontaneous bacterial peritonitis [93,94].

Finally, Qin et al. reported a difference of 75,245 microbial genes between liver cirrhosis patients and healthy subjects using the newest quantitative metagenomic methods; about 50% of the bacterial species were of buccal origin thus justifying the hypothesis that oral bacteria could invade the gut of liver cirrhosis patients [95] (Table 1).

Hepatocellular carcinoma is a common complication of liver cirrhosis and, in some contexts (as NASH), also of non-liver cirrhosis conditions. The pathogenesis of this malignancy involves chronic liver inflammation, with continuous cell death and regeneration processes [96]. Genetic TLR4 inactivation, gut microbial deprivation or germ-free status decrease the development of hepatocellular carcinoma hepatocellular carcinoma in almost 80% of cases [97]. However, pathogenic changes in the immune system have been implicated in hepatocellular carcinoma development. These include leucocyte dysfunction with reduced phagocytic activity of reticulo-endothelial cells (that is, Kupffer cells) [98–100], reduced antibody- and complement-mediated bacterial killing [101] and reduced proliferation of intraepithelial lymphocytes [102]. Altogether, these mechanisms explain the dysbiosis occurring in the cirrhotic patients that, in turn, enhances hepatocellular carcinoma progression (Table 1).

Despite substantial improvements in short-term outcome, liver cirrhosis, in the very last stages, continues to have a poor prognosis [103]. Thus, liver transplantation remains the only treatment option for end-stage liver disease [103]. Immunosuppression and an altered entero-hepatic bile recirculation due to anatomical changes, however, after transplant may both play a significant role in reshuffling intestinal microbial populations. In fact, in cynologous monkeys, the immunosuppressant alemtuzumab induced a complete alteration of gut microbiota with reduction of predominant Bacteroides species and increase of Enterobacteriaceae [104].

In humans, fecal microbial diversity assessment in both the pre- and post-transplant period, by immune profiling, revealed poor microbial diversity, with reduction in several commensal species and increase in pathogenic ones, such as *Enterobacteriaceae* and *Enterococcus* species. Surprisingly, this dysbiosis resolved overtime after transplantation, especially when bacterial prophylaxis was stopped and immunosuppressive regimens were reduced [105] (Table 1).

3.5. Gut Virome and Liver Diseases at the Time of SARS-COV-2 Pandemic

The existence of a gut virome has been very recently recognised despite the fact that pathogens (such as Norwalk virus, Rotavirus and Enterovirus) have been long-known to be found in the human intestine [106–108]. With advances in metagenomic technologies, novel enteric eukaryotic viruses such as *Adenoviridae*, *Picornaviridae*, *Reoviridae* families, were found to be responsible for acute diarrhoea in children's small bowel enteropathy in developing areas of Australia [109,110]. Giant DNA viruses that infect human intestinal parasites (namely, amoebae) are mainly represented by *Mimiviridae, Mamaviridae, Marseilleviridae*. Mimiviruses have been sometimes associated with pneumonitis and diarrhoea in humans [111]. Plant-derived viruses are also present in human faeces. They are represented by pepper mild mottle virus (PMMV), oat blue dwarf virus, grapevine asteroid mosaic associated virus, maize chlorotic mottle virus, oat chlorotic stunt virus, panicum mosaic virus, and tobacco mosaic virus [112].

Intestinal bacteriophages account for around 90% of the entire gut virome [106,107]. They are commonly described as viruses of bacteria or bacterial parasites due to the ability to inject their genome into their host, integrating with its genetic material (prophage state) and inducing other phage particle synthesis resulting in bacterial cell lysis (lytic state) [106,113]. Bacteriophages have double-stranded DNA (dsDNA) [113], although single-stranded DNA (ssDNA) types are found amongst the *Microviridae* family [112]. *Microviridae* are small icosahedral viruses with circular ssDNA genomes and their members are divided into microviruses (genus *Microvirus*), gokushoviruses (subfamily *Gokushovirinae*) and *Alpavirinae* [114].

The human gut virome maintains stability and generates diversity of the human gut microbiome in dynamic equilibrium with the host via immune system tolerance [114]. Gut virome genes are also implicated in human metabolism, inflammation and carcinogenesis modulation [114]. Recent evidence points out to a new role of bacteriophages in liver metabolism and immune response regulation in humans [115].

As previously mentioned, gut microbiota promotes ethanol- induced liver disease in mice but little is known about the specific microbial factors that are responsible for this process. The presence of *E. faecalis* correlates with the severity of liver disease and with mortality in patients with alcoholic liver disease. Duan et al. recently showed that bacteriophages were able to decrease cytolysin expression in the liver and abolished ethanol-induced liver disease in humanized mice [116]. Cytolysin is a bacterial exotoxin (or bacteriocin) that is produced by *E. faecalis* but also by eukaryotic cells [117,118]. Alcoholic liver disease can be transmitted via faecal microbiota. Duan et al. found no multi-collinearity between the detection of faecal cytolysin-encoding genes and other cofactors in mice. This indicates that cytolysin may be considered an independent predictor of mortality for alcoholic liver disease. Moreover, cytolysin production is a transportable trait among *E. faecalis* isolates. Indeed, it includes both chromosomally encoded pathogenicity islands and plasmids [119]. These results confirm that the presence of cytolysin-producing *E. faecalis*, rather than the total number of bacteria, determines the severity of alcoholic liver disease and associated mortality.

Ethanol-induced changes in the gut barrier are necessary for the translocation of cytolytic *E. faecalis* from the intestine to the liver, suggesting that this bacterium may promote ethanol-induced liver disease after abnormalities of IP, as reported in mice [116]. Cytolysin-induced hepatocyte cell death may be mediated by pore formation resulting in cell lysis, independently of ethanol [116,119].

E. faecalis bacteriophages are highly strain-specific, can be easily isolated and, in the perspective of future therapeutic implications, present a potential for direct editing of gut microbiota [120]. Duan et al. isolated four distinct phages from sewage water. These phages can lyse the cytolytic *E. faecalis* strain isolated from Atp4aSl/Sl mice. All four phages were podophages of the virulent Picovirinae group. Importantly, administration of *E. faecalis* phages significantly reduced levels of hepatic cytolysin and faecal concentration of *Enterococcus*. Furthermore, phages administration (with siphophage or myophage morphology) did not affect the overall composition of the faecal microbiome, intestinal absorption or hepatic metabolism of ethanol [116].

In mice, the phages against cytolytic *E. faecalis* abolished ethanol-induced liver injury and steatosis, lowering the levels of transaminases (ALT), the percentages of hepatic cells positive for terminal deoxynucleotide transferase-mediated dUTP nick-end labelling, and reducing the levels of hepatic triglycerides and oil red O-staining, compared to control phages (namely, against *C. crescentus*) [116]. It can be hypothesized that treatment with lytic phages can attenuate the ethanol-induced liver disease also in humans. However, since phages can induce a strong immune reaction, safety studies are required [121]. Overall, these data are promising and suggest that cytolysin may be used as a predictive biomarker of alcoholic liver disease shifting to alcoholic steatohepatitis.

In AIH, patients are typically treated with steroids and show a good response profile. In cases where immunosuppressive therapy does not offer any benefit, and the side effects are seriousleading to the development of malignancies, bacteriophage-based approaches have been considered. Bacteriophages have been increasingly recognized as immunomodulators contributing to immune homeostasis and curbing inflammation [122]. Phages have been shown to down-regulate the expression and/or production and activity of factors associated with hepatic injury (e.g., reactive oxygen species, TLR-4 and NF-kB activation, pro-inflammatory and pro-coagulant activities of platelets) and up-regulate the expression and/or production of protective factors (e.g., IL-10, IL-1 receptor antagonist) [121]. Phages may modulate the immune response, contributing to maintenance of immune homeostasis in the GI tract and, possibly, in other sites [123,124]. Furthermore, they can diminish T cell activation, alloantigen-induced Ig production in vitro and extend the skin allograft survival in naive and sensitized mice [123,124]. In addition, phages may reduce autoimmune reaction in a mouse model of autoimmunity (namely collagen-induced arthritis) [125]. Skin and organ inflammatory infiltration induced by alloantigens and endotoxin can also be reduced markedly by phage or a phage protein administration [126]. More importantly, phages do not impair the ability of granulocytes and monocytes to kill bacteria. Clinical phage therapy decreased inflammatory markers (e.g., C-reactive protein [CRP], erythrocyte sedimentation rate, leukocytosis), even though eradication of pathogens was not achieved [127].

Liver macrophages or Kupffer cells are of paramount importance for maintenance of liver and immune systemic homeostasis [128]. In fact, deletion of Kupffer cells in experimentally-induced hepatitis suppresses liver damage and, also, collagen-induced autoimmune arthritis in mice [129,130]. Kupffer cells may modulate liver allograft tolerance implicating that transplanted subject survival may be accomplished without concurrent immunosuppression [131]. Moreover, when liver and kidney are transplanted simultaneously the liver becomes immunoprotective for the kidney [132].

Targeting pathogenic Kupffer cells may be a novel promising approach in acute and chronic liver diseases. From seventy to ninety per cent of phages administered intravenously in mice are taken up by liver [133]. Liver Kupffer cells are primarily responsible for this uptake and are unable to prime lymphocytes for antibody responses against phages. In contrast, almost the entire humoral response to phages is attributable to spleen [134].

If enhanced phagocytosis by Kupffer cells may translate into attenuation of autoimmune-mediated hepatitis, it may be expected that phage uptake by Kuppfer cells may also mediate similar effects [133]. Specifically, phage-induced decrease of reactive oxygen species and enhancement of IL-10 production by these cells may also contribute significantly to achieving immune homeostasis.

Phages induce IL-10 production by human mononuclear cells [135]. This cytokine, known for its anti-inflammatory action, plays a protective role against hepatic injury. It also has anti-fibrotic properties [136]. IL-10-producing T cells prevent liver damage in chronic hepatitis C virus infection [137]. Phages can have a moderate inhibitory effect on the activation of NF-kB, thus inhibiting liver inflammation and injury [138].

Biliary epithelial cells express TLR-4. There is increasing evidence that this receptor plays a key role in HCV infection and replication. TLR-4 has been identified as a factor associated with a high risk of developing cirrhosis in patients with chronic hepatitis C. Moreover, TLR-4 activation has been associated with the progression of other chronic liver diseases, such as AIH, PBC and PSC. Inhibitors of TLR-4 are being tested in the hope that they might prevent the progression of chronic hepatitis [139,140]. In addition, purified phages may down-regulate TLR-4, leading to lower hepatic injury with subsequent lowered hepato-carcinogenesis [141]. Of note, antiplatelet therapy prevents the development of hepatocellular carcinoma. Phages may also be part of this process, as they inhibit platelet adhesion to fibrinogen [142]. Finally, phages could also be used for the development of vaccine against hepatitis B virus and production of nanomolecules displaying peptides that could interfere with attachment of pathogenic viruses and their entry into liver cells [143].

To date, SARS-CoV-2 is responsible for a tremendous pandemic that has changed clinical as well as social behaviours. The relative collection of clinical manifestations, namely COVID-19, includes not only pulmonary abnormalities but is a systemic disease, involving the heart, liver, pancreas and kidneys. SARS-CoV-2 also affects circulating lymphocytes and the immune system [144–146]. Liver damage can occur during disease progression and/or as consequence of COVID-19 treatment in patients with or without pre-existing liver diseases [146]. Overall, the incidence of elevated serum transaminases in hospitalized COVID-19 patients, and, less frequently, bilirubin, ranges from 14% to 53% [147]. Moreover, liver derangement is observed more commonly in male patients and in those with more severe disease [148].

Hitherto, there is no evidence of acute or acute on chronic liver failure in COVID-19 patients [147,148]. Retrospective studies, with large cohorts, have shown that a small percentage had pre-existing hepatitis B [148]. Histopathologically, the liver of COVID-19-affected patients shows moderate microvascular steatosis and mild lobular and portal activity, indicating that the injury could have been caused by either SARS-CoV-2 infection or drugs [149]. Due to the novelty of COVID-19, we can only report putative mechanisms leading to liver damage: immune-mediated injury due to the dramatic inflammatory storm following the first week of SARS-CoV-2 infection [150]; direct cytotoxic damage due to viral replication within hepatic cells through ACE-2 receptor binding [151]; viral-induced endothelial injury and/or microthrombotic events; anoxia due to respiratory failure; drug-induced liver injury (DILI) (e.g., due to use of lopinavir/ritonavir, remdesivir, chloroquine, tocilizumab, uminefovir, Chinese traditional medicine which are potentially hepatotoxic in some patients) [146,151]. It is also noteworthy that drugs like tocilizumab and baricitinib can cause HBV reactivation, thus leading to liver failure.

It is not yet clear whether COVID-19 impairs cholestasis in patients with pre-existing cholestatic liver diseases [152]. However, the outcome of patients with liver injury is generally favourable as alterations of liver transaminases are transient and often without fatal exitus. Thus, COVID-19 liver features and preliminary evidence reported in literature raise open issues: disease evolution history will provide details about the exact pathogenesis of liver manifestations following COVID-19; the putative role for biliary tract cells in shedding the infection to the intestinal cells (also expressing ACE2); the real incidence of DILI during the treatment of COVID-19; the eventual susceptibility of patients with pre-existing liver disease to COVID-19 disease (e.g., the possible protective role of immunosuppressant *versus* disease severity); the prognostic weight of pre-existing liver disease on COVID-19 survival.

3.6. An Example of Gut Microbiota Modulation through Immune Interaction in Liver Disease: The Case of Probiotics

Evidence on the efficacy of gut microbiota modulation in liver cirrhosis natural history comes from studies on the use of prebiotics. Prebiotics, usually plant fibres and other non-digestible fermentable carbohydrates that lead to preferential intestinal microbial growth, have been first used in liver cirrhosis patients [153]. Lactulose is able to reverse and improve hepatic encephalopathy and the add-on positive effect on the usage of rifaximin, an antibiotic poorly absorbed at the intestinal level, support its enormous therapeutic potential in altering intestinal microbial communities to revert disease progression [3]. Moreover, lactulose, as a non-absorbable disaccharide, lowers colonic pH, improves excretion of ammonia, stimulates growth of *Bifidobacterium* and *Lactobacillus* [154].

Probiotics are defined as "live microorganisms beneficially affecting human health" [155]. Symbiotics are a combination of the prebiotics and probiotics [156]. alcoholic liver disease has been linked to an over-population of Gram-negative microbial species in the gut [157]. Studies on animal models showed the potential of *Lactobacillus GG* in reducing the severity of alcoholic hepatitis. The latter is linked to the complex mechanism of action of this probiotic that causes a reduction in gut leakiness, oxidative stress and liver inflammation [158].

In human studies, the add-on use of other probiotics, namely *Bifidobacterium bifidum* and *Lactobacillus plantarum*, was able to reverse the intestinal microbial dysbiosis with a simultaneous improvement in alcoholic liver disease features [159]. From an immunological point of view, Stadlbauer et al. showed the immune-modulator effect of *Lactobacillus casei Shirota* that was able to restore neutrophils' phagocytic capacity, inversely correlated with an increased risk of mortality in alcoholic liver disease patients [160].

NAFLD and NASH are the most studied models in which gut microbiota and immune system dysfunction are strictly linked in determining liver damages until liver cirrhosis and hepatocellular carcinoma development [161]. In fact, data from animal studies have provided indications on the efficacy of prebiotics, probiotics and symbiotics in NAFLD treatment. Li et al. showed that 4 weeks of treatment with VSL#3, containing *lactobacillus, bifidobacterium* species and a streptococcal strain, was associated with improved NAFLD histology, with a reduction in hepatic total fatty acid content, and reduced serum aminotransferases levels in *ob/ob* mice fed with a high fat diet. These effects paralleled a significant reduction in Jun-Kinase (JNK) activity and DNA-binding activity of NF-kB [162]. In humans, a study by Loguercio et al. confirmed the capability of VSL#3 to reduce these parameters, especially with a significant decrease in lipid peroxidation, in NAFLD patients [163]. In addition, recent data supported the efficacy of gut microbiota modulation in changing not only the GALT-associated immunity but also the systemic inflammatory response. Reduced levels of LPS were found after probiotic administration in patients with NAFLD [164,165]. Malaguarnera et al. also showed that probiotics and fructooligosaccharides administration was superior to lifestyle changes in NAFLD subjects in reducing inflammatory marker levels. Levels of TNFα, endotoxin and the NASH activity index were significantly reduced by probiotics add-on use [166]. However, evidence supporting a curative role for probiotics in NAFLD, NASH and its subsiding systemic micro-inflammation process has not yet been confirmed by larger population-based studies [167].

Within the array of biliary tract liver diseases, PSC is one of the most studied autoimmune liver diseases in terms of gut microbiota modulation. In a pilot study by Vleggaar et al., patients with PSC and IBD received a multi-strain probiotic for three months without benefits in terms of symptoms relief or improvement in both liver function indexes and bile salt levels [168–170].

As reported above, gut microbiota and its interaction with immune system have been implicated in the pathophysiology of major complications of liver cirrhosis. Thus, research focused on microbial re-modulation, in order to reverse liver cirrhosis natural course [171]. A symbiotic preparation was used by Liu et al., who reported a significant improvement in Child-Pugh class (that is associated with prognosis) staging in about half of the patients treated, accompanied by reduction in the levels of circulating endotoxin [172].

Probiotics may have a potential as add-on treatments to prevent spontaneous bacterial peritonitis occurrence, to promote the growth of protective anaerobic organisms, but also to reduce IP [172] and GALT activation [59]. However, neither preliminary animal studies [173] nor clinical data support the efficacy of probiotics add-on to antibiotics in preventing primary or secondary spontaneous bacterial peritonitis [174]. On the contrary, the potential efficacy of probiotics in hepatic encephalopathy treatment is supported by the evidence of the beneficial effect on colonic non-urease producing bacteria that can reduce the total amount of ammonia reaching the portal system [175]. Thus, high oral doses of *Lactobacillus acidophilus* have been shown to be beneficial in improving hepatic encephalopathy [176,177]. These findings were confirmed in patients refractory to neomicyn treatment [177]. Furthermore, Malaguarnera [166] and Liu [172] confirmed these effects by using a combination of prebiotics and probiotics (a symbiotic approach) in the treatment of minimal hepatic encephalopathy. Bacterial translocation is also responsible for the increased portal pressure at the basis of hyperdynamic circulatory state and increased hepatic vascular resistance [178]. Probiotics can decrease blood portal pressure and bleeding risk [179]. These promising but not yet uniform results [180,181] were confirmed by Rincon et al., who after 6 weeks VSL#3 administration, reported reduced hepatic venous pressure gradient in liver cirrhosis patients [182].

The final and most dramatic stage of liver cirrhosis evolution can be hepatocellular carcinoma. There are a few promising studies on the role of probiotics in reducing the carcinogenetic process of hepatocellular carcinoma. An in vivo study reported that rats exposed to aflatoxin had a lower expression of *c-myc, bcl2, cyclin D1* and *rasp21* after *Lactobacillus rhamnosus GG* administration [183]. On the other hand, administration of a multistrain probiotic (namely, *Lactobacillus* and *Propionobacterium* species) did not change the urinary excretion of aflatoxin metabolite in healthy volunteers. These data suggest that probiotics administration might reduce the effects of aflatoxin and have a chemopreventive role in hepatocellular carcinoma [184]. However, further studies are required to clarify these limited data.

4. Conclusions

The increasing evidence of the role of gut microbiota in the development, maintenance and disruption of the immune system comes from animal and human studies. The liver, as a key organ in local and systemic immunity maintenance, is in strict contact with microbial antigens and gut microbiota derangement has a direct or indirect causative role on the development and progression of several liver diseases (Table 1). Thus, microbiota modulation consisting in the use of probiotics seems an appealing instrument for a safe immunity re-shaping in liver diseases.

Gut virome modulation on liver and systemic immunity for the treatment of viral- and immune-mediated hepatitis and hepatocellular carcinoma are more than promising. However, randomized controlled trials are needed to confirm animal and preliminary human studies. Understanding in depth the immunomodulatory role of the gut microbiota and virome in health and disease is also of prime importance to counteract pandemics such as that caused by the ongoing

SARS-CoV-2 infection, as COVID-19-affected patients show not only respiratory distress syndrome but also multiorgan dysfunction including the liver.

Author Contributions: L.A. and E.S. had the original idea for the review article; L.A. and E.S. performed the review of literature; C.R., E.R., T.L. and F.L. reviewed the literature findings; E.S. and L.A. wrote the manuscript; S.F., P.R. and I.A. critically revised the manuscript; S.F. revised the English form. All authors have read and agreed to the published version of the manuscript.

Funding: This research received no external funding.

Conflicts of Interest: Authors declare no financial conflict of interests.

References

1. Rinninella, E.; Raoul, P.; Cintoni, M.; Franceschi, F.; Miggiano, G.A.D.; Gasbarrini, A.; Mele, M.C. What is the Healthy Gut Microbiota Composition? A Changing Ecosystem across Age; Environment; Diet; and Diseases. *Microorganisms* **2019**, *7*, 14. [CrossRef] [PubMed]
2. Butel, M.J.; Waligora-Dupriet, A.J.; Wydau-Dematteis, S. The developing gut microbiota and its consequences for health. *J. Dev. Orig. Health Dis.* **2018**, *9*, 590–597. [CrossRef] [PubMed]
3. Preveden, T.; Scarpellini, E.; Milić, N.; Luzza, F.; Abenavoli, L. Gut microbiota changes and chronic hepatitis C virus infection. *Expert Rev. Gastroenterol. Hepatol.* **2017**, *11*, 813–819. [CrossRef] [PubMed]
4. Maroni, L.; Ninfole, E.; Pinto, C.; Benedetti, A.; Marzioni, M. Gut-Liver Axis and Inflammasome Activation in Cholangiocyte Pathophysiology. *Cells* **2020**, *9*, 736. [CrossRef]
5. Jia, W.; Xie, G.; Jia, W. Bile acid-microbiota crosstalk in gastrointestinal inflammation and carcinogenesis. *Nat. Rev. Gastroenterol. Hepatol.* **2018**, *15*, 111–128. [CrossRef]
6. Testino, G.; Bottaro, L.C.; Patussi, V.; Scafato, E.; Addolorato, G.; Leone, S.; Renzetti, D.; Balbinot, P.; Greco, G.; Fanucchi, T.; et al. Study Committee of SIA (Società Italiana di Alcologia). Addiction disorders: A need for change. Proposal for a new management. Position paper of SIA, Italian Society on Alcohol. *Minerva. Med.* **2018**, *109*, 369–385. [CrossRef]
7. Saracco, G.M.; Evangelista, A.; Fagoonee, S.; Ciccone, G.; Bugianesi, E.; Caviglia, G.P.; Abate, M.L.; Rizzetto, M.; Pellicano, R.; Smedile, A. Etiology of chronic liver diseases in the Northwest of Italy, 1998 through 2014. *World J. Gastroenterol.* **2016**, *22*, 8187–8193. [CrossRef]
8. Liberati, A.; Altman, D.G.; Tetzlaff, J.; Mulrow, C.; Gøtzsche, P.C.; Ioannidis, J.P.; Clarke, M.; Devereaux, P.J.; Kleijnen, J.; Moher, D. The PRISMA statement for reporting systematic reviews and meta-analyses of studies that evaluate health care interventions: Explanation and elaboration. *J. Clin. Epidemiol.* **2009**, *62*, e1–e34. [CrossRef]
9. Arumugam, M.; Raes, J.; Pelletier, E.; Le Paslier, D.; Yamada, T.; Mende, D.R.; Fernandes, G.R.; Tap, J.; Bruls, T.; Batto, J.M.; et al. Enterotypes of the human gut microbiome. *Nature* **2011**, *473*, 174–180. [CrossRef]
10. Qin, J.; Li, R.; Raes, J.; Arumugam, M.; Burgdorf, K.S.; Manichanh, C.; Nielsen, T.; Pons, N.; Levenez, F.; Yamada, T.; et al. A human gut microbial gene catalogue established by metagenomic sequencing. *Nature* **2010**, *464*, 59–65. [CrossRef]
11. Tap, J.; Mondot, S.; Levenez, F.; Pelletier, E.; Caron, C.; Furet, J.P.; Ugarte, E.; Muñoz-Tamayo, R.; Paslier, D.L.; Nalin, R.; et al. Towards the human intestinal microbiota phylogenetic core. *Environ. Microbiol.* **2009**, *11*, 2574–2584. [CrossRef] [PubMed]
12. Zhuang, L.; Chen, H.; Zhang, S.; Zhuang, J.; Li, Q.; Feng, Z. Intestinal Microbiota in Early Life and Its Implications on Childhood Health. *Genom. Proteom. Bioinform.* **2019**, *17*, 13–25. [CrossRef]
13. Yatsunenko, T.; Rey, F.E.; Manary, M.J.; Trehan, I.; Dominguez-Bello, M.G.; Contreras, M.; Magris, M.; Hidalgo, G.; Baldassano, R.N.; Anokhin, A.P.; et al. Human gut microbiome viewed across age and geography. *Nature* **2012**, *486*, 222–227. [CrossRef] [PubMed]
14. Biagi, E.; Franceschi, C.; Rampelli, S.; Severgnini, M.; Ostan, R.; Turroni, S.; Consolandi, C.; Quercia, S.; Scurti, M.; Monti, D.; et al. Gut Microbiota and Extreme Longevity. *Curr. Biol.* **2016**, *26*, 1480–1485. [CrossRef] [PubMed]
15. Rooks, M.G.; Garrett, W.S. Gut microbiota; metabolites and host immunity. *Nat. Rev. Immunol.* **2016**, *16*, 341–352. [CrossRef] [PubMed]

16. Maynard, C.L.; Elson, C.O.; Hatton, R.D.; Weaver, C.T. Reciprocal interactions of the intestinal microbiota and immune system. *Nature* **2012**, *489*, 231–241. [CrossRef]
17. Brandl, K.; Plitas, G.; Schnabl, B.; DeMatteo, R.P.; Pamer, E.G. MyD88-mediated signals induce the bactericidal lectin RegIII gamma and protect mice against intestinal Listeria monocytogenes infection. *J. Exp. Med.* **2007**, *204*, 1891–1900. [CrossRef]
18. Johansson, M.E.; Sjovall, H.; Hansson, G.C. The gastrointestinal mucus system in health and disease. *Nat. Rev. Gastroenterol. Hepatol.* **2013**, *10*, 352–361. [CrossRef]
19. Federico, A.; Dallio, M.; Caprio, G.G.; Ormando, V.M.; Loguercio, C. Gut microbiota and the liver. *Minerva. Gastroenterol. Dietol.* **2017**, *63*, 385–398. [CrossRef]
20. Weber, C.R.; Nalle, S.C.; Tretiakova, M.; Rubin, D.T.; Turner, J.R. Claudin-1 and 6claudin-2 expression is elevated in inflammatory bowel disease and may contribute to early neoplastic transformation. *Lab. Investig.* **2008**, *88*, 1110–1120. [CrossRef]
21. Ahmad, R.; Sorrell, M.F.; Batra, S.K.; Dhawan, P.; Singh, A.B. Gut permeability and mucosal inflammation: Bad; good or context dependent. *Mucosal. Immunol.* **2017**, *10*, 307–317. [CrossRef] [PubMed]
22. Wang, F.; Graham, W.V.; Wang, Y.; Witkowski, E.D.; Schwarz, B.T.; Turner, J.R. Interferon-gamma and tumor necrosis factor-alpha synergize to induce intestinal epithelial barrier dysfunction by up-regulating myosin light chain kinase expression. *Am. J. Pathol.* **2005**, *166*, 409–419. [CrossRef]
23. Smith, K.; McCoy, K.D.; Macpherson, A.J. Use of axenic animals in studying the adaptation of mammals to their commensal intestinal microbiota. *Semin. Immunol.* **2007**, *19*, 59–69. [CrossRef] [PubMed]
24. Ahluwalia, B.; Magnusson, M.K.; Öhman, L. Mucosal immune system of the gastrointestinal tract: Maintaining balance between the good and the bad. *Scand. J. Gastroenterol.* **2017**, *52*, 1185–1193. [CrossRef]
25. Eberl, G.; Lochner, M. The development of intestinal lymphoid tissues at the interface of self and microbiota. *Mucosal. Immunol.* **2009**, *2*, 478–485. [CrossRef]
26. Sawa, S.; Cherrier, M.; Lochner, M.; Satoh-Takayama, N.; Fehling, H.J.; Langa, F.; Di Santo, J.P.; Eberl, G. Lineage relationship analysis of RORgammat+ innate lymphoid cells. *Science* **2010**, *330*, 665–669. [CrossRef]
27. Fagarasan, S.; Muramatsu, M.; Suzuki, K.; Nagaoka, H.; Hiai, H.; Honjo, T. Critical Roles of Activation-Induced Cytidine Deaminase in the Homeostasis of Gut Flora. *Science* **2002**, *298*, 1424–1427. [CrossRef]
28. Takahashi, K.; Yano, A.; Watanabe, S.; Langella, P.; Bermúdez-Humarán, L.G.; Inoue, N. M cell-targeting strategy enhances systemic and mucosal immune responses induced by oral administration of nuclease-producing L. lactis. *Appl. Microbiol. Biotechnol.* **2018**, *102*, 10703–10711. [CrossRef]
29. Bouskra, D.; Brézillon, C.; Bérard, M.; Werts, C.; Varona, R.; Boneca, I.G.; Eberl, G. Lymphoid tissue genesis induced by commensals through NOD1 regulates intestinal homeostasis. *Nature* **2008**, *456*, 507–510. [CrossRef]
30. Larsson, E.; Tremaroli, V.; Lee, Y.S.; Koren, O.; Nookaew, I.; Fricker, A.; Nielsen, J.; Ley, R.E.; Bäckhed, F. Analysis of gut microbial regulation of host gene expression along the length of the gut and regulation of gut microbial ecology through MyD88. *Gut* **2012**, *61*, 1124–1131. [CrossRef]
31. Biswas, A.; Wilmanski, J.; Forsman, H.; Hrncir, T.; Hao, L.; Tlaskalova-Hogenova, H.; Kobayashi, K.S. Negative regulation of Toll-like receptor signaling plays an essential role in homeostasis of the intestine. *Eur. J. Immunol.* **2011**, *41*, 182–194. [CrossRef] [PubMed]
32. Kanneganti, T.D.; Lamkanfi, M.; Nunez, G. Intracellular NOD-like receptors in host defense and disease. *Immunity* **2007**, *27*, 549–559. [CrossRef] [PubMed]
33. Claes, A.K.; Zhou, J.Y.; Philpott, D.J. NOD-Like Receptors: Guardians of Intestinal Mucosal Barriers. *Physiology (Bethesda)* **2015**, *30*, 241–250. [CrossRef] [PubMed]
34. Lebeis, S.L.; Powell, K.R.; Merlin, D.; Sherman, M.A.; Kalman, D. Interleukin-1 receptor signaling protects mice from lethal intestinal damage caused by the attaching and effacing pathogen Citrobacter rodentium. *Infect. Immun.* **2009**, *77*, 604–614. [CrossRef] [PubMed]
35. Li, X.V.; Leonardi, I.; Iliev, I.D. Gut Mycobiota in Immunity and Inflammatory Disease. *Immunity* **2019**, *50*, 1365–1379. [CrossRef] [PubMed]
36. Chung, H.; Pamp, S.J.; Hill, J.A.; Surana, N.K.; Edelman, S.M.; Troy, E.B.; Reading, N.C.; Villablanca, E.J.; Wang, S.; Mora, J.R.; et al. Gut immune maturation depends on colonization with a host-specific microbiota. *Cell* **2012**, *149*, 1578–1593. [CrossRef]
37. Okada, H.; Kuhn, C.; Feillet, H.; Bach, J.F. The 'hygiene hypothesis' for autoimmune and allergic diseases: An update. *Clin. Exp. Immunol.* **2010**, *160*, 1–9. [CrossRef]

38. Ivanov, I.I.; Atarashi, K.; Manel, N.; Brodie, E.L.; Shima, T.; Karaoz, U.; Wei, D.; Goldfarb, K.C.; Santee, C.A.; Lynch, S.V.; et al. Induction of intestinal Th17 cells by segmented filamentous bacteria. *Cell* **2009**, *139*, 485–498. [CrossRef]
39. Shi, Y.; Liu, X.F.; Zhuang, Y.; Zhang, J.Y.; Liu, T.; Yin, Z.; Wu, C.; Mao, X.H.; Jia, K.R.; Wang, F.J.; et al. Helicobacter pylori-induced Th17 responses modulate Th1 cell responses; benefit bacterial growth; and contribute to pathology in mice. *J. Immunol.* **2010**, *184*, 5121–5129. [CrossRef]
40. Atarashi, K.; Nishimura, J.; Shima, T.; Umesaki, Y.; Yamamoto, M.; Onoue, M.; Yagita, H.; Ishii, N.; Evans, R.; Honda, K.; et al. ATP drives lamina propria T(H)17 cell differentiation. *Nature* **2008**, *455*, 808–812. [CrossRef]
41. Kim, S.C.; Tonkonogy, S.L.; Karrasch, T.; Jobin, C.; Sartor, R.B. Dual-association of gnotobiotic IL-10-/- mice with 2 nonpathogenic commensal bacteria induces aggressive pancolitis. *Inflamm. Bowel. Dis.* **2007**, *13*, 1457–1466. [CrossRef] [PubMed]
42. Barnes, M.J.; Powrie, F. Regulatory T cells reinforce intestinal homeostasis. *Immunity* **2009**, *31*, 401–411. [CrossRef] [PubMed]
43. Safinia, N.; Sagoo, P.; Lechler, R.; Lombardi, G. Adoptive regulatory T cell therapy: Challenges in clinical transplantation. *Curr. Opin. Organ. Transplant.* **2010**, *15*, 427–434. [CrossRef] [PubMed]
44. Sakaguchi, S.; Sakaguchi, N.; Asano, M.; Itoh, M.; Toda, M. Immunologic self tolerance maintained by activated T cells expressing IL-2 receptor alpha chains (CD25). Breakdown of a single mechanism of self-tolerance causes various autoimmune diseases. *J. Immunol.* **1995**, *155*, 1151–1164. [PubMed]
45. Battaglia, M.; Gianfrani, C.; Gregori, S.; Roncarolo, M.G. IL-10-producing T regulatory type 1 cells and oral tolerance. *Ann. N. Y. Acad. Sci.* **2004**, *1029*, 142–153. [CrossRef] [PubMed]
46. Walker, L.S. Treg and CTLA-4: Two intertwining pathways to immune tolerance. *J. Autoimm.* **2013**, *45*, 49–57. [CrossRef]
47. Hara, M.; Kingsley, C.I.; Niimi, M.; Read, S.; Turvey, S.E.; Bushell, A.R.; Morris, P.J.; Powrie, F.; Wood, K.J. IL-10 is required for regulatory T cells to mediate tolerance to alloantigens in vivo. *J. Immunol.* **2001**, *166*, 3789–3796. [CrossRef]
48. Atarashi, K.; Tanoue, T.; Shima, T.; Imaoka, A.; Kuwahara, T.; Momose, Y.; Cheng, G.; Yamasaki, S.; Saito, T.; Ohba, Y.; et al. Induction of colonic regulatory T cells by indigenous Clostridium species. *Science* **2011**, *331*, 337–341. [CrossRef]
49. Chinen, T.; Rudensky, A.Y. The effects of commensal microbiota on immune cell subsets and inflammatory responses. *Immunol. Rev.* **2012**, *245*, 45–55. [CrossRef]
50. Narushima, S.; Sugiura, Y.; Oshima, K.; Atarashi, K.; Hattori, M.; Suematsu, M.; Honda, K. Characterization of the 17 strains of regulatory T cell-inducing human-derived Clostridia. *Gut Microbes* **2014**, *5*, 333–339. [CrossRef]
51. Smith, P.M.; Howitt, M.R.; Panikov, N.; Michaud, M.; Gallini, C.A.; Bohlooly-Y, M.; Glickman, J.N.; Garrett, W.S. The microbial metabolites; short-chain fatty acids; regulate colonic Treg cell homeostasis. *Science* **2013**, *341*, 569–573. [CrossRef] [PubMed]
52. Peng, G.; Guo, Z.; Kiniwa, Y.; Voo, K.S.; Peng, W.; Fu, T.; Wang, D.Y.; Li, Y.; Wang, H.Y.; Wang, R.F. Toll-like receptor 8-mediated reversal of CD4+ regulatory T cell function. *Science* **2005**, *309*, 1380–1384. [CrossRef]
53. Wesemann, D.R.; Portuguese, A.J.; Meyers, R.M.; Gallagher, M.P.; Cluff-Jones, K.; Magee, J.M.; Panchakshari, R.A.; Rodig, S.J.; Kepler, T.B.; Alt, F.W. Microbial colonization influences early B-lineage development in the gut lamina propria. *Nature* **2013**, *501*, 112–115. [CrossRef] [PubMed]
54. Vossenkämper, A.; Blair, P.A.; Safinia, N.; Fraser, L.D.; Das, L.; Sanders, T.J.; Stagg, A.J.; Sanderson, J.D.; Taylor, K.; Chang, F.; et al. A role for gut-associated lymphoid tissue in shaping the human B cell repertoire. *J. Exp. Med.* **2013**, *210*, 1665–1674. [CrossRef] [PubMed]
55. Alhabbab, R.; Blair, P.; Elgueta, R.; Stolarczyk, E.; Marks, E.; Becker, P.D.; Ratnasothy, K.; Smyth, L.; Safinia, N.; Sharif-Paghaleh, E.; et al. Diversity of gut microflora is required for the generation of B cell with regulatory properties in a skin graft model. *Sci. Rep.* **2015**, *5*, 11554. [CrossRef] [PubMed]
56. Rosser, E.C.; Oleinika, K.; Tonon, S.; Doyle, R.; Bosma, A.; Carter, N.A.; Harris, K.A.; Jones, S.A.; Klein, N.; Mauri, C. Regulatory B cells are induced by gut microbiota-driven interleukin-1β and interleukin-6 production. *Nat. Med.* **2014**, *20*, 1334–1339. [CrossRef] [PubMed]
57. Wiest, R.; Albillos, A.; Trauner, M.; Bajaj, J.S.; Jalan, R. Targeting the gut-liver axis in liver disease. *J. Hepatol.* **2017**, *67*, 1084–1103. [CrossRef]

58. Catala, M.; Anton, A.; Portoles, M.T. Characterization of the simultaneous binding of Escherichia coli endotoxin to Kupffer and endothelial liver cells by flow cytometry. *Cytometry* **1999**, *36*, 123–130. [CrossRef]
59. Kobyliak, N.; Abenavoli, L.; Mykhalchyshyn, G.; Kononenko, L.; Boccuto, L.; Kyriienko, D.; Dynnyk, O. A Multi-strain Probiotic Reduces the Fatty Liver Index; Cytokines and Aminotransferase levels in NAFLD Patients: Evidence from a Randomized Clinical Trial. *J. Gastrointest. Liver Dis.* **2018**, *27*, 41–49. [CrossRef]
60. Ahlawat, S.; Sharma, K.K. Gut-organ axis: A microbial outreach and networking. *Lett. Appl. Microbiol.* **2020**. Epub ahead of print. [CrossRef] [PubMed]
61. Phillips, G.B.; Schwartz, R.; Gabuzda, G.J., Jr.; Davidson, C.S. The syndrome of impending hepatic coma in patients with cirrhosis of the liver given certain nitrogenous substances. *New Engl. J. Med.* **1952**, *247*, 239–246. [CrossRef] [PubMed]
62. Roh, Y.S.; Seki, E. Toll-like receptors in alcoholic liver disease; non-alcoholic steatohepatitis and carcinogenesis. *J. Gastroenterol. Hepatol.* **2013**, *28*, 38–42. [CrossRef] [PubMed]
63. Scarpellini, E.; Forlino, M.; Lupo, M.; Rasetti, C.; Fava, G.; Abenavoli, L.; De Santis, A. Gut Microbiota and Alcoholic Liver Disease. *Rev. Recent Clin. Trials* **2016**, *11*, 213–219. [CrossRef] [PubMed]
64. Abenavoli, L.; Masarone, M.; Federico, A.; Rosato, V.; Dallio, M.; Loguercio, C.; Persico, M. Alcoholic Hepatitis: Pathogenesis; Diagnosis and Treatment. *Rev. Recent Clin. Trials* **2016**, *11*, 159–166. [CrossRef]
65. Yan, A.W.; Fouts, D.E.; Brandl, J.; Stärkel, P.; Torralba, M.; Schott, E.; Tsukamoto, H.; Nelson, K.E.; Brenner, D.A.; Schnabl, B. Enteric dysbiosis associated with a mouse model of alcoholic liver disease. *Hepatology* **2011**, *53*, 96–105. [CrossRef]
66. Yang, A.M.; Inamine, T.; Hochrath, K.; Chen, P.; Wang, L.; Llorente, C.; Bluemel, S.; Hartmann, P.; Xu, J.; Koyama, Y.; et al. Intestinal fungi contribute to development of alcoholic liver disease. *J. Clin. Investig.* **2017**, *127*, 2829–2841. [CrossRef]
67. Thomas, H. Gut microbiota: Intestinal fungi fuel the inflammatory fire in alcoholic liver disease. *Nat. Rev. Gastroenterol. Hepatol.* **2017**, *14*, 385. [CrossRef]
68. Dyson, J.K.; Beuers, U.; Jones, D.E.J.; Lohse, A.W.; Hudson, M. Primary sclerosing cholangitis. *Lancet* **2018**, *391*, 2547–2559. [CrossRef]
69. Sibley, D.; Jerrells, T.R. Alcohol consumption by C57BL/6 mice is associated with depletion of lymphoid cells from the gut-associated lymphoid tissues and altered resistance to oral infections with Salmonella typhimurium. *J. Infect Dis.* **2000**, *182*, 482–489. [CrossRef]
70. Kim, R.; Lee, D.H.; Subramanian, S.V. Understanding the obesity epidemic. *BMJ* **2019**, *366*, l4409. [CrossRef]
71. Friedman, S.L.; Neuschwander-Tetri, B.A.; Rinella, M.; Sanyal, A.J. Mechanisms of NAFLD development and therapeutic strategies. *Nat. Med.* **2018**, *24*, 908–922.
72. Abenavoli, L.; Milic, N.; Di Renzo, L.; Preveden, T.; Medić-Stojanoska, M.; De Lorenzo, A. Metabolic aspects of adult patients with nonalcoholic fatty liver disease. *World J. Gastroenterol.* **2016**, *22*, 7006–7016. [CrossRef] [PubMed]
73. Gomes, A.C.; Hoffmann, C.; Mota, J.F. The human gut microbiota: Metabolism and perspective in obesity. *Gut Microbes* **2018**, *9*, 308–325. [CrossRef] [PubMed]
74. Kang, Y.; Cai, Y. Gut microbiota and obesity: Implications for fecal microbiota transplantation therapy. *Hormones (Athens)* **2017**, *16*, 223–234. [CrossRef] [PubMed]
75. Wigg, A.J.; Roberts-Thomson, I.C.; Dymock, R.B.; McCarthy, P.J.; Grose, R.H.; Cummins, A.G. The role of small intestinal bacterial overgrowth; intestinal permeability; endotoxaemia; and tumour necrosis factor alpha in the pathogenesis of non-alcoholic steatohepatitis. *Gut* **2001**, *48*, 206–211. [CrossRef]
76. Kim, H.N.; Joo, E.J.; Cheong, H.S.; Kim, Y.; Kim, H.L.; Shin, H.; Chang, Y.; Ryu, S.J. Gut Microbiota and Risk of Persistent Nonalcoholic Fatty Liver Diseases. *J. Clin. Med.* **2019**, *8*, 1089. [CrossRef] [PubMed]
77. Iruzubieta, P.; Medina, J.M.; Fernández-López, R.; Crespo, J.; de la Cruz, F.A. Role for Gut Microbiome Fermentative Pathways in Fatty Liver Disease Progression. *J. Clin. Med.* **2020**, *9*, 1369. [CrossRef] [PubMed]
78. Miele, L.; Valenza, V.; La Torre, G.; Montalto, M.; Cammarota, G.; Ricci, R.; Masciàna, R.; Forgione, A.; Gabrieli, M.L.; Perotti, G.; et al. Increased intestinal permeability and tight junction alterations in nonalcoholic fatty liver disease. *Hepatology* **2009**, *49*, 1877–1887. [CrossRef]
79. Kirsch, R.; Clarkson, V.; Verdonk, R.C.; Marais, A.D.; Shephard, E.G.; Ryffel, B.; de la M Hall, P.A.U.L.I.N.E. Rodent nutritional model of steatohepatitis: Effects of endotoxin (lipopolysaccharide) and tumor necrosis factor alpha deficiency. *J. Gastroenterol. Hepatol.* **2006**, *21*, 174–182. [CrossRef]

80. Saad, M.J.; Santos, A.; Prada, P.O. Linking Gut Microbiota and Inflammation to Obesity and Insulin Resistance. *Physiology (Bethesda)* **2016**, *31*, 283–293. [CrossRef]
81. Engel, B.; Taubert, R.; Jaeckel, E.; Manns, M.P. The future of autoimmune liver diseases—Understanding pathogenesis and improving morbidity and mortality. *Liver Int.* **2020**, *40*, 149–153. [CrossRef]
82. Bossen, L.; Gerussi, A.; Lygoura, V.; Mells, G.F.; Carbone, M.; Invernizzi, P. Support of precision medicine through risk-stratification in autoimmune liver diseases—histology; scoring systems; and non-invasive markers. *Autoimmun. Rev.* **2018**, *17*, 854–865. [CrossRef] [PubMed]
83. Cherrier, M.; Eberl, G. The development of LTi cells. *Curr. Opin. Immunol.* **2012**, *24*, 178–183. [CrossRef] [PubMed]
84. Washington, M.K. Autoimmune liver disease: Overlap and outliers. *Mod. Pathol.* **2007**, *20*, S15–S30. [CrossRef] [PubMed]
85. Hopf, U.; Möller, B.; Stemerowicz, R.; Lobeck, H.; Rodloff, A.; Freudenberg, M.; Galanos, C.; Huhn, D. Relation between Escherichia coli R(rough)-forms in gut; lipid A in liver; and primary biliary cirrhosis. *Lancet* **1989**, *2*, 1419–1422. [CrossRef]
86. Tripathi, A.; Debelius, J.; Brenner, D.A.; Karin, M.; Loomba, R.; Schnabl, B.; Knight, R. The gut-liver axis and the intersection with the microbiome. *Nat. Rev. Gastroenterol. Hepatol.* **2018**, *15*, 397–411. [CrossRef] [PubMed]
87. Yu, L.X.; Schwabe, R.F. The gut microbiome and liver cancer: Mechanisms and clinical translation. *Nat. Rev. Gastroenterol. Hepatol* **2017**, *14*, 527–539. [CrossRef]
88. Weng, M.T.; Chiu, Y.T.; Wei, P.Y.; Chiang, C.W.; Fang, H.L.; Wei, S.C. Microbiota and gastrointestinal cancer. *J. Formos. Med. Assoc.* **2019**, *118*, S32–S41. [CrossRef]
89. Such, J.; Francés, R.; Muñoz, C.; Zapater, P.; Casellas, J.A.; Cifuentes, A.; Rodríguez-Valera, F.; Pascual, S.; Sola-Vera, J.; Carnicer, F.; et al. Detection and identification of bacterial DNA in patients with cirrhosis and culture-negative; nonneutrocytic ascites. *Hepatology* **2002**, *36*, 135–141. [CrossRef]
90. Papp, M.; Norman, G.L.; Vitalis, Z.; Tornai, I.; Altorjay, I.; Foldi, I.; Udvardy, M.; Shums, Z.; Dinya, T.; Orosz, P.; et al. Presence of anti-microbial antibodies in liver cirrhosis–a tell-tale sign of compromised immunity? *PLoS ONE* **2010**, *5*, e12957. [CrossRef]
91. Ridlon, J.M.; Kang, D.J.; Hylemon, P.B. Bile salt biotransformations by human intestinal bacteria. *J. Lipid Res.* **2006**, *47*, 241–259. [CrossRef] [PubMed]
92. Kakiyama, G.; Pandak, W.M.; Gillevet, P.M.; Hylemon, P.B.; Heuman, D.M.; Daita, K.; Takei, H.; Muto, A.; Nittono, H.; Ridlon, J.M.; et al. Modulation of the fecal bile acid profile by gut microbiota in cirrhosis. *J. Hepatol.* **2013**, *58*, 949–955. [CrossRef] [PubMed]
93. Guarner, C.; Soriano, G. Spontaneous bacterial peritonitis. *Semin. Liv. Dis.* **1997**, *17*, 203–217. [CrossRef] [PubMed]
94. Chen, Y.; Yang, F.; Lu, H.; Wang, B.; Chen, Y.; Lei, D.; Wang, Y.; Zhu, B.; Li, L. Characterization of fecal microbial communities in patients with liver cirrhosis. *Hepatology* **2011**, *54*, 562–572. [CrossRef]
95. Qin, N.; Yang, F.; Li, A.; Prifti, E.; Chen, Y.; Shao, L.; Guo, J.; Le Chatelier, E.; Yao, J.; Wu, L.; et al. Alterations of the human gut microbiome in liver cirrhosis. *Nature* **2014**, *513*, 59–64. [CrossRef]
96. Huang, B.; Zhao, J.; Unkeless, J.C.; Feng, Z.H.; Xiong, H. TLR signaling by tumor and immune cells: A double-edged sword. *Oncogene* **2008**, *27*, 218–224. [CrossRef]
97. Dapito, D.H.; Mencin, A.; Gwak, G.Y.; Pradere, J.P.; Jang, M.K.; Mederacke, I.; Caviglia, J.M.; Khiabanian, H.; Adeyemi, A.; Bataller, R.; et al. Promotion of hepatocellular carcinoma by the intestinal microbiota and TLR4. *Cancer Cell* **2012**, *21*, 504–516. [CrossRef]
98. Garcia-Gonzalez, M.; Boixeda, D.; Herrero, D.; Burgaleta, C. Effect of granulocyte-macrophage colony-stimulating factor on leukocyte function in cirrhosis. *Gastroenterology* **1993**, *105*, 527–531. [CrossRef]
99. Rajkovic, I.A.; Williams, R. Abnormalities of neutrophil phagocytosis; intracellular killing and metabolic activity in alcoholic cirrhosis and hepatitis. *Hepatology* **1986**, *6*, 252–262. [CrossRef]
100. Rimola, A.; Soto, R.; Bory, F.; Arroyo, V.; Piera, C.; Rodes, J. Reticuloendothelial system phagocytic activity in cirrhosis and its relation to bacterial infections and prognosis. *Hepatology* **1984**, *4*, 53–58. [CrossRef]
101. Lamontagne, A.; Long, R.E.; Comunale, M.A.; Hafner, J.; Rodemich-Betesh, L.; Wang, M.; Marrero, J.; Di Bisceglie, A.M.; Block, T.; Mehta, A. Altered functionality of anti-bacterial antibodies in patients with chronic hepatitis C virus infection. *PLoS ONE* **2013**, *8*, e64992. [CrossRef] [PubMed]

102. Inamura, T.; Miura, S.; Tsuzuki, Y.; Hara, Y.; Hokari, R.; Ogawa, T.; Teramoto, K.; Watanabe, C.; Kobayashi, H.; Nagata, H.; et al. Alteration of intestinal intraepithelial lymphocytes and increased bacterial translocation in a murine model of cirrhosis. *Immunol. Lett.* **2003**, *90*, 3–11. [CrossRef] [PubMed]
103. Germani, G.; Becchetti, C. Liver transplantation for non-alcoholic fatty liver disease. *Minerva. Gastroenterol. Dietol.* **2018**, *64*, 138–146. [CrossRef] [PubMed]
104. Li, Q.R.; Wang, C.Y.; Tang, C.; He, Q.; Li, N.; Li, J.S. Reciprocal interaction between intestinal microbiota and mucosal lymphocyte in cynomolgus monkeys after alemtuzumab treatment. *Am. J. Transpl.* **2013**, *13*, 899–910. [CrossRef]
105. Wu, Z.W.; Ling, Z.X.; Lu, H.F.; Zuo, J.; Sheng, J.F.; Zheng, S.S.; Li, L.J. Changes of gut bacteria and immune parameters in liver transplant recipients. *Hepatobiliary Pancreat Dis. Int.* **2012**, *11*, 40–50. [CrossRef]
106. Reyes, A.; Semenkovich, N.P.; Whiteson, K.; Rohwer, F.; Gordon, J.I. Going viral: Next-generation sequencing applied to phage populations in the human gut. *Nat. Rev. Microbiol.* **2012**, *10*, 607–617. [CrossRef]
107. Lozupone, C.A.; Stombaugh, J.I.; Gordon, J.I.; Jansson, J.K.; Knight, R. Diversity; stability and resilience of the human gut microbiota. *Nature* **2012**, *489*, 220–230. [CrossRef]
108. Scarpellini, E.; Ianiro, G.; Attili, F.; Bassanelli, C.; De Santis, A.; Gasbarrini, A. The human gut microbiota and virome: Potential therapeutic implications. *Dig. Liver Dis.* **2015**, *47*, 1007–1012. [CrossRef]
109. Lagier, J.C.; Million, M.; Hugon, P.; Armougom, F.; Raoult, D. Human gut microbiota: Repertoire and variations. *Front. Cell Infect Microbiol.* **2012**, *2*, 136. [CrossRef]
110. Holtz, L.R.; Cao, S.; Zhao, G.; Bauer, I.K.; Denno, D.M.; Klein, E.J.; Antonio, M.; Stine, O.C.; Snelling, T.L.; Kirkwood, C.D.; et al. Geographic variation in the eukaryotic virome of human diarrhea. *Virology* **2014**, *468–470*, 556–564. [CrossRef]
111. Colson, P.; Fancello, L.; Gimenez, G.; Armougom, F.; Desnues, C.; Fournous, G.; Yoosuf, N.; Million, M.; La Scola, B.; Raoult, D. Evidence of the megavirome in humans. *J. Clin. Virol.* **2013**, *57*, 191–200. [CrossRef] [PubMed]
112. Zhang, T.; Breitbart, M.; Lee, W.H.; Run, J.Q.; Wei, C.L.; Soh, S.W.; Hibberd, M.L.; Liu, E.T.; Rohwer, F.; Ruan, Y. RNA viral community in human feces: Prevalence of plant pathogenic viruses. Version 2. *PLoS Biol.* **2006**, *4*, e3. [CrossRef] [PubMed]
113. Sutton, T.D.S.; Hill, C. Gut Bacteriophage: Current Understanding and Challenges. *Front. Endocrinol. (Lausanne)* **2019**, *10*, 784. [CrossRef] [PubMed]
114. Roux, S.; Krupovic, M.; Poulet, A.; Debroas, D.; Enault, F. Evolution and diversity of the Microviridae viral family through a collection of 81 new complete genomes assembled from virome reads. *PLoS ONE* **2012**, *7*, e40418. [CrossRef]
115. Vemuri, R.; Shankar, E.M.; Chieppa, M.; Eri, R.; Kavanagh, K. Beyond Just Bacteria: Functional Biomes in the Gut Ecosystem Including Virome; Mycobiome; Archaeome and Helminths. *Microorganisms* **2020**, *8*, 483. [CrossRef]
116. Duan, Y.; Llorente, C.; Lang, S.; Brandl, K.; Chu, H.; Jiang, L.; White, R.C.; Clarke, T.H.; Nguyen, K.; Torralba, M.; et al. Bacteriophage targeting of gut bacterium attenuates alcoholic liver disease. *Nature* **2019**, *575*, 505–511. [CrossRef]
117. Gilmore, M.S.; Segarra, R.A.; Booth, M.C.; Bogie, C.P.; Hall, L.R.; Clewell, D.B. Genetic structure of the Enterococcus faecalis plasmid pAD1-encoded cytolytic toxin system and its relationship to lantibiotic determinants. *J. Bacteriol.* **1994**, *176*, 7335–7344. [CrossRef]
118. Cox, C.R.; Coburn, P.S.; Gilmore, M.S. Enterococcal cytolysin: A novel two component peptide system that serves as a bacterial defense against eukaryotic and prokaryotic cells. *Curr. Protein Pept. Sci.* **2005**, *6*, 77–84. [CrossRef]
119. Van Tyne, D.; Martin, M.J.; Gilmore, M.S. Structure; function; and biology of the Enterococcus faecalis cytolysin. *Toxins* **2013**, *5*, 895–911. [CrossRef]
120. Chatterjee, A.; Johnson, C.N.; Luong, P.; Hullahalli, K.; McBride, S.W.; Schubert, A.M.; Palmer, K.L.; Carlson, P.E., Jr.; Duerkop, B.A. Bacteriophage Resistance Alters Antibiotic-Mediated Intestinal Expansion of Enterococci. *Infect Immun.* **2019**, *87*, e00085-19. [CrossRef]
121. Górski, A.; Dąbrowska, K.; Międzybrodzki, R.; Weber-Dąbrowska, B.; Łusiak-Szelachowska, M.; Jończyk-Matysiak, E.; Borysowski, J. Phages and immunomodulation. *Future Microbiol.* **2017**, *12*, 905–914. [CrossRef] [PubMed]

122. Górski, A.; Jończyk-Matysiak, E.; Łusiak-Szelachowska, M.; Weber-Dąbrowska, B.; Międzybrodzki, R.; Borysowski, J. Therapeutic potential of phages in autoimmune liver diseases. *Clin. Exp. Immunol.* **2018**, *192*, 1–6. [CrossRef] [PubMed]
123. Barr, J.J.; Auro, R.; Furlan, M.; Whiteson, K.L.; Erb, M.L.; Pogliano, J.; Stotland, A.; Wolkowicz, R.; Cutting, A.S.; Doran, K.S.; et al. Bacteriophage adhering to mucus provide a non-host-derived immunity. *Proc. Natl. Acad. Sci. USA* **2013**, *110*, 10771–10776. [CrossRef]
124. Gorski, A.; Weber-DaBrowska, B. The potential role of endogenous phages in controlling invading pathogens. *Cell Mol. Life Sci.* **2005**, *62*, 511–519. [CrossRef] [PubMed]
125. Międzybrodzki, R.; Borysowski, J.; Kłak, M.; Jończyk-Matysiak, E.; Obmińska-Mrukowicz, B.; Suszko-Pawłowska, A.; Bubak, B.; Weber-Dąbrowska, B.; Górski, A. In Vivo Studies on the Influence of Bacteriophage Preparations on the Autoimmune Inflammatory Process. *Biomed. Res. Int.* **2017**, *2017*, 3612015. [CrossRef] [PubMed]
126. Miernikiewicz, P.; Kłopot, A.; Soluch, R.; Szkuta, P.; Kęska, W.; Hodyra-Stefaniak, K.; Konopka, A.; Nowak, M.; Lecion, D.; Kaźmierczak, Z.; et al. T4 Phage Tail Adhesin Gp12 Counteracts LPS-Induced Inflammation In Vivo. *Front. Microbiol.* **2016**, *7*, 1112. [CrossRef]
127. Miedzybrodzki, R.; Fortuna, W.; Weber-Dabrowska, B.; Górski, A. A retrospective analysis of changes in inflammatory markers in patients treated with bacterial viruses. *Clin. Exp. Med.* **2009**, *9*, 303–312. [CrossRef]
128. Krenkel, O.; Tacke, F. Liver macrophages in tissue homeostasis and disease. *Nat. Rev. Immunol.* **2017**, *17*, 306–321. [CrossRef]
129. de Araújo, R.F., Jr.; Reinaldo, M.P.; Brito, G.A.; Cavalcanti Pde, F.; Freire, M.A.; de Medeiros, C.A.; de Araújo, A.A. Olmesartan decreased levels of IL-1β and TNF-α; down-regulated MMP-2; MMP-9; COX-2; RANK/RANKL and up-regulated SOCs-1 in an intestinal mucositis model. *PLoS ONE* **2014**, *9*, e114923. [CrossRef]
130. Kakinuma, Y.; Kimura, T.; Watanabe, Y. Possible Involvement of Liver Resident Macrophages (Kupffer Cells) in the Pathogenesis of Both Intrahepatic and Extrahepatic Inflammation. *Can. J. Gastroenterol. Hepatol.* **2017**, *2017*, 2896809. [CrossRef]
131. Baroja-Mazo, A.; Revilla-Nuin, B.; Parrilla, P.; Martínez-Alarcón, L.; Ramírez, P.; Pons, J.A. Tolerance in liver transplantation: Biomarkers and clinical relevance. *World J. Gastroenterol.* **2016**, *22*, 7676–7691. [CrossRef] [PubMed]
132. Ruiz, R.; Kunitake, H.; Wilkinson, A.H.; Danovitch, G.M.; Farmer, D.G.; Ghobrial, R.M.; Yersiz, H.; Hiatt, J.R.; Busuttil, R.W. Long-term analysis of combined liver and kidney transplantation at a single center. *Arch. Surg.* **2006**, *141*, 735–741. [CrossRef] [PubMed]
133. Inchley, C.J. The activity of mouse Kupffer cells following intravenous injection of bacteriophage. *Clin. Exp. Immunol.* **1969**, *5*, 173–187. [PubMed]
134. Inchley, C.J.; Howard, J.G. The immunogenicity of phagocytosed T4 bacteriophage: Cell replacement studies with splenectomised and irradiated mice. *Clin. Exp. Immunol.* **1969**, *5*, 189–198. [PubMed]
135. Van Belleghem, J.D.; Clement, F.; Merabishvili, M.; Lavigne, R.; Vaneechoutte, M. Pro- and anti-inflammatory responses of peripheral blood mononuclear cells induced by Staphylococcus aureus and Pseudomonas aeruginosa phages. *Sci. Rep.* **2017**, *7*, 8004. [CrossRef]
136. Zhang, L.J.; Wang, X.Z. Interleukin-10 and chronic liver disease. *World J. Gastroenterol.* **2006**, *12*, 1681–1685. [CrossRef]
137. Abel, M.; Sène, D.; Pol, S.; Bourlière, M.; Poynard, T.; Charlotte, F.; Cacoub, P.; Caillat-Zucman, S. Intrahepatic virus-specific IL-10-producing CD8 T cells prevent liver damage during chronic hepatitis C virus infection. *Hepatology* **2006**, *44*, 1607–1616. [CrossRef]
138. Luedde, T.; Schwabe, R.F. NF-kappa B in liver injury; fibrosis and hepatocellular carcinoma. *Nat. Rev. Gastroenterol. Hepatol.* **2011**, *8*, 108–118. [CrossRef]
139. Soares, J.B.; Pimentel-Nunes, P.; Roncon-Albuquerque, R.; Leite-Moreira, A. The role of lipopolysaccharide/Toll-like receptor 4 signaling in chronic liver diseases. *Hepatol. Int.* **2010**, *4*, 659–672. [CrossRef]
140. Kiziltas, S. Toll-like receptors in pathophysiology of liver diseases. *World J. Hepatol.* **2016**, *8*, 1354–1369. [CrossRef]
141. Chauhan, A.; Adams, D.H.; Watson, S.P.; Lalor, P.F. Platelets: No longer bystanders in liver disease. *Hepatology* **2016**, *64*, 1774–1784. [CrossRef] [PubMed]

142. Chang, L.; Wang, G.; Jia, T.; Zhang, L.; Li, Y.; Han, Y.; Zhang, K.; Lin, G.; Zhang, R.; Li, J.; et al. Armored long non-coding RNA MEG3 targeting EGFR based on recombinant MS2 bacteriophage virus-like particles against hepatocellular carcinoma. *Oncotarget* **2016**, *7*, 23988–24004. [CrossRef] [PubMed]
143. Bakhshinejad, B.; Sadeghizadeh, M. Bacteriophages and their applications in the diagnosis and treatment of hepatitis B virus infection. *World J. Gastroenterol.* **2014**, *20*, 11671–11683. [CrossRef] [PubMed]
144. Gentile, I.; Abenavoli, L. COVID-19: Perspectives on the Potential Novel Global Threat. *Rev. Recent Clin. Trials* **2020**. [CrossRef] [PubMed]
145. National Institute for Health and Care Excellence (NICE) in collaboration with NHS England and NHS Improvement. Managing COVID-19 symptoms (including at the end of life) in the community: Summary of NICE guidelines. *BMJ* **2020**, *369*, m1461. [CrossRef]
146. Méndez-Sánchez, N.; Valencia-Rodríguez, A.; Qi, X.; Yoshida, E.M.; Romero-Gómez, M.; George, J.; Eslam, M.; Abenavoli, L.; Xie, W.; Teschke, R.; et al. What Has the COVID-19 Pandemic Taught Us so Far? Addressing the Problem from a Hepatologist's Perspective. *J. Clin. Transl. Hepatol.* **2020**, *8*, 0024. [CrossRef] [PubMed]
147. Huang, C.; Wang, Y.; Li, X.; Ren, L.; Zhao, J.; Hu, Y.; Zhang, L.; Fan, G.; Xu, J.; Gu, X.; et al. Clinical features of patients infected with 2019 novel coronavirus in Wuhan; China. *Lancet* **2020**, *395*, 497–506. [CrossRef]
148. Zhang, C.; Shi, L.; Wang, F.S. Liver injury in COVID-19: Management and challenges. *Lancet Gastroenterol. Hepatol.* **2020**, *5*, 428–430. [CrossRef]
149. Xu, Z.; Shi, L.; Wang, Y.; Zhang, J.; Huang, L.; Zhang, C.; Liu, S.; Zhao, P.; Liu, H.; Zhu, L.; et al. Pathological findings of COVID-19 associated with acute respiratory distress syndrome. *Lancet Respir. Med.* **2020**, *8*, 420–422. [CrossRef]
150. Mehta, P.; McAuley, D.F.; Brown, M.; Sanchez, E.; Tattersall, R.S.; Manson, J.J. HLH Across Speciality Collaboration; UK. COVID-19: Consider cytokine storm syndromes and immunosuppression. *Lancet* **2020**, *395*, 1033–1034. [CrossRef]
151. Pirola, C.J.; Sookoian, S. SARS-CoV-2 virus and liver expression of host receptors: Putative mechanisms of liver involvement in COVID-19. *Liver Int.* **2020**, in press. [CrossRef] [PubMed]
152. Mantovani, A.; Beatrice, G.; Dalbeni, A. Coronavirus disease 2019 (COVID-19) and prevalence of chronic liver disease: A meta-analysis. *Liver Int.* **2020**, in press. [CrossRef] [PubMed]
153. Zacharias, H.D.; Zacharias, A.P.; Gluud, L.L.; Morgan, M.Y. Pharmacotherapies that specifically target ammonia for the prevention and treatment of hepatic encephalopathy in adults with cirrhosis. *Cochrane Database Syst. Rev.* **2019**, *6*, CD012334. [CrossRef] [PubMed]
154. Panesar, P.S.; Kumari, S. Lactulose: Production; purification and potential applications. *Biotechnol. Adv.* **2011**, *29*, 940–948. [CrossRef]
155. Markowiak, P.; Śliżewska, K. Effects of Probiotics; Prebiotics; and Synbiotics on Human Healh. *Nutrients* **2017**, *9*, 1021. [CrossRef]
156. Bengmark, S. Bioecologic control of the gastrointestinal tract: The role of flora and supplemented probiotics and synbiotics. *Gastroenterol. Clin. North Am.* **2005**, *34*, 413–436. [CrossRef]
157. Bajaj, J.S. Alcohol; liver disease and the gut microbiota. *Nat. Rev. Gastroenterol. Hepatol.* **2019**, *16*, 235–246. [CrossRef]
158. Forsyth, C.B.; Farhadi, A.; Jakate, S.M.; Tang, Y.; Shaikh, M.; Keshavarzian, A. Lactobacillus GG treatment ameliorates alcohol-induced intestinal oxidative stress; gut leakiness; and liver injury in a rat model of alcoholic steatohepatitis. *Alcohol* **2009**, *43*, 163–172. [CrossRef]
159. Kirpich, I.A.; Solovieva, N.V.; Leikhter, S.N.; Shidakova, N.A.; Lebedeva, O.V.; Sidorov, P.I.; Bazhukova, T.A.; Soloviev, A.G.; Barve, S.S.; McClain, C.J.; et al. Probiotics restore bowel flora and improve liver enzymes in human alcohol-induced liver injury: A pilot study. *Alcohol* **2008**, *42*, 675–682. [CrossRef]
160. Stadlbauer, V.; Mookerjee, R.P.; Hodges, S.; Wright, G.A.; Davies, N.A.; Jalan, R. Effect of probiotic treatment on deranged neutrophil function and cytokine responses in patients with compensated alcoholic cirrhosis. *J. Hepatol.* **2008**, *48*, 945–951. [CrossRef]
161. Kolodziejczyk, A.A.; Zheng, D.; Shibolet, O.; Elinav, E. The role of the microbiome in NAFLD and NASH. *EMBO Mol. Med.* **2019**, *11*, e9302. [CrossRef] [PubMed]

162. Li, Z.; Yang, S.; Lin, H.; Huang, J.; Watkins, P.A.; Moser, A.B.; Desimone, C.; Song, X.Y.; Diehl, A.M. Probiotics and antibodies to TNF inhibit inflammatory activity and improve nonalcoholic fatty liver disease. *Hepatology* **2003**, *37*, 343–350. [CrossRef] [PubMed]
163. Loguercio, C.; Federico, A.; Tuccillo, C.; Terracciano, F.; D'Auria, M.V.; De Simone, C.; Del Vecchio Blanco, C. Beneficial effects of a probiotic VSL#3 on parameters of liver dysfunction in chronic liver diseases. *J. Clin. Gastroenterol.* **2005**, *39*, 540–543. [CrossRef] [PubMed]
164. Aller, R.; De Luis, D.A.; Izaola, O.; Conde, R.; Gonzalez Sagrado, M.; Primo, D.; De La Fuente, B.; Gonzalez, J. Effect of a probiotic on liver aminotransferases in nonalcoholic fatty liver disease patients: A double blind randomized clinical trial. *Eur. Rev. Med. Pharmacol. Sci.* **2011**, *15*, 1090–1095. [PubMed]
165. Vajro, P.; Mandato, C.; Licenziati, M.R.; Franzese, A.; Vitale, D.F.; Lenta, S.; Caropreso, M.; Vallone, G.; Meli, R. Effects of Lactobacillus rhamnosus strain GG in pediatric obesity-related liver disease. *J. Pediatr. Gastroenterol. Nutr.* **2011**, *52*, 740–743. [CrossRef]
166. Malaguarnera, M.; Vacante, M.; Antic, T.; Giordano, M.; Chisari, G.; Acquaviva, R.; Mastrojeni, S.; Malaguarnera, G.; Mistretta, A.; Li Volti, G.; et al. Bifidobacterium longum with fructo-oligosaccharides in patients with non alcoholic steatohepatitis. *Dig. Dis. Sci.* **2012**, *57*, 545–553. [CrossRef]
167. Ma, Y.Y.; Li, L.; Yu, C.H.; Shen, Z.; Chen, L.H.; Li, Y.M. Effects of probiotics on nonalcoholic fatty liver disease: A meta-analysis. *World J. Gastroenterol.* **2013**, *19*, 6911–6918. [CrossRef]
168. Vleggaar, F.P.; Monkelbaan, J.F.; van Erpecum, K.J. Probiotics in primary sclerosing cholangitis: A randomized placebo-controlled crossover pilot study. *Eur. J. Gastroenterol. Hepatol.* **2008**, *20*, 688–692. [CrossRef]
169. Tsochatzis, E.A.; Bosch, J.; Burroughs, A.K. Liver cirrhosis. *Lancet* **2014**, *383*, 1749–1761. [CrossRef]
170. Tilg, H.; Cani, P.D.; Mayer, E.A. Gut microbiome and liver diseases. *Gut* **2016**, *65*, 2035–2044. [CrossRef]
171. Acharya, C.; Bajaj, J.S. Gut Microbiota and Complications of Liver Disease. *Gastroenterol. Clin. N. Am.* **2017**, *46*, 155–169. [CrossRef] [PubMed]
172. Liu, Q.; Duan, Z.P.; Ha, D.K.; Bengmark, S.; Kurtovic, J.; Riordan, S.M. Symbiotic modulation of gut flora: Effect on minimal hepatic encephalopathy in patients with cirrhosis. *Hepatology* **2004**, *39*, 1441–1449. [CrossRef] [PubMed]
173. Lachar, J.; Bajaj, J.S. Changes in the Microbiome in Cirrhosis and Relationship to Complications: Hepatic Encephalopathy; Spontaneous Bacterial Peritonitis; and Sepsis. *Semin. Liver Dis.* **2016**, *36*, 327–330. [CrossRef] [PubMed]
174. Bauer, T.M.; Fernandez, J.; Navasa, M.; Vila, J.; Rodes, J. Failure of Lactobacillus spp. to prevent bacterial translocation in a rat model of experimental cirrhosis. *J. Hepatol.* **2002**, *36*, 501–506. [CrossRef]
175. Pande, C.; Kumar, A.; Sarin, S.K. Addition of probiotics to norfloxacin does not improve efficacy in the prevention of spontaneous bacterial peritonitis: A double-blind placebo-controlled randomized-controlled trial. *Eur. J. Gastroenterol. Hepatol.* **2012**, *24*, 831–839. [CrossRef]
176. Macbeth, W.A.; Kass, E.H.; McDermott, W.V., Jr. Treatment of Hepatic Encephalopathy by Alteration of Intestinal Flora with Lactobacillus Acidophilus. *Lancet* **1965**, *1*, 399–403. [CrossRef]
177. Read, A.E.; McCarthy, C.F.; Heaton, K.W.; Laidlaw, J. Lactobacillus acidophilus (enpac) in treatment of hepatic encephalopathy. *BMJ* **1966**, *1*, 1267–1269. [CrossRef]
178. Arab, J.P.; Martin-Mateos, R.M.; Shah, V.H. Gut-liver axis; cirrhosis and portal hypertension: The chicken and the egg. *Hepatol. Int.* **2018**, *12*, 24–33. [CrossRef]
179. De Santis, A.; Famularo, G.; De Simone, C. Probiotics for the hemodynamic alterations of patients with liver cirrhosis. *Am. J. Gastroenterol.* **2000**, *95*, 323–324. [CrossRef]
180. Jayakumar, S.; Carbonneau, M.; Hotte, N.; Befus, A.D.; St Laurent, C.; Owen, R.; McCarthy, M.; Madsen, K.; Bailey, R.J.; Ma, M.; et al. VSL#3® probiotic therapy does not reduce portal pressures in patients with decompensated cirrhosis. *Liver Int.* **2013**, *33*, 1470–1477. [CrossRef]
181. Tandon, P.; Moncrief, K.; Madsen, K.; Arrieta, M.C.; Owen, R.J.; Bain, V.G.; Wong, W.W.; Ma, M.M. Effects of probiotic therapy on portal pressure in patients with cirrhosis: A pilot study. *Liver Int.* **2009**, *29*, 1110–1115. [CrossRef] [PubMed]
182. Rincón, D.; Vaquero, J.; Hernando, A.; Galindo, E.; Ripoll, C.; Puerto, M.; Salcedo, M.; Francés, R.; Matilla, A.; Catalina, M.V.; et al. Oral probiotic VSL#3 attenuates the circulatory disturbances of patients with cirrhosis and ascites. *Liver Int.* **2014**, *34*, 1504–1512. [CrossRef] [PubMed]

183. Vaikunthanathan, T.; Safinia, N.; Lombardi, G.; Lechler, R.I. Microbiota; immunity and the liver. *Immunol. Lett.* **2016**, *171*, 36–49. [CrossRef] [PubMed]
184. El-Nezami, H.S.; Polychronaki, N.N.; Ma, J.; Zhu, H.; Ling, W.; Salminen, E.K.; Juvonen, R.O.; Salminen, S.J.; Poussa, T.; Mykkänen, H.M. Probiotic supplementation reduces a biomarker for increased risk of liver cancer in young men from Southern China. *Am. J. Clin. Nutr.* **2006**, *83*, 1199–1203. [CrossRef]

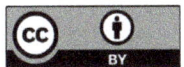

© 2020 by the authors. Licensee MDPI, Basel, Switzerland. This article is an open access article distributed under the terms and conditions of the Creative Commons Attribution (CC BY) license (http://creativecommons.org/licenses/by/4.0/).

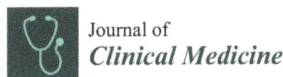

Review

Gut Microbiota: Implications in Alzheimer's Disease

Yixi He [1], Binyin Li [1], Dingya Sun [2] and Shengdi Chen [1,*]

[1] Department of Neurology and Institute of Neurology, Ruijin Hospital affiliated to Shanghai Jiao Tong University School of Medicine, Shanghai 200025, China; heyixiheyixi@163.com (Y.H.); libinyin@126.com (B.L.)

[2] Institute of Neuroscience, Key Laboratory of Molecular Neurobiology of the Ministry of Education, Second Military Medical University, Shanghai 200433, China; dingyasun@163.com

* Correspondence: chensd@rjh.com.cn

Received: 30 March 2020; Accepted: 15 June 2020; Published: 29 June 2020

Abstract: Alzheimer's disease (AD), the most common cause of dementia, is a neurodegenerative disease that seriously threatens human health and life quality. The main pathological features of AD include the widespread deposition of amyloid-beta and neurofibrillary tangles in the brain. So far, the pathogenesis of AD remains elusive, and no radical treatment has been developed. In recent years, mounting evidence has shown that there is a bidirectional interaction between the gut and brain, known as the brain–gut axis, and that the intestinal microbiota are closely related to the occurrence and development of neurodegenerative diseases. In this review, we will summarize the laboratory and clinical evidence of the correlation between intestinal flora and AD, discuss its possible role in the pathogenesis, and prospect its applications in the diagnosis and treatment of AD.

Keywords: Alzheimer's disease; gut microbiota; microbiota–gut–brain axis; neurodegenerative disease; intestinal flora

1. Introduction

Alzheimer's disease (AD), a neurodegenerative disease, as well as the most common cause of dementia in the elderly population, is a serious threat to human health and quality of life. Currently, there are 30 million cases of AD worldwide, and the number is expected to rise to 90 million by 2050 as the population ages [1]. China has the largest population of dementia patients in the world, which brings great pressure to its society [2]. AD usually has three stages: preclinical, mild cognitive impairment and dementia. Mild cognitive impairment, characterized mainly by forgetting, is the most common and most likely to develop into dementia. The pathological manifestations of AD mainly include extensive plaques formed by extracellular amyloid beta (Aβ) aggregation and intracellular neurofibrillary tangles formed by over-phosphorylated TAU protein, which are the gold standard for the pathological diagnosis of AD [3–5]. However, the deposits of Aβ and Tau have been shown to appear in the brain 10–20 years before the onset of clinical symptoms of dementia [3]. As for the clinical diagnosis of AD, although these biomarkers can be detected by positron emission tomography for Pittsburgh compound B (PiB) or lumbar puncture for CSF biochemical tests, few can accept radioactive or invasive testing when the patient is in very mild cognitive dysfunction, and diagnosing mainly depends on the evaluation of clinical symptoms. In terms of treatment, there is still a lack of effective drugs that can change the pathological process of AD despite the huge investment made by the industry [6]. Therefore, it is necessary to further clarify the pathological mechanism of AD, explore novel non-traumatic early biomarkers and develop new effective treatment strategies.

There are billions of microbes colonizing the human gut. Growing evidences suggest that there is a bidirectional connection between the gut microbiota and the brain, which is called the Microbiota–Gut–Brain Axis [7]. Gut dysbiosis has been revealed to be associated with neurodegenerative diseases, such as Parkinson's disease and Huntington's disease [8–10]. Currently, accumulating evidence supports the hypothesis that gut microbiota are closely related to the occurrence and development of many neurological diseases [7,11]. Experimental studies have shown that intestinal flora regulate brain functions such as learning and memory [12]. The intestinal microbiota can secrete a large amount of amyloids and lipopolysaccharide, which may lead to changes in signaling pathways and the production of pro-inflammatory factors, leading to Aβ deposition [13]. More importantly, the composition and function of gut microbiota can affect the pathophysiology of age-related cognitive impairment and dementia, suggesting that changes of intestinal flora may be one of the causes of AD [14–17]. Despite the fact that many excellent reviews have discussed the associations between gut microbiota and their role in AD and other neurodegenerative disorders [18–22], an in-depth comprehensive literature revision on the gut microbiota implications in AD is still greatly needed in order to understand the pathogenesis and to develop possible therapeutic and diagnostic strategies. Here, we intend to summarize gut microbiota alterations in AD patients and discuss their possible roles in the pathogenesis, and prospect its clinical implications.

2. Gut Microbiota Alterations in AD Patients

The studies of gut microbiota alterations in AD patients are summarized in Table 1. Analysis of intestinal flora in patients with AD-related cognitive dysfunction was first conducted by Cattaneo A and his colleagues [23]. In patients with cognitive impairment and brain amyloidosis ($n = 40$), patients with cognitive impairment without brain amyloidosis ($n = 33$) and healthy controls ($n = 10$), they measured the abundance of selected bacterial gut microbiota taxa in the feces, as well as the levels of cytokines and inflammatory factors in the blood. The characteristics of AD patients and healthy controls were of no significant difference regarding age, gender and body mass index. They found an increased abundance of the pro-inflammatory species Escherichia/Shigella in the intestinal flora of people with cognitive impairment and brain amyloidosis, while the abundance of anti-inflammatory species E. Rectale decreased. Moreover, the levels of pro-inflammatory cytokines IL-1β, NLRP3 and CXCL2 were positively correlated with inflammatory Escherichia/Shigella abundance and negatively correlated with anti-inflammatory E. Rectale. Haran JP and his colleagues recruited AD patients ($n = 24$, with average age 84.7 years) and gender-matched controls ($n = 51$, with average age 83.0 years), in which there were no significant difference in age, gender or medical history between the groups. They showed that the proportion of bacteria capable of synthesizing butyrate in the microbiota of AD patients' feces decreased, while the abundance of pro-inflammatory bacteria increased [24]. They also found that fecal samples from elderly patients with AD could induce lower expression level of p-glycoprotein (a key mediator of intestinal homeostasis) in intestinal epithelial cells in vitro, and p-glycoprotein dysregulation would contribute directly to inflammatory disorders of the intestine. These studies suggest that disturbance in the gut microbiota, which leads to loss of intestinal homeostasis and inflammation, may underlie neurodegenerative disease.

Table 1. Gut microbiota alterations in patients with Alzheimer's disease.

Cases	Age	Clinical Evaluation	Phylum	Class	Order	Family	Genus	References
33	74.85 (11.37)	MMSE; MoCA	↑Proteobacteria ↓Firmicutes	↑Gammaproteobacteria ↓Clostridia	↑Enterobacteriales ↓Clostridiales	↑Enterobacteriaceae ↓Clostridiaceae, Lachnospiraceae, Ruminococcaceae	↓Blautia, Ruminococcus	Liu, et al. 2019
30	66.3 (5.1)	MMSE; MTA	/	/	/	/	↑Bifidobacterium, Blautia, Dorea, Escherichia, Lactobacillus, Streptococcus ↓Alistipes, Bacteroides, Parabacteroides, Paraprevotella, Sutterella	Li, et al. 2019
24	84.7 (8.1)	CDR	/	/	/	/	↑Alistipes, Bacteroides, Barnesiella, Collinsella, Odoribacter ↓Eubacterium, Lachnoclostridium, Roseburia	Haran, et al. 2019
43	70.12 (8.78)	MMSE; ADL; CDR; PiB	↑Actinobacteria ↓Bacteroidetes	↑Actinobacteria, Bacilli ↓Bacteroidia, Negativicutes	↑Lactobacillales ↓Bacteroidales, Selenomonadales	↑Enterococcaceae, Lactobacillaceae, Ruminococcaceae ↓Bacteroidaceae, Lanchnospiraceae, Veillonellaceae	↑Subdoligranulum ↓Bacteroides, Lachnoclostridium	Zhuang et al. 2018
40	71 (7.0)	MMSE; Amyloid PET	/	/	/	/	↑Escherichia/Shigella ↓Bacteroides fragilis, Eubacterium rectale	Cattaneo, et al. 2017
25	71.3 (7.3)	CDR; CSF marker	↑Bacteroidetes ↓Firmicutes, Actinobacteria			↑Bacteroidaceae, Rikenellaceae, Gemellaceae ↓Ruminococcaceae, Bifidobacteriaceae, Clostridiaceae, Mogibacteriaceae, Turicibacteraceae, Peptostreptococcaceae	↑Alistipes, Bacteroides, Bilophila, Blautia, Gemella, Phascolarctobacterium ↓Adlercreutzia, Bifidobacterium, cc115, Clostridium, Dialister, SMB53, Turicibacter	Vogt, et al. 2017

Abbreviations: Age, years (SD); MMSE, Mini-Mental State Examination; ADL, Activities of Daily Living; CDR, Clinical Dementia Rating; MoCA, Montreal Cognitive Assessment; Amyloid PET, amyloid positron-emission tomography (PET) with 18 F-Florbetapir; PiB, Positron emission tomography for Pittsburgh compound B to detect and quantify Aβ deposition; MTA, Medial temporal atrophy score measured by structural MRI; CSF marker, CSF biochemical tests including Aβ42, Aβ40, phosphorylated tau. ↑, increased abundance; ↓, decreased abundance.

Vogt et al. examined the composition of intestinal microbiota of AD patients ($n = 25$) and controls ($n = 25$). The characteristics of patients with AD and healthy controls were of no significant differences in age, gender, ethnicity, body mass index or diabetes status [25]. The results showed that the intestinal microbial diversity decreased in AD patients. Compared with the control group, the abundance of Firmicutes and Actinobacteria in AD patients was lower, while the abundance of Bacteroidetes was higher. They also analyzed the correlation between the levels of genera abundance and the cerebrospinal fluid biomarkers for AD, and suggested that AD should be included in the list of diseases associated with microbial changes in the gut. Zhuang ZQ et al. collected fecal samples from AD patients ($n = 43$) and normal controls ($n = 43$), and analyzed the fecal flora composition [26]. There was no significant difference in education and comorbidities of hypertension, diabetes mellitus, hypercholesterolemia and coronary heart disease between AD patients and normal controls. They found that several bacteria taxa in AD patients were changed at taxonomic levels. They further demonstrated that the decreased abundance of Bacteroides and Lachnoclostridium at genus level may represent the alterations at the family level in the intestinal bacteria of AD patients.

Cognitive dysfunction is the clinical characteristic of AD. Although studies have suggested changes in the intestinal flora of AD, it is unclear whether these changes are related to patients' cognitive dysfunction. Liu P et al. recruited a total of 97 subjects (33 AD, 32 aMCI and 32 healthy controls), in which all were right-handed, aged 50 to 85 years, with at least six years of education. They found a decrease in fecal microbial diversity and significant differences in microbial composition in AD patients compared to aMCI patients and healthy controls [27]. Compared with the control group, in the feces of AD patients, the proportion of Firmicutes decreased significantly, while the abundance of Proteobacteria increased. Gammaproteobacteria, Enterobacteriales and Enterobacteriaceae were shown to have an enriched prevalence from aMCI to AD patients. There was a significant correlation between clinical severity score and changes in microflora abundance in patients with AD. In our study, a total of 90 subjects (30 AD, 30 aMCI and 30 healthy controls) were recruited, and the characteristics of patients with AD and MCI and healthy controls were of no significant differences in age, gender, education, body mass index or constipation. The mini-mental State Examination (MMSE) scale was evaluated, and the composition of gut and blood bacterial communities was determined by 16S ribosomal RNA gene sequencing [28]. Our results showed that patients with AD have similar intestinal flora to those with MCI. Compared with the control group, the abundance of Alistipes, Bacteroides, Parabacteroides, Sutterella and Paraprevotella in the fecal samples of AD patients was decreased. Notably, the reduction of Bacteroides has been reported in another report [26], which suggests that this genus may be a protective factor of AD. The proportion of Dorea, Lactobacillus, Streptococcus, Escherichia, Bifidobacterium and Blautia in the fecal samples of AD patients was increased, among which the increased abundance of Blautia and Dorea was correlated with a decreased MMSE score, suggesting that they were risk factors for the development of AD. The abundance of Escherichia in the blood and stool samples of AD and MCI patients was increased, suggesting that Escherichia may be involved in the pathogenesis of AD, given that the deposition of Aβ in the brain of AD patients may be associated with central bacterial infection and inflammation.

3. The Pathogenic Role of Gut Microbiota in AD

3.1. Gut Microbiota Alterations in AD Models

Many studies have shown that changes in intestinal flora composition lead to increased intestinal barrier permeability and systemic inflammation, which impairs the blood–brain barrier, promotes neuroinflammation, and ultimately results in neurodegeneration (Figure 1). It is proposed that the alterations in the network composed of intestinal flora, mucosal immune system and enteric nervous system could represent a common path driving the onset of neurodegenerative diseases [29–31].

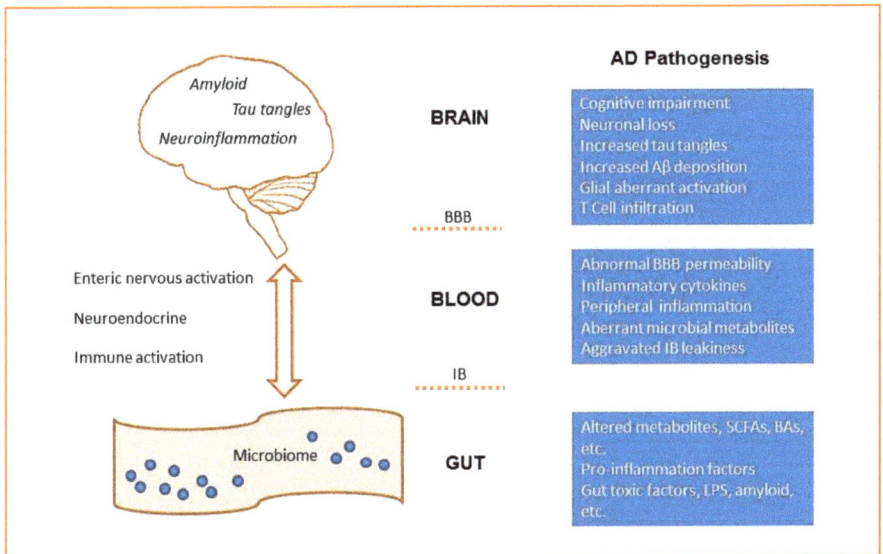

Figure 1. The microbiota–gut–brain axis in AD. The microbiota–gut–brain axis is a bidirectional communication system that includes neural, immune, endocrine and metabolic pathways. Dysbiosis of gut microbiota would affect the permeability of the intestinal barrier (IB), induce the leak of the brain–blood–barrier (BBB), and aggravate neuroinflammation and AD pathologies.

Many studies have shown significant alterations in gut microbiota in AD mouse models (Table 2). Peng W et al. compared the intestinal flora composition of AD model SAMP8 mice and control SAMR1 mice by 16S rRNA gene and metagenomic sequencing analysis. The results showed that the characteristic composition of intestinal microbiota of SAMP8 mice was significantly different from that of SAMR1 mice. Network analysis showed that the correlation density and clustering of operational taxonomic units in the intestinal flora of SAMP8 mice decreased [32]. Importantly, they observed that the abundance of *norank f Lachnospiraceae* and *unclassified f Lachnospiraceae* were increased in SAMP8 mice, which is consistent with a report showing the upregulation of *Lachnospiraceae* in AD patients [25]. Moreover, the abundance of *Alistipes* increased in SAMP8 mice, which have also been found to be more abundant in AD patients [25]. These consistent alterations in patients and animal models suggest the importance of theses taxa on AD pathogenesis. Zhan G. et al. found that 27 intestinal bacteria at 6 phylogenetic levels in SAMP8 mice were different from those in SAMR1 mice [33]. The pseudo germ-free mice showed significantly reduced cognitive function, and they showed improved behavioral and α, β diversity indices after being transplanted with the fecal bacteria of SAMR1 mice instead of SAMP8 mice. These results suggest that cognitive dysfunction in SAMP8 mice is associated with the abnormal composition of intestinal flora. Studies by Shen L. et al. on APP/PS1 transgenic mice, another AD mouse model, showed that the mice at 6 months had spatial learning and memory impairment, which was further worsened at 8 months [34]. They found that with the growth of age, the microbial diversity of APP/PS1 mice decreased. The abundance of Helicobacaceae and Desulfovibrionaceae at the family level, and Odoribacter and Helicobacter at the genus level were significantly increased in APP/PS1 mice, while the abundance of Prevotella was significantly decreased [34]. Interestingly, *Prevotellaceae* showed increasing abundance from 3.05% at 3 months old, 5.03% at 6 months old, to 10.30% at 8 months old, suggesting the association of this bacterial taxon with aging in APP/PS1 mice. Some studies on AD mouse models have shown increased levels of pro-inflammatory bacteria in the intestinal flora. For example, Bauerl C et al. compared the intestinal flora of APP/PS1 mice with their wild-type littermates. They found that the bacterial profiles were similar at 3 months, but the populations were different at 6 months. As age increases, Turicibacteriaceae and Rikenellaceae increased in all groups, although total Bacteroidetes remained stable. Proteobacteria, especially of the genus Sutterella, were specifically increased at 6 months in APP/PS1 mice. Moreover, the inflammation related family Erysipelotrichaceae was more abundant in APP/PS1 mice at 24 months, which suggested that AD pathology in mice shifts the gut microbiota towards profiles like inflammatory disorders [35].

Table 2. Gut microbiota alterations in AD mice.

AD Model	Control	Age	Alterations of Abundance	References
APP/PS1	WT	3, 6 and 8 months	At 3, 6 and 8 months: ↑ Helicobacteraceae, Desulfovibrionaceae, Odoribacter, Helicobacter; ↓ Prevotella. At 6 and 8 months: ↑Coriobacteriaceae; ↓Ruminococcus.	Shen et al. 2017
APP/PS1	WT	6 and 24 months	At 6 and 24 months: ↑Proteobacteria, Sutterella; ↓Rikenellaceae. At 24 months: ↑Erysilopetrichaceae.	Bauerl et al. 2018
5xFAD	WT	9 weeks	↑Firmicutes, Clostridium leptum group; ↓Bacteroidetes.	Brandscheid C. et al. 2017
SAMP8	SAMR1	7 months	↓Deferribacteres, Deferribacteres, Deltaproteobacteria, Deferribacterales, Desulfovibrionales, Mollicutes RF9, Clostridiales vadinBB60 group, Desulfovibrionaceae, Christensenellaceae, Family XIII, Deferribacteraceae, Ruminococcaceae, Mucispirillum, Serratia, Family XIII AD3011 group, Christensenellaceae R-7 group, Subdoligranulum, Desulfovibrio, Ruminiclostridium 9, Coprococcus 1, Ruminococcaceae UCG 004, Lachnospiraceae NK4A136 group, Lachnospiraceae oscillibacter	Zhan et al. 2018
SAMP8	SAMR1	8 months	↑norank f Lachnospiraceae, Alistipes, Odoribacter, unclassified f Lachnospiraceae, Akkermansia in SAMP8; ↑ norank_f Bacteroidales S24-7 group, Prevotella 9, Parasutterella, Butyrivibrio in SAMR1.	Peng et al. 2018

Abbreviations SAMP8: senescence accelerated mouse prone 8 mice; SAMR1: senescence-accelerated mouse resistant 1 mice; APP/PS1: APPswe/PS1dE9 mice; 5xFAD: 5xFAD (APP K670N, M671L, I716V, PS1 M146L, L286V) mice; WT: wild type; ↑, increased abundance; ↓, decreased abundance.

3.2. Gut Microbiota and Neuroinflammation

Intestinal flora is closely associated with neuroinflammation, and this is crucial for the pathogenesis of AD [36,37]. Gram-negative facultative anaerobe Bacteroides fragilis constitutes a considerable proportion of the microbial community in the human gastrointestinal tract. Like most gram-negative bacilli, Bacteroides fragilis secretes an unusual mixture of neurotoxins, including pro-inflammatory lipopolysaccharides (LPS). Zhao Y et al. reported that the level of LPS of AD patients increased by two times in the neocortex and three times in the hippocampus compared with the control group of the same age, and LPS mainly existed around the nucleus [38,39]. Notably, Bacteroides fragilis and the neurotropic herpes simplex virus 1 share a common final pathway after activating NF-κB (p50/p65) [40,41]. Using the co-culture system of human neuronal-glial cells, Zhao Y et al. found that when lipopolysaccharide BF-LPS was added, presynaptic neurexin-1 (NRXN-1), synaptosomal-associated phosphoprotein-25 (SNAP-25), phosphoprotein synapsin-2 (SYN-2), postsynaptic protein neuroligin (NLGN), the sh3-ankyrin repeat domain and proline-rich cytoskeletal scaffolding protein (SHANK3) were all significantly down-regulated [42]. Moreover, the DNA transcription products in the culture cells were reduced when stimulated by LPS [43]. These studies suggest that pro-inflammatory toxins secreted by gastrointestinal bacteria may "leak" into the circulation and then enter the brain, causing neuroinflammation and affecting neuronal function.

Using the 5XFAD AD mouse model, Wang X et al. found that intestinal flora composition changed and led to the peripheral accumulation of phenylalanine and isoleucine, which further stimulated the differentiation and proliferation of pro inflammatory T helper 1 (Th1) cells [44]. The peripheral Th1 cells infiltrating into the brain are associated with microglia M1 activation, which lead to neuroinflammation. They also found that the levels of phenylalanine and isoleucine and the quantity of Th1 cells were elevated in the blood of patients with mild cognitive impairment. These results suggest that neuroinflammation caused by metabolic abnormalities due to intestinal flora imbalance may be associated with AD. Inflammation of the brain is not always a response to local primary insults in the periphery. However, by using a drosophila AD model, Wu SC et al. demonstrated that intestinal bacterial infection can stimulate immune cell recruitment into the brain, thus aggravating the progress of AD. This work emphasized the importance of gut–brain crosstalk in neurodegenerative diseases [45]. Minter MR et al. found that long-term combinatorial broad-spectrum antibiotic treatment would change the composition and diversity of gut microbes in APPSWE/PS1ΔE9 mice, reduce Aβ plaque deposits and attenuate glial activation, suggesting the diversity of gut microbiota can regulate the host's innate immunity and affect Aβ amyloidosis [46].

3.3. Intestinal Metabolites

Changes in intestinal flora can cause alterations in intestinal metabolites. By using stable isotope labeling combined with liquid chromatography-tandem mass spectrometry, Zheng J et al. found that the contents of nine short-chain fatty acids (SCFAs) were significantly different between AD and wild type mouse fecal samples [47]. The level of propionic acid, isobutyric acid, 3-hydroxy butyric acid and 3-hydroxy isopropyl acid were reduced, while lactic acid, 2-hydroxy butyric acid, 2-hydroxy isobutyric acid, levulinic acid and valproic acid were increased. SCFAs are metabolites produced mainly by the intestinal flora from undigested fibers and proteins. As these molecules can act as G-protein-coupled receptor activators and histone deacetylase inhibitors, the changes of SCFAs in the feces of AD mice may be associated with the pathology of AD [47]. SCFAs have been shown to be able to inhibit the aggregation of Aβ in vitro [48]. Zhang L et al. compared the fecal microbiota and fecal SCFAs composition of wild-type and AD mice at different ages [49]. The results showed that the composition and diversity of the microbiota in AD mice were disturbed, and SCFAs levels were decreased, which may be related to the amyloid deposition and ultrastructural abnormalities in AD mouse intestines [49]. Tran TTT studied the relationship between the apolipoprotein E gene and gut microbes using APOE-targeted replacement (TR) transgenic mice [50]. They found the proportion of Prevotellaceae, Ruminococcaceae and several butyrate-producing genera changed. Metabolomics analysis of mouse feces revealed significant differences in microbial-related amino acids and short-chain fatty acids, suggesting that the most common genetic risk factor for AD is associated with specific intestinal microbiota profiles and metabolites changes. Yuan BF et al. synthesized stable isotopic labeling reagents to label metabolites with different chemical groups, including carboxyl, carbonyl, amine and sulfhydryl, and then combined these with liquid chromatography-mass spectrometry to analyze the mouse fecal metabolomics, and established the database of mouse fecal metabolomics [51]. They found significant differences in 211 fecal metabolites between AD and wild-type mice. It would be important to determine whether these metabolites are also changed in the feces of AD patients, as they could be new biomarkers for the diagnosis of AD. Trimethylamine N-oxide (TMAO) is a small molecule produced by the metabolism of dietary choline. CSF TMAO was shown to be higher in individuals with MCI and AD compared to healthy controls, and the elevated CSF TMAO was associated with AD pathological markers phosphorylated tau and Aβ42 [52]. Bile acids (BAs) are the end products of human cholesterol metabolism, which is produced by human and gut microbiota co-metabolism. In a 1562 case study, Nho K measured 20 kinds of primary and secondary BAs metabolites at the serum level, which were found to be related with amyloid proteins and tau in the cerebrospinal fluid of AD patients, as well as with brain atrophy and cerebral glucose metabolism dysfunction, thus providing further support for the role of this pathway in AD pathophysiology [53].

4. Clinical Implications of Gut Microbiota in AD

A large number of studies have shown that the composition and functionality of intestinal microbiota can affect the pathophysiology of age-related cognitive impairment and dementia, so it is highly possible to use fecal microbiota-related parameters and microbiota-derived metabolites as biomarkers for these cognitive-related diseases [16]. Based on the 20 kinds of typical predominant genera model, Liu P et al. could effectively distinguish AD and MCI from healthy controls [27]. They also found that the models based on the abundance of the Enterobacteriaceae family could distinguish AD from both MCI and healthy controls. Our research also showed that 93% of MCI patients could be distinguished by established random forest models with all different fecal genera [28]. These studies have facilitated the possibilities of finding clinically specific biomarkers for AD. However, gut microbes can be influenced by many factors, such as living region and diet. Although much evidence has been found supporting a close relationship between AD and gut microbes, no specific intestinal flora have been identified in AD patients; hence, large-scale sample screening and analysis is undoubtedly necessary.

Many studies have attempted to combat neurodegenerative disease by modifying the gut microbiota [11,54]. The studies to modify the gut microbiota in AD patients and models are summarized in Table 3. Amyloid and neurofibrillary tangles transgenic (ADLPAPT) mice show amyloid deposits, neurofibrillary tangles, reactive gliosis and memory defects. Kim MS et al. found that fecal transplantation from wild-type mice to ADLPAPT mice reduced the formation of amyloid plaques and neuronal tangles, and alleviated glial responses and cognitive impairment [55]. Sun J et al. used APPswe/PS1dE9 transgenic mice, another AD model, and found that fecal microbiota transplantation alleviated the cognitive decline and decreased the deposition of Aβ in the brain [56]. Further analysis showed tau phosphorylation, and that the level of Aβ40 and Aβ42, and COX-2 or CD11b positive cells decreased, while synaptic plasticity increased, indicating an overall improved pathological condition.

Bifidobacterium longum (NK46), a probiotic isolated from human intestinal flora, was found to have a strong inhibitory effect on the production of intestinal microbial endotoxin and the activation of NF-κB in BV-2 cells after LPS stimulation [57]. Using 5xFAD-Tg mice, an AD model, they demonstrated that oral administration of NK46 could change the composition of gut microbiota, especially the proportion of Proteobacteria, reduce the level of LPS in the feces and blood, and increase the colon tight junction protein expression. Moreover, administration of NK46 inhibited amyloid-β, β/γ-secretase and caspase-3 expression in the hippocampus, and alleviated the cognitive decline [57]. Kobayashi Y et al. studied the effects of oral administration of Bifidobacterium breve strain A1 (B. breve A1) on the behavior and pathophysiological process of mice injected with Aβ25-35 in the lateral ventricle [58]. They found that B. breve A1 reversed the impairment on alternate behavior in a Y maze experiment, and reduced the latency in a passive avoidance experiment. Gene expression profile analysis showed that B. breve A1 could suppress the expressions of inflammationrelated genes induced by Aβ in the hippocampus [58]. The mixed probiotics (Lactobacillus acidophilus, Bifidobacterium bifidum and Bifidobacterium longum) treatment was also found to improve the impaired spatial cognition ability and restore synaptic plasticity in the rats injected with Aβ in lateral ventricle [59]. Bonfili L et al. studied the role of a probiotic (SLAB51) in combating AD-associated oxidative brain damage [60]. By using a 3xTg-AD model mouse, they found that SLAB51 affected the composition of intestinal flora and its metabolites, as well as plasma concentrations of inflammatory cytokines and key metabolic hormones. They observed a partial recovery of damaged neuronal proteolytic pathways and less amyloid accumulation; thus, the cognitive impairment was alleviated [60]. They also found that administration of SLAB51 significantly reduced oxidative stress in the brains of AD mice by activating sirt1-dependent mechanisms [61]. Hoffman JD et al. reported that inulin, a non-digestible carbohydrate fiber fermented in the gastrointestinal tract, could increase the beneficial microbiota, reduce the harmful microbiota, and enhance peripheral and brain metabolism in APOE4 transgenic mice. Inulin also reduced inflammatory gene expression in the hippocampus, suggesting that a prebiotic diet may help reduce the risk of AD in asymptomatic APOE4 carriers [62]. Westfall S et al. examined the effects of synbiotic formula (containing three metabolically active probiotics and a polyphenol-rich prebiotic) on an AD drosophila model, and they found that synbiotic treatment could improve the animal survival rate and mobility, and reverse amyloid deposition and acetyl cholinesterase activity [63]. Taken together, these findings suggest that a diet supplement of probiotics may provide a promising adjuvant therapy for AD.

Dietary habits are closely related to the composition of intestinal bacteria. A ketogenic diet has been reported to increase the abundance of intestinal beneficial taxa (Akkermansia muciniphila and Lactobacillus) and reduce the abundance of intestinal pro-inflammatory taxa (Desulfovibrio and Turicibacter) [64]. It also increased the cerebral blood flow and p-glycoprotein transports on the blood–brain barrier to facilitate the clearance of Aβ, suggesting that a ketogenic diet may reduce the risk of AD. Nagpal R et al. compared the differences of intestinal flora between elderly people with mild cognitive impairment and elderly people with normal cognition, and found that, in MCI subjects, Proteobacteria was positively correlated with the ratio of Aβ1-42/Aβ1-40, and fecal propionate and butyrate were negatively correlated with Aβ1-42. After adopting the mediterranean-ketogenic diet (MMKD), the abundance of Enterobacteriaceae, Akkermansia, Slackia, Christensenellaceae and Erysipelotriaceae increased, while the abundance of Bifidobacterium and Lachnobacterium decreased. MMKD also increased the level of propionate and butyrate while slightly decreasing the level of lactic acid and acetate in feces. These results suggest that a ketogenic diet regulates intestinal microbiota and metabolites, and is associated with improvement of AD pathology [65].

Some compounds derived from plants with anti-AD effects were found to regulate intestinal flora in animal studies. Silymarin and its main active component silybin administration could alleviate the memory deficits and reduce amyloid plaques in APP/PS1 mice [15]. Meanwhile, the diversity of the bacterial community decreased, and the abundance of several key bacterial species associated with AD changed, suggesting that the regulation of gut microbiota is involved in their effects against AD [15]. Pomegranate extract administration significantly reduced the expression of inflammatory biomarkers in the hippocampus of transgenic AD R1.40 mice [66]. Yuan et al. found that urolithin (6H-dibenzo [b,d]pyran-6-one derivatives), an intestinal metabolite of ellagitannins from pomegranate, which can pass through the blood–brain barrier, could prevent fibrosis of Aβ in vitro. Urolithin significantly reduced the levels of nitric oxide, interleukin 6, prostaglandin E2 and tumor necrosis factor in LPS-stimulated BV-2 cells. Furthermore, Methyl-urolithin B (3-methoxy-6h-dibenzo [B, d] pyran-6-one) had protective effects on the neurotoxicity and paralysis of Caenorhabditis induced by Aβ1-42 [67]. This result indicates that the intestinal metabolites derived from plant elements may have protective effects against AD.

Table 3. Summary of studies to modify the gut microbiota in AD models and patients.

Intervention	Subjects	Main Effects	References
Faecal microbiota transfer	ADLPAPT	Reduction of the Aβ deposition, neurofibrillary tangle formation, and glial activation; reversed abnormalities in the colonic expression of genes related to inflammatory responses; ameliorated cognitive impairment.	Kim MS et al. 2019
Faecal microbiota transfer	APP/PS1	Reduction of the Aβ deposition and decreased phosphorylation of tau protein; reduced expression of COX-2 and CD11b, and increased expression of PSD-95 and synapsin I; improvement of cognitive deficits.	Sun J et al. 2019.
Bifidobacterium longum	5XFAD	Shifted gut microbiota composition and reduced fecal and blood LPS levels; suppressed NF-κB activation, decreased expression of TNF-α, and upregulated expression of tight junction protein in the colon; suppressed caspase-3 expression and Aβ accumulation in the hippocampus; alleviated cognitive decline.	Lee HJ et al. 2019
Bifidobacterium breve strain A1	Aβ treated mice	Suppressed hippocampal expressions of inflammation and immune-reactive genes; improved behavior in a Y maze test and the reduced latency time in a passive avoidance test.	Kobayashi Y et al. 2017
Mixed probiotics	Aβ treated rats	Improvement of the anti-oxidant/oxidant biomarkers; restored LTP and improved the maze navigation.	Rezae Asl Z et al. 2019
SLAB51	3xTg-AD	Shifted plasma concentration of inflammatory cytokines and key metabolic hormones; reduced oxidative stress and restoration of impaired neuronal proteolytic pathways; alleviated cognitive decline.	Bonfili L et al. 2017; Bonfili L et al. 2018
Inulin	E4FAD	Increased abundance of beneficial microbiota and reduced harmful microbiota in the feces; higher levels of SCFAs, tryptophan-derived metabolites, bile acids and glycolytic metabolites; suppressed the hippocampal expressions of inflammatory genes.	Hoffman JD et al. 2019
Symbiotic formulation	AD-drosophila	Rescued Aβ deposition and acetylcholinesterase activity; increased survivability and motility.	Westfall S et al. 2019
MMKD	MCI patients	Modified gut microbiota composition and metabolites; improved AD biomarkers in CSF.	Nagpal R et al. 2019

Table 3. Cont.

Intervention	Subjects	Main Effects	References
Silymarin and silibinin	APP/PS1	Regulative effect in abundances on bacterial species associated with AD development; reduce the amyloid plaque burden; alleviated memory deficits.	Shen L et al. 2019
Urolithins	AD-elegans	Suppressed Aβ fibrillation in vitro; protective effects against Aβ-induced neurotoxicity; increased the maximum survival/mobility.	Yuan T et al. 2016
Fructooligosaccharides	APP/PS1	Reversed the alteration of microbial composition; increased expression of glucagon-like peptide-1 in the gut; up-regulated expression of synapsin I and PSD-95.	Sun et al. 2019
OMO	APP/PS1	Regulative effect on the composition and metabolism of the gut microbiota; suppressed brain tissue swelling and neuronal apoptosis and downregulated expression of Aβ; ameliorated memory deficits.	Xin Y et al. 2018
OMO	Aβ treated rats	Regulated the composition and metabolism of gut microbiota; suppressed oxidative stress and inflammation; improvement of the learning and memory abilities.	Chen D et al. 2017
CA-30	SAMP8	Beneficial effects on the gastrointestinal microbiota dysbiosis; delayed aging processes; ameliorated cognitive impairments.	Wang J et al. 2016; Wang J et al. 2019.
Probiotic preparation	AD patients	Changes in the composition of intestinal bacteria, with the increased abundance of Faecalibacterium prausnitzii and decreased abundance of the inflammation-related bacteria; decline of fecal zonulin concentrations, and increased serum kynurenine concentrations.	Leblhuber F et al. 2018; Leblhuber F et al. 2019
Probiotic preparation	AD patients	No pronounced changes in scores of Test Your Memory and levels of serum biomarkers (TNF-α, IL-6, IL-10, TAC, GSH, NO, MDA, and 8-OHdG).	Agahi A et al. 2018
GV-971	AD patients; 5XFAD; APP/PS1	Suppress of gut dysbiosis; harnesses of blood phenylalanine/isoleucine accumulation and neuroinflammation; cognition improvement in a phase 3 clinical trial.	Wang X et al. 2019

Abbreviations ADLPAPT: AD-like pathology with amyloid and neurofibrillary tangles transgenic mice; AD-drosophila: drosophila expressing human BACE1 and the 695 amino acid isoform of human APP; AD-elegans: Caenorhabditis elegans treated with Aβ1-42; APP/PS1: APPswe/PS1df9 mice; E4FAD: asymptomatic APOE4 transgenic mice; SAMP8: senescence accelerated mouse prone 8 mice; 3xTg-AD: 129-Psen1tm1Mpm Tg (APPSwe, tauP301L)1Lfa/J transgenic mice; 5XFAD: 5XFAD transgenic (Tg) mouse model. Probiotic formulation and supplements: CA-30 (an oligosaccharide fraction derived from Liuwei Dihuang decoction); GV-971(a mixture of oligosaccharides with the degree of polymerization from 2 to 10); Mixed probiotics (Lactobacillus acidophilus, Bifidobacterium bifidum and Bifidobacterium longum); MMKD (a modified Mediterranean-ketogenic diet); OMO (an oligosaccharide from Morinda officinalis); SLAB51 (lactic acid bacteria and b fidobacterial); Probiotic preparation (Lactobacillus casei W56, Lactococcus lactis W19, Lactobacillus acidophilus W22, Bifidobacterium lactis W52, Lactobacillus paracasei W20, Lactobacillus plantarum W62 Bifidobacterium bifidum W23 and Lactobacillus salivarius W24); Symbiotic formulation (Lactobacillus plantarum, L. fermentum, Bifidobacteria longum spp. infantis and a polyphenol rich polyphenol plant extract from the gastrointestinal tonic Triphala); Urolithins: gut microbiota-derived metabolites of pomegranate extract.

There is emerging evidence that oligosaccharides could regulate the intestinal microflora, which may be developed as drugs to treat AD. Sun et al. examined the effect of fructooligosaccharides (FOS) on AD using Apse/PSEN 1dE9 (APP/PS1) mice, and found that treatment with FOS for 6 weeks reversed the changes in intestinal microbial composition and alleviated cognitive dysfunction and pathological changes. FOS significantly up-regulated the expression levels of synapsin 1 and PSD-95 whilst decreasing the phosphorylation level of JNK [68]. Oligosaccharide (OMO) is an oligosaccharide derived from Morinda officinalis. OMO was shown to improve memory behavior, reduce neuronal cell apoptosis and down-regulate the expression of Aβ 1-42 in both APP/PS1 transgenic mice and Aβ1-42-induced deficient rats [69,70].The CA-30, an oligosaccharide fraction derived from Liuwei Dihuang decoction, was shown to be able to modulate intestinal microbiota, rebalance the gut microbe-neuroendocrine immune regulatory network and ameliorate the cognitive deterioration of SAMP8 mice [71,72]. By using a 5XFAD AD mouse model, Wang X et al. found that GV-971, a sodium oligomannate, could inhibit peripheral phenylalanine/isolucine accumulation, control neuroinflammation and reverse cognitive impairment [44].

5. Future Perspectives

Although there is growing evidence supporting the close relationship between the intestinal flora and cognitive dysfunction in AD patients, more cautious evaluation and analysis of the data are greatly needed. Firstly, it is necessary to collect samples from patients on a large scale and in multiple centers, as gut microbiota are easily affected by patient's location, diet, living habits and gastrointestinal tract infection. For instance, the reduced abundance of Bacteroides was found in the fecal samples of AD patients from Chinese cohorts [26,28]. On the contrary, intestinal Bacteroides have been reported to be increased in AD patients from the USA [24,25]. In addition, we found a higher abundance of *Blautia* in AD patients [28], which is consistent with a previous report [25]. However, another study showed that the relative abundance of *Blautia* was dramatically decreased [27]. These inconsistent results warrant further validation and investigation. Secondly, the diagnosis standardization of AD needs to be strengthened. Beside cognitive scale assessment, CSF biomarker analysis and brain imaging are required. The most exciting part of intestinal flora analysis in AD patients is the possibility to provide a non-invasive, patient-compliant diagnostic approach. Therefore, the intestinal flora spectra of AD patients should be compared not only with healthy controls, but also with those of patients with other neurodegenerative diseases (such as PD, MSA, etc.). This could not only reveal the specificity of AD intestinal flora, but also provide new clues for its etiological research.

Currently, there are still no effective treatments for AD; thus, the strategy of regulating intestinal microbial flora to treat AD has attracted great attention. The probiotic preparation (Lactobacillus casei W56, Lactococcus lactis W19, Lactobacillus acidophilus W22, Bifidobacterium lactis W52, Lactobacillus paracasei W20, Lactobacillus plantarum W62 Bifidobacterium lactis W51, Bifidobacterium bifidum W23 and Lactobacillus salivarius W24) was tested in 20 AD patients for 4 weeks. Administration of the probiotics affected the composition of intestinal bacteria in AD patients, with an increased abundance of Faecalibacterium prausnitzii and decreased abundance of the inflammation-related bacteria. Since the study was only observed for 4 weeks, to avoid variability in repeated tests, they did not compare changes in cognitive scales [73,74]. However, after finishing a trial of 96 patients with severe AD treated with probiotics for 12 weeks, they concluded that the AD patients were insensitive to probiotics based on cognitive scale assessment and serum biomarker evaluation. [75]. Undoubtedly, more rigorous clinical trials are needed to assess the efficacy of this probiotic preparation on the treatment of AD patients. Recently, in a phase 3 clinical trial in China, GV-971 (a mixture of acidic oligosaccharides) was shown to improve cognition in AD patients by suppressing gut dysbiosis and the associated phenylalanine/isoleucine accumulation, and was conditionally approved as a therapeutic drug for AD [44]. However, large-scale, multicenter, prudent clinical efficacy tests are extremely necessary.

Many studies on animal models of AD have revealed changes in intestinal flora, providing evidence for the role of gut microbiota in the pathogenesis of AD. However, up to now, most of the experimental evidence has come from correlation research; many studies still remain to describe the alterations of intestinal flora, and rigorous sufficient and necessary proof is still lacking. The microbiota–gut–brain axis is a bidirectional communication system that includes neural, immune, endocrine and metabolic pathways (Figure 1). Dysbiosis of gut microbiota can affect the permeability of the intestine and the blood–brain barrier, which contributes to AD pathologies. On the other hand, the brain may also regulate the intestinal flora through vagus nerve activity and neuroendocrine. For example, it was found that Aβ was not only expressed in the brain, but also in the intestinal tissues in 5xFAD mice. Fecal protein analysis revealed reduced trypsin levels in this mouse model compared to wild-type mice [76]. Therefore, the pathological changes in the intestinal tract of AD mice may also result from the neurological function variation caused by Aβ abnormal expression. In addition, the secreted miRNAs are able to enter microbial organisms, and the host's miRNA might affect the intestinal microbial ecosystem [77]. Therefore, it is likely that AD-related miRNAs may enter intestinal bacteria and produce diseased microbiota. It should be taken into consideration that changes in gut flora may be the result of AD rather than the cause, although in vivo validation is greatly needed.

The underlying mechanism of how microbiota affect host neuronal activity and behavior is a very interesting question. Recent studies by Chu C et al. have found that manipulation of the microbiota in antibiotic-treated or germ-free adult mice resulted in significant deficits in fear extinction learning, which was associated with defective learning-related remodeling of postsynaptic dendritic spines and decreased activity in cue-encoding neurons in the medial prefrontal cortex [12]. Further metabolomics analysis identified four metabolites that were significantly down-regulated in germ-free mice and have been reported to be associated with neuropsychiatric disorders in both mouse models and humans, suggesting that compounds derived from the microbiota may directly affect brain function and behavior. Certainly, it would be interesting to further examine the levels of these metabolites in the blood and CSF of AD patients. To examine whether microbiota from AD patients would affect animal behavior, Fujii Y et al. transplanted fecal samples from a healthy control and an AD patient to germ-free C57BL/6N mice [78]. They found that, compared with the former, the latter performed significantly worse on an object location test and an object recognition test at 55 weeks of age, suggesting that the intestinal microbiota transplanted from the patients do affect the behavior of the mice. Further studies with samples from more AD patients are greatly needed. Moreover, investigations to clarify the molecular mechanism underlying this phenomenon are undoubtedly helpful for understanding the etiology of AD.

In conclusion, accumulating evidence of the association between gut microbiota and AD has been revealed. Further study on the role of intestinal flora in the pathogenesis of AD may develop new strategies for the diagnosis and treatment of the disease.

Author Contributions: Y.H. and S.C. conceived the manuscript. Y.H., B.L. and D.S. drafted the paper. S.C. and D.S. supervised and edited the manuscript. All authors have read and agreed to the published version of the manuscript.

Funding: This work was funded by Shanghai Municipal Science and Technology Major Project, grant number 2018SHZDZX05; the Innovation Program of Shanghai Municipal Education Commission, grant number 2017-01-07-00-01-E00046 and Shanghai Jiao Tong University School of Medicine, grant number DLY201603, 2017NKX001. And the APC was funded by Shanghai Municipal Science and Technology Major Project, grant number 2018SHZDZX05.

Conflicts of Interest: The authors declare no conflict of interest.

References

1. Prince, M.; Wimo, A.; Guerchet, M.; Ali, G.C.; Wu, Y.T.; Prina, M. *World Alzheimer Report 2015: The Global Impact of Dementia. An Analysis of Prevalence, Incidence, Costs and Trends*; Alzheimer Disease International: London, UK, 2019.
2. Jia, L.; Quan, M.; Fu, Y.; Zhao, T.; Li, Y.; Wei, C.; Tang, Y.; Qin, Q.; Wang, F.; Qiao, Y.; et al. Dementia in China: Epidemiology, clinical management, and research advances. *Lancet Neurol.* **2020**, *19*, 81–92. [CrossRef]

3. Long, J.M.; Holtzman, D.M. Alzheimer Disease: An Update on Pathobiology and Treatment Strategies. *Cell* **2019**, *179*, 312–339. [CrossRef] [PubMed]
4. Huang, Y.; Mucke, L. Alzheimer mechanisms and therapeutic strategies. *Cell* **2012**, *148*, 1204–1222. [CrossRef] [PubMed]
5. Zhang, H.; Ng, K.P.; Therriault, J.; Kang, M.S.; Pascoal, T.A.; Rosa-Neto, P.; Gauthier, S. Cerebrospinal fluid phosphorylated tau, visinin-like protein-1, and chitinase-3-like protein 1 in mild cognitive impairment and Alzheimer's disease. *Transl. Neurodegener.* **2018**, *7*, 23. [CrossRef] [PubMed]
6. Kodamullil, A.T.; Zekri, F.; Sood, M.; Hengerer, B.; Canard, L.; McHale, D.; Hofmann-Apitius, M. Trial watch: Tracing investment in drug development for Alzheimer disease. *Nat. Rev. Drug Discov.* **2017**, *16*, 819. [CrossRef]
7. Cryan, J.F.; O'Riordan, K.J.; Cowan, C.S.M.; Sandhu, K.V.; Bastiaanssen, T.F.S.; Boehme, M.; Codagnone, M.G.; Cussotto, S.; Fulling, C.; Golubeva, A.V.; et al. The Microbiota-Gut-Brain Axis. *Physiol. Rev.* **2019**, *99*, 1877–2013. [CrossRef] [PubMed]
8. Scheperjans, F.; Aho, V.; Pereira, P.A.; Koskinen, K.; Paulin, L.; Pekkonen, E.; Haapaniemi, E.; Kaakkola, S.; Eerola-Rautio, J.; Pohja, M.; et al. Gut microbiota are related to Parkinson's disease and clinical phenotype. *Mov. Disord.* **2015**, *30*, 350–358. [CrossRef]
9. Vizcarra, J.A.; Wilson-Perez, H.E.; Espay, A.J. The power in numbers: Gut microbiota in Parkinson's disease. *Mov. Disord.* **2015**, *30*, 296–298. [CrossRef] [PubMed]
10. Kong, G.; Cao, K.L.; Judd, L.M.; Li, S.; Renoir, T.; Hannan, A.J. Microbiome profiling reveals gut dysbiosis in a transgenic mouse model of Huntington's disease. *Neurobiol. Dis.* **2020**, *135*, 104268. [CrossRef]
11. Sasmita, A.O. Modification of the gut microbiome to combat neurodegeneration. *Rev. Neurosci.* **2019**, *30*, 795–805. [CrossRef] [PubMed]
12. Chu, C.; Murdock, M.H.; Jing, D.; Won, T.H.; Chung, H.; Kressel, A.M.; Tsaava, T.; Addorisio, M.E.; Putzel, G.G.; Zhou, L.; et al. The microbiota regulate neuronal function and fear extinction learning. *Nature* **2019**, *574*, 543–548. [CrossRef] [PubMed]
13. Du, X.; Wang, X.; Geng, M. Alzheimer's disease hypothesis and related therapies. *Transl. Neurodegener.* **2018**, *7*, 2. [CrossRef] [PubMed]
14. Jiang, C.; Li, G.; Huang, P.; Liu, Z.; Zhao, B. The Gut Microbiota and Alzheimer's Disease. *J. Alzheimers Dis.* **2017**, *58*, 1–15. [CrossRef] [PubMed]
15. Shen, L.; Ji, H.F. Associations Between Gut Microbiota and Alzheimer's Disease: Current Evidences and Future Therapeutic and Diagnostic Perspectives. *J. Alzheimers Dis.* **2019**, *68*, 25–31. [CrossRef] [PubMed]
16. Ticinesi, A.; Nouvenne, A.; Tana, C.; Prati, B.; Meschi, T. Gut Microbiota and Microbiota-Related Metabolites as Possible Biomarkers of Cognitive Aging. *Adv. Exp. Med. Biol.* **2019**, *1178*, 129–154. [PubMed]
17. Szablewski, L. Human Gut Microbiota in Health and Alzheimer's Disease. *J. Alzheimers Dis.* **2018**, *62*, 549–560. [CrossRef] [PubMed]
18. Chandra, S.; Alam, M.T.; Dey, J.; Chakrapani, P.S.B.; Ray, U.; Srivastava, A.K.; Gandhi, S.; Tripathi, P.P. Healthy Gut, Healthy Brain: The Gut Microbiome in Neurodegenerative Disorders. *Curr. Top. Med. Chem.* **2020**, *20*, 1142–1153. [CrossRef] [PubMed]
19. Gubert, C.; Kong, G.; Renoir, T.; Hannan, A.J. Exercise, diet and stress as modulators of gut microbiota: Implications for neurodegenerative diseases. *Neurobiol. Dis.* **2020**, *134*, 104621. [CrossRef] [PubMed]
20. Pluta, R.; Ułamek-Kozioł, M.; Januszewski, S.; Czuczwar, S.J. Gut microbiota and pro/prebiotics in Alzheimer's disease. *Aging (Albany NY)* **2020**, *12*, 5539–5550. [PubMed]
21. Sun, M.; Ma, K.; Wen, J.; Wang, G.; Zhang, C.; Li, Q.; Bao, X.; Wang, H. A Review of the Brain-Gut-Microbiome Axis and the Potential Role of Microbiota in Alzheimer's Disease. *J. Alzheimers Dis.* **2020**, *73*, 849–865. [CrossRef]
22. Cerovic, M.; Forloni, G.; Balducci, C. Neuroinflammation and the Gut Microbiota: Possible Alternative Therapeutic Targets to Counteract Alzheimer's Disease? *Front. Aging Neurosci.* **2019**, *11*, 284. [CrossRef] [PubMed]
23. Cattaneo, A.; Cattane, N.; Galluzzi, S.; Provasi, S.; Lopizzo, N.; Festari, C.; Ferrari, C.; Guerra, U.P.; Paghera, B.; Muscio, C.; et al. Association of brain amyloidosis with pro-inflammatory gut bacterial taxa and peripheral inflammation markers in cognitively impaired elderly. *Neurobiol. Aging* **2017**, *49*, 60–68. [CrossRef] [PubMed]

24. Haran, J.P.; Bhattarai, S.K.; Foley, S.E.; Dutta, P.; Ward, D.V.; Bucci, V.; McCormick, B.A. Alzheimer's Disease Microbiome Is Associated with Dysregulation of the Anti-Inflammatory P-Glycoprotein Pathway. *MBio* **2019**, *10*, e00632-19. [CrossRef] [PubMed]
25. Vogt, N.M.; Kerby, R.L.; Dill-McFarland, K.A.; Harding, S.J.; Merluzzi, A.P.; Johnson, S.C.; Carlsson, C.M.; Asthana, S.; Zetterberg, H.; Blennow, K.; et al. Gut microbiome alterations in Alzheimer's disease. *Sci. Rep.* **2017**, *7*, 13537. [CrossRef]
26. Zhuang, Z.Q.; Shen, L.L.; Li, W.W.; Fu, X.; Zeng, F.; Gui, L.; Lü, Y.; Cai, M.; Zhu, C.; Tan, Y.L.; et al. Gut Microbiota is Altered in Patients with Alzheimer's Disease. *J. Alzheimers Dis.* **2018**, *63*, 1337–1346. [CrossRef]
27. Liu, P.; Wu, L.; Peng, G.; Han, Y.; Tang, R.; Ge, J.; Zhang, L.; Jia, L.; Yue, S.; Zhou, K.; et al. Altered microbiomes distinguish Alzheimer's disease from amnestic mild cognitive impairment and health in a Chinese cohort. *Brain. Behav. Immun.* **2019**, *80*, 633–643. [CrossRef]
28. Li, B.; He, Y.; Ma, J.; Huang, P.; Du, J.; Cao, L.; Wang, Y.; Xiao, Q.; Tang, H.; Chen, S. Mild cognitive impairment has similar alterations as Alzheimer's disease in gut microbiota. *Alzheimer's Dement. J. Alzheimer's Assoc.* **2019**, *15*, 1357–1366. [CrossRef]
29. Pellegrini, C.; Antonioli, L.; Colucci, R.; Blandizzi, C.; Fornai, M. Interplay among gut microbiota, intestinal mucosal barrier and enteric neuro-immune system: A common path to neurodegenerative diseases? *Acta Neuropathol.* **2018**, *136*, 345–361. [CrossRef]
30. Kowalski, K.; Mulak, A. Brain-Gut-Microbiota Axis in Alzheimer's Disease. *J. Neurogastroenterol. Motil.* **2019**, *25*, 48–60. [CrossRef]
31. Lin, L.; Zheng, L.J.; Zhang, L.J. Neuroinflammation, Gut Microbiome, and Alzheimer's Disease. *Mol. Neurobiol.* **2018**, *55*, 8243–8250. [CrossRef]
32. Peng, W.; Yi, P.; Yang, J.; Xu, P.; Wang, Y.; Zhang, Z.; Huang, S.; Wang, Z.; Zhang, C. Association of gut microbiota composition and function with a senescence-accelerated mouse model of Alzheimer's Disease using 16S rRNA gene and metagenomic sequencing analysis. *Aging (Albany NY)* **2018**, *10*, 4054–4065. [CrossRef]
33. Zhan, G.; Yang, N.; Li, S.; Huang, N.; Fang, X.; Zhang, J.; Zhu, B.; Yang, L.; Yang, C.; Luo, A. Abnormal gut microbiota composition contributes to cognitive dysfunction in SAMP8 mice. *Aging (Albany NY)* **2018**, *10*, 1257–1267. [CrossRef]
34. Shen, L.; Liu, L.; Ji, H.F. Alzheimer's Disease Histological and Behavioral Manifestations in Transgenic Mice Correlate with Specific Gut Microbiome State. *J. Alzheimers Dis.* **2017**, *56*, 385–390. [CrossRef] [PubMed]
35. Bäuerl, C.; Collado, M.C.; Diaz Cuevas, A.; Viña, J.; Pérez Martínez, G. Shifts in gut microbiota composition in an APP/PSS1 transgenic mouse model of Alzheimer's disease during lifespan. *Lett. Appl. Microbiol.* **2018**, *66*, 464–471. [CrossRef] [PubMed]
36. Sochocka, M.; Donskow-Łysoniewska, K.; Diniz, B.S.; Kurpas, D.; Brzozowska, E.; Leszek, J. The Gut Microbiome Alterations and Inflammation-Driven Pathogenesis of Alzheimer's Disease-a Critical Review. *Mol. Neurobiol.* **2019**, *56*, 1841–1851. [CrossRef]
37. De De-Paula, V., Jr.; Forlenza, A.S.; Forlenza, O.V. Relevance of gutmicrobiota in cognition, behaviour and Alzheimer's disease. *Pharmacol. Res.* **2018**, *136*, 29–34. [CrossRef] [PubMed]
38. Zhao, Y.; Jaber, V.; Lukiw, W.J. Secretory Products of the Human GI Tract Microbiome and Their Potential Impact on Alzheimer's Disease (AD): Detection of Lipopolysaccharide (LPS) in AD Hippocampus. *Front. Cell. Infect. Microbiol.* **2017**, *7*, 318. [CrossRef] [PubMed]
39. Zhao, Y.; Cong, L.; Jaber, V.; Lukiw, W.J. Microbiome-Derived Lipopolysaccharide Enriched in the Perinuclear Region of Alzheimer's Disease Brain. *Front. Immunol.* **2017**, *8*, 1064. [CrossRef] [PubMed]
40. Zhao, Y.; Lukiw, W.J. Microbiome-Mediated Upregulation of MicroRNA-146a in Sporadic Alzheimer's Disease. *Front. Neurol.* **2018**, *9*, 145. [CrossRef] [PubMed]
41. Zhao, Y.; Lukiw, W.J. Bacteroidetes Neurotoxins and Inflammatory Neurodegeneration. *Mol. Neurobiol.* **2018**, *55*, 9100–9107. [CrossRef]
42. Zhao, Y.; Sharfman, N.M.; Jaber, V.R.; Lukiw, W.J. Down-Regulation of Essential Synaptic Components by GI-Tract Microbiome-Derived Lipopolysaccharide (LPS) in LPS-Treated Human Neuronal-Glial (HNG) Cells in Primary Culture: Relevance to Alzheimer's Disease (AD). *Front. Cell. Neurosci.* **2019**, *13*, 314. [CrossRef] [PubMed]

43. Zhao, Y.; Cong, L.; Lukiw, W.J. Lipopolysaccharide (LPS) Accumulates in Neocortical Neurons of Alzheimer's Disease (AD) Brain and Impairs Transcription in Human Neuronal-Glial Primary Co-cultures. *Front. Aging Neurosci.* **2017**, *9*, 407. [CrossRef] [PubMed]
44. Wang, X.; Sun, G.; Feng, T.; Zhang, J.; Huang, X.; Wang, T.; Xie, Z.; Chu, X.; Yang, J.; Wang, H.; et al. Sodium oligomannate therapeutically remodels gut microbiota and suppresses gut bacterial amino acids-shaped neuroinflammation to inhibit Alzheimer's disease progression. *Cell Res.* **2019**, *29*, 787–803. [CrossRef] [PubMed]
45. Wu, S.C.; Cao, Z.S.; Chang, K.M.; Juang, J.L. Intestinal microbial dysbiosis aggravates the progression of Alzheimer's disease in Drosophila. *Nat. Commun.* **2017**, *8*, 24. [CrossRef] [PubMed]
46. Minter, M.R.; Zhang, C.; Leone, V.; Ringus, D.L.; Zhang, X.; Oyler-Castrillo, P.; Musch, M.W.; Liao, F.; Ward, J.F.; Holtzman, D.M.; et al. Antibiotic-induced perturbations in gut microbial diversity influences neuro-inflammation and amyloidosis in a murine model of Alzheimer's disease. *Sci. Rep.* **2016**, *6*, 30028. [CrossRef] [PubMed]
47. Zheng, J.; Zheng, S.J.; Cai, W.J.; Yu, L.; Yuan, B.F.; Feng, Y.Q. Stable isotope labeling combined with liquid chromatography-tandem mass spectrometry for comprehensive analysis of short-chain fatty acids. *Anal. Chim. Acta* **2019**, *1070*, 51–59. [CrossRef]
48. Ho, L.; Ono, K.; Tsuji, M.; Mazzola, P.; Singh, R.; Pasinetti, G.M. Protective roles of intestinal microbiota derived short chain fatty acids in Alzheimer's disease-type beta-amyloid neuropathological mechanisms. *Expert Rev. Neurother.* **2018**, *18*, 83–90. [CrossRef] [PubMed]
49. Zhang, L.; Wang, Y.; Xiayu, X.; Shi, C.; Chen, W.; Song, N.; Fu, X.; Zhou, R.; Xu, Y.F.; Huang, L.; et al. Altered Gut Microbiota in a Mouse Model of Alzheimer's Disease. *J. Alzheimers Dis.* **2017**, *60*, 1241–1257. [CrossRef]
50. Tran, T.T.T.; Corsini, S.; Kellingray, L.; Hegarty, C.; Le Gall, G.; Narbad, A.; Müller, M.; Tejera, N.; O'Toole, P.W.; Minihane, A.M.; et al. APOE genotype influences the gut microbiome structure and function in humans and mice: Relevance for Alzheimer's disease pathophysiology. *FASEB J.* **2019**, *33*, 8221–8231. [CrossRef]
51. Yuan, B.F.; Zhu, Q.F.; Guo, N.; Zheng, S.J.; Wang, Y.L.; Wang, J.; Xu, J.; Liu, S.J.; He, K.; Hu, T.; et al. Comprehensive Profiling of Fecal Metabolome of Mice by Integrated Chemical Isotope Labeling-Mass Spectrometry Analysis. *Anal. Chem.* **2018**, *90*, 3512–3520. [CrossRef] [PubMed]
52. Vogt, N.M.; Romano, K.A.; Darst, B.F.; Engelman, C.D.; Johnson, S.C.; Carlsson, C.M.; Asthana, S.; Blennow, K.; Zetterberg, H.; Bendlin, B.B.; et al. The gut microbiota-derived metabolite trimethylamine N-oxide is elevated in Alzheimer's disease. *Alzheimers Res. Ther.* **2018**, *10*, 124. [CrossRef] [PubMed]
53. Nho, K.; Kueider-Paisley, A.; MahmoudianDehkordi, S.; Arnold, M.; Risacher, S.L.; Louie, G.; Blach, C.; Baillie, R.; Han, X.; Kastenmüller, G.; et al. Altered bile acid profile in mild cognitive impairment and Alzheimer's disease: Relationship to neuroimaging and CSF biomarkers. *Alzheimer's Dement. J. Alzheimer's Assoc.* **2019**, *15*, 232–244. [CrossRef] [PubMed]
54. Mancuso, C.; Santangelo, R. Alzheimer's disease and gut microbiota modifications: The long way between preclinical studies and clinical evidence. *Pharmacol. Res.* **2018**, *129*, 329–336. [CrossRef] [PubMed]
55. Kim, M.S.; Kim, Y.; Choi, H.; Kim, W.; Park, S.; Lee, D.; Kim, D.K.; Kim, H.J.; Choi, H.; Hyun, D.W.; et al. Transfer of a healthy microbiota reduces amyloid and tau pathology in an Alzheimer's disease animal model. *Gut* **2020**, *69*, 283–294. [CrossRef] [PubMed]
56. Sun, J.; Xu, J.; Ling, Y.; Wang, F.; Gong, T.; Yang, C.; Ye, S.; Ye, K.; Wei, D.; Song, Z.; et al. Fecal microbiota transplantation alleviated Alzheimer's disease-like pathogenesis in APP/PS1 transgenic mice. *Transl. Psychiatry* **2019**, *9*, 189. [CrossRef] [PubMed]
57. Lee, H.J.; Lee, K.E.; Kim, J.K.; Kim, D.H. Suppression of gut dysbiosis by Bifidobacterium longum alleviates cognitive decline in 5XFAD transgenic and aged mice. *Sci. Rep.* **2019**, *9*, 11814. [CrossRef] [PubMed]
58. Kobayashi, Y.; Sugahara, H.; Shimada, K.; Mitsuyama, E.; Kuhara, T.; Yasuoka, A.; Kondo, T.; Abe, K.; Xiao, J.Z. Therapeutic potential of Bifidobacterium breve strain A1 for preventing cognitive impairment in Alzheimer's disease. *Sci. Rep.* **2017**, *7*, 13510. [CrossRef]
59. Rezaei Asl, Z.; Sepehri, G.; Salami, M. Probiotic treatment improves the impaired spatial cognitive performance and restores synaptic plasticity in an animal model of Alzheimer's disease. *Behav. Brain Res.* **2019**, *376*, 112183. [CrossRef] [PubMed]
60. Bonfili, L.; Cecarini, V.; Berardi, S.; Scarpona, S.; Suchodolski, J.S.; Nasuti, C.; Fiorini, D.; Boarelli, M.C.; Rossi, G.; Eleuteri, A.M. Microbiota modulation counteracts Alzheimer's disease progression influencing neuronal proteolysis and gut hormones plasma levels. *Sci. Rep.* **2017**, *7*, 2426. [CrossRef]

61. Bonfili, L.; Cecarini, V.; Cuccioloni, M.; Angeletti, M.; Berardi, S.; Scarpona, S.; Rossi, G.; Eleuteri, A.M. SLAB51 Probiotic Formulation Activates SIRT1 Pathway Promoting Antioxidant and Neuroprotective Effects in an AD Mouse Model. *Mol. Neurobiol.* **2018**, *55*, 7987–8000. [CrossRef]
62. Hoffman, J.D.; Yanckello, L.M.; Chlipala, G.; Hammond, T.C.; McCulloch, S.D.; Parikh, I.; Sun, S.; Morganti, J.M.; Green, S.J.; Lin, A.L. Dietary inulin alters the gut microbiome, enhances systemic metabolism and reduces neuroinflammation in an APOE4 mouse model. *PLoS ONE* **2019**, *14*, e0221828. [CrossRef] [PubMed]
63. Westfall, S.; Lomis, N.; Prakash, S. A novel synbiotic delays Alzheimer's disease onset via combinatorial gut-brain-axis signaling in Drosophila melanogaster. *PLoS ONE* **2019**, *14*, e0214985. [CrossRef] [PubMed]
64. Ma, D.; Wang, A.C.; Parikh, I.; Green, S.J.; Hoffman, J.D.; Chlipala, G.; Murphy, M.P.; Sokola, B.S.; Bauer, B.; Hartz, A.M.S.; et al. Ketogenic diet enhances neurovascular function with altered gut microbiome in young healthy mice. *Sci. Rep.* **2018**, *8*, 6670. [CrossRef] [PubMed]
65. Nagpal, R.; Neth, B.J.; Wang, S.; Craft, S.; Yadav, H. Modified Mediterranean-ketogenic diet modulates gut microbiome and short-chain fatty acids in association with Alzheimer's disease markers in subjects with mild cognitive impairment. *EBioMedicine* **2019**, *47*, 529–542. [CrossRef] [PubMed]
66. DaSilva, N.A.; Nahar, P.P.; Ma, H.; Eid, A.; Wei, Z.; Meschwitz, S.; Zawia, N.H.; Slitt, A.L.; Seeram, N.P. Pomegranate ellagitannin-gut microbial-derived metabolites, urolithins, inhibit neuroinflammation in vitro. *Nutr. Neurosci.* **2019**, *22*, 185–195. [CrossRef]
67. Yuan, T.; Ma, H.; Liu, W.; Niesen, D.B.; Shah, N.; Crews, R.; Rose, K.N.; Vattem, D.A.; Seeram, N.P. Pomegranate's Neuroprotective Effects against Alzheimer's Disease Are Mediated by Urolithins, Its Ellagitannin-Gut Microbial Derived Metabolites. *ACS Chem. Neurosci.* **2016**, *7*, 26–33. [CrossRef]
68. Sun, J.; Liu, S.; Ling, Z.; Wang, F.; Ling, Y.; Gong, T.; Fang, N.; Ye, S.; Si, J.; Liu, J. Fructooligosaccharides Ameliorating Cognitive Deficits and Neurodegeneration in APP/PS1 Transgenic Mice through Modulating Gut Microbiota. *J. Agric. Food Chem.* **2019**, *67*, 3006–3017. [CrossRef] [PubMed]
69. Xin, Y.; Diling, C.; Jian, Y.; Ting, L.; Guoyan, H.; Hualun, L.; Xiaocui, T.; Guoxiao, L.; Ou, S.; Chaoqun, Z.; et al. Effects of Oligosaccharides From Morinda officinalis on Gut Microbiota and Metabolome of APP/PS1 Transgenic Mice. *Front. Neurol.* **2018**, *9*, 412. [CrossRef]
70. Chen, D.; Yang, X.; Yang, J.; Lai, G.; Yong, T.; Tang, X.; Shuai, O.; Zhou, G.; Xie, Y.; Wu, Q. Prebiotic Effect of Fructooligosaccharides from Morinda officinalis on Alzheimer's Disease in Rodent Models by Targeting the Microbiota-Gut-Brain Axis. *Front. Aging Neurosci.* **2017**, *9*, 403. [CrossRef]
71. Wang, J.; Lei, X.; Xie, Z.; Zhang, X.; Cheng, X.; Zhou, W.; Zhang, Y. CA-30, an oligosaccharide fraction derived from Liuwei Dihuang decoction, ameliorates cognitive deterioration via the intestinal microbiome in the senescence-accelerated mouse prone 8 strain. *Aging (Albany NY)* **2019**, *11*, 3463–3486. [CrossRef]
72. Wang, J.; Ye, F.; Cheng, X.; Zhang, X.; Liu, F.; Liu, G.; Ni, M.; Qiao, S.; Zhou, W.; Zhang, Y. The Effects of LW-AFC on Intestinal Microbiome in Senescence-Accelerated Mouse Prone 8 Strain, a Mouse Model of Alzheimer's Disease. *J. Alzheimers Dis.* **2016**, *53*, 907–919. [CrossRef] [PubMed]
73. Leblhuber, F.; Steiner, K.; Schuetz, B.; Fuchs, D.; Gostner, J.M. Probiotic Supplementation in Patients with Alzheimer's Dementia—An Explorative Intervention Study. *Curr. Alzheimer Res.* **2018**, *15*, 1106–1113. [CrossRef] [PubMed]
74. Leblhuber, F.; Steiner, K.; Schuetz, B.; Fuchs, D. Commentary: Does Severity of Alzheimer's Disease Contribute to Its Responsiveness to Modifying Gut Microbiota? A Double Blind Clinical Trial. *Front. Neurol.* **2019**, *10*, 667. [CrossRef] [PubMed]
75. Agahi, A.; Hamidi, G.A.; Daneshvar, R.; Hamdieh, M.; Soheili, M.; Alinaghipour, A.; Esmaeili Taba, S.M.; Salami, M. Does Severity of Alzheimer's Disease Contribute to Its Responsiveness to Modifying Gut Microbiota? A Double Blind Clinical Trial. *Front. Neurol.* **2018**, *9*, 662. [CrossRef] [PubMed]
76. Brandscheid, C.; Schuck, F.; Reinhardt, S.; Schäfer, K.H.; Pietrzik, C.U.; Grimm, M.; Hartmann, T.; Schwiertz, A.; Endres, K. Altered Gut Microbiome Composition and Tryptic Activity of the 5xFAD Alzheimer's Mouse Model. *J. Alzheimers Dis.* **2017**, *56*, 775–788. [CrossRef]

77. Hewel, C.; Kaiser, J.; Wierczeiko, A.; Linke, J.; Reinhardt, C.; Endres, K.; Gerber, S. Common miRNA Patterns of Alzheimer's Disease and Parkinson's Disease and Their Putative Impact on Commensal Gut Microbiota. *Front. Neurosci.* **2019**, *13*, 113. [CrossRef] [PubMed]
78. Fujii, Y.; Nguyen, T.T.T.; Fujimura, Y.; Kameya, N.; Nakamura, S.; Arakawa, K.; Morita, H. Fecal metabolite of a gnotobiotic mouse transplanted with gut microbiota from a patient with Alzheimer's disease. *Biosci. Biotechnol. Biochem.* **2019**, *83*, 2144–2152. [CrossRef] [PubMed]

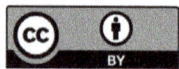

© 2020 by the authors. Licensee MDPI, Basel, Switzerland. This article is an open access article distributed under the terms and conditions of the Creative Commons Attribution (CC BY) license (http://creativecommons.org/licenses/by/4.0/).

MDPI
St. Alban-Anlage 66
4052 Basel
Switzerland
Tel. +41 61 683 77 34
Fax +41 61 302 89 18
www.mdpi.com

Journal of Clinical Medicine Editorial Office
E-mail: jcm@mdpi.com
www.mdpi.com/journal/jcm

www.ingramcontent.com/pod-product-compliance
Lightning Source LLC
LaVergne TN
LVHW070422100526
838202LV00014B/1510